Public Health Advocacy and Tobacco Control: Making Smoking History

This book is dedicated to my mother Margaret, who died from cancer aged just 64.

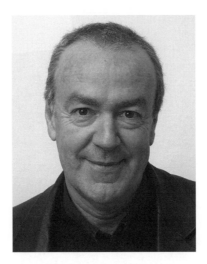

Simon Chapman

Public Health Advocacy and Tobacco Control: Making Smoking History

Simon Chapman
School of Public Health
University of Sydney
NSW, Australia

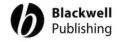

Blackwell Publishing editorial offices:
Blackwell Publishing Ltd, 9600 Garsington Road, Oxford OX4 2DQ, UK
   Tel: +44 (0)1865 776868
Blackwell Publishing Inc., 350 Main Street, Malden, MA 02148-5020, USA
   Tel: +1 781 388 8250
Blackwell Publishing Asia Pty Ltd, 550 Swanston Street, Carlton, Victoria 3053, Australia
   Tel: +61 (0)3 8359 1011

First published 2007 by Blackwell Publishing Ltd

2   2008

ISBN: 978-1-4051-6163-3

Library of Congress Cataloging-in-Publication Data
Chapman, Simon.
    Public health advocacy and tobacco control : making smoking history / Simon Chapman.
          p. ; cm.
    Includes bibliographical references and index.
    ISBN: 978–1–4051–6163–3 (pbk. : alk. paper)
    1. Tobacco use—Prevention.   2. Smoking—Prevention.   3. Health promotion.
4. Tobacco industry.   I. Title.
    [DNLM: 1. Smoking Cessation.   2. Consumer Advocacy.   3. Tobacco Industry.
WM 290 C466p 2007]
    HV5732.C435 2007
    362.29′66—dc22

                                                            2007010861

A catalogue record for this title is available from the British Library

Set in 11/13pt Bembo
by Graphicraft Limited, Hong Kong
Printed and bound in Singapore
by Fabulous Printers Pte Ltd

For further information on Blackwell Publishing, visit our website:
www.blackwellpublishing.com

Contents

Preface

This is a revised, updated and in its entire first part, a very different version of a book I wrote with Deborah Lupton in 1994: *The Fight for Public Health: Principles and Practice of Media Advocacy*[1]. Those who know that book will recognise that Part II of this book – An A–Z of Tobacco Control Advocacy Strategy – contains much that is similar, although many new sections and more recent case studies have been added and some long-redundant ones cut.

Part I of the first book was an attempt to explore the concept of advocacy and its applications in the broad field of public health, particularly as these related to media advocacy. In this book, I have chosen to take a different approach and to focus on two related objectives. First, I want to explore what needs to be done in tobacco control in the first decades of the twenty-first century if we are to accelerate the decline in smoking that has long been experienced in those nations that have adopted comprehensive tobacco control policies. Next, I want to apply the principles of public health advocacy to tobacco control. As the subtitle of the book suggests, in some nations with advanced histories of tobacco control, we may well be nearing a point when we can be confident that within two decades – perhaps earlier – we will see tobacco use wane to such a point that it will be almost "history": an uncommon, marginal behaviour, largely disappearing from public sight in much the same way that public spitting did in many nations early in the twentieth century[2].

But in most nations today, smoking remains depressingly and avoidably common, legislative controls rudimentary, and the public culture surrounding smoking one that sees it as very normal, accommodated and unexceptional. The future of the global tobacco epidemic, which will see 10 million deaths a year by the year 2030[3], will be increasingly played out in less developed nations. There are important reasons why some key forms of advocacy will not readily transfer (for example) from advanced, industrialised, fully democratic nations to less developed nations with centrally controlled news media. However, there are also many case studies of the successful transfer of strategy that show that tobacco control can become a vital and energetically adopted part of the government of low-income nations.

I have been fortunate to live in Australia for most of my life, and to have spent nearly 30 years working in tobacco control. During this time I have seen huge and extraordinary changes in the social and political climate surrounding tobacco use and efforts to control it. In 2001, I was leaked a staff training DVD from British American Tobacco (Australia). Five senior executives sat in front of the camera blubbing about the inexorable fall in smoking in Australia and how it would only get worse. They tried to inspire their staff by talking up hopes that as the remaining water drained from the pool, they might still snatch profit from brands they might inspire smokers to believe were at the "luxury" end of the market. Luxurious carcinogens. It was desperate stuff, but very heartening all the same. In the early 1960s, nearly 60% of men and 30% of women smoked in Australia[4]. Today, daily smoking by people aged 14 and over is now 17.4%[5] and shows no signs of having bottomed out. Lung cancer in men has been falling since the early 1980s and female lung cancer appears to have stopped rising[6]. Death rates from coronary heart disease fell by 59% in men and 55% in women between 1980 and 2000, in large part because of changes in risk factors like smoking[7]. Such gains in reducing smoking rank with vaccine uptake, the fall in the road toll and the arresting of the AIDS epidemic as being among the major public health achievements of the last 50 years in Australia. Similar stories can be told about tobacco control for a growing number of nations.

Today smokers huddle in doorways, quietly excuse themselves from meetings and slip out of your house to smoke during visits. Increasingly, to smoke today in many nations is to wear a badge that says "I am either an immature youth, have little education or life aspiration, or am a resigned addict". Thirty years ago it was very different. Through advertising, the tobacco industry had infected smokers with the idea that they had a monopoly on all that was interesting, convivial and sensual. The revelations of epidemiology about smoking and disease rather ruined all that, but it has been advocacy that has ensured the epidemiologists' conclusions became translated into policy, mass outreach programmes and law reform rather than languishing in scholarly journals read by few.

In the late 1970s I was becoming bored in my first job as a community health educator. While I gave interminable talks to Rotarians and teachers' staff development courses about the "drug problem", tobacco advertising wallpapered every conceivable public space. As the then head of the Victorian Anti-Cancer Council, Nigel Gray, once wrote to a newspaper, drug pushers were very publicly jailed while tobacco company directors were quietly knighted. With a few colleagues in 1978, I formed MOP UP (Movement Opposed to the Promotion of Unhealthy Products). We put out a precocious press release and the next week were profiled by the *Sydney Morning Herald* as the latest pebble in the shoe of sin industries[8]. We engineered the removal of the actor Paul Hogan from the hugely successful *Winfield* cigarette advertising campaign[9] ("MOP UP's slingshot cuts down the advertising ogre" read the headline) and re-energized the debate about tobacco advertising that Nigel Gray and Cotter Harvey, the founder of the Australian Council on Smoking and Health, had started in the 1960s.

At our first meeting – held in the lecture theatre of the Sydney morgue in Camperdown – someone stood and declared impatiently that our political letter writing plans were pathetic, and if we had courage, we would take more direct action. BUGA UP, the graffiti movement, was born and over the next eight years revolutionised ordinary Australians' understanding of the politics of tobacco control[10]. My modest involvement was to take on-going responsibility for the billboard on a shop directly opposite the entrance to News Ltd where several Murdoch newspapers were printed, but my admiration for the dozens of courageous people who risked much over a decade of civil disobedience is boundless. We held a 20-year reunion in October 2003.

When I first started in tobacco control, people at parties would occasionally give me wide berth as a probable teetotal morals crusader who would soon move to turn the music down at your party and pluck sweets from children's mouths. MOP UP and especially BUGA UP changed all that. Understanding that the tobacco industry is a pariah of the corporate world rapidly became a litmus test of a whole set of values. Today, one very rarely reads, hears or sees a tobacco industry executive in the media: they have vanished from public discourse, knowing that their credibility is rock bottom[11] with every public appearance promising further humiliation. As my colleague Stan Glantz from the University of California, San Francisco, has said, "they are like cockroaches. They spread disease and don't like to be seen in the light". No respectable politician would today ever risk open public association with them and this has facilitated the incremental adoption of a legislative programme that puts Australia at the forefront of nations trying to reduce tobacco's toll.

Those heady days and my first degree in media sociology gave me a taste for the nature and importance of understanding news values. They blooded me for a career in which I have tried to translate epidemiologists' conclusions into public discourses that gel with community concerns and taught me how these must be truncated into soundbite-length summations if they have any hope of making the news. I have always had enormous respect for the power of the news media to influence the way that communities think about issues. My honours thesis on imagery in advertising for psychotropic drugs in medical journals was tabled into the Australian Senate Hansard in 1979[12], teaching me that academic work could climb out of its mostly cosseted sanctuary and influence political debates.

Since 1976, I have published over 330 research papers, editorials, letters and commentaries in peer-reviewed journals and another 100 in throwaway journals. I have written twelve books and large reports. A few of these have been cited reasonably well. But if I was to nominate my most influential contributions, without hesitation, I would name some of my 130 newspaper opinion pieces, my letters to newspapers or some of my extended radio and TV interviews during critical periods of advocacy for change like the tumultuous period of advocacy that was required after the Port Arthur gun massacre in 1996 to secure tough gun laws[13].

Years of watching my citation rate splutter upwards and 16 years of editing an international research journal (*Tobacco Control*) have taught me that scholarship, for all its importance, exists in political backwaters and seldom influences practice, public or political opinion. Colleagues boast of a paper being cited a few hundred times or of speaking to 5000 like-minded people at an international conference. I am always aware that a gloves-off opinion piece in a morning newspaper followed by a round of interviews on breakfast radio on the morning of a vital political decision about public health will be read and often discussed by incomparably more people than those who would encounter the same arguments in a journal.

The structure of the book

The book has two parts. Part I addresses *what* needs to be done in the twenty-first century to arrest smoking and the diseases it causes, when the goal is to reduce those risks across whole populations of thousands, millions or hundreds of millions of people. Part II is devoted to the *how* – it describes strategies and tactics of public health advocacy that can assist in ensuring that tobacco remains in the public and political eye as a priority issue in public health, deserving of appropriate laws and regulations, and of funding support.

According to data from the Tobacco Merchants Association, in 2005 an estimated 5.494 trillion cigarettes were consumed by the world's 1.3 billion smokers[14]. Making significant inroads into a phenomenon of that scale is what effective tobacco control must do. Part I pulls few punches, because over 30 years I have seen a huge amount of effort described as tobacco control that collectively counts for little. It would not really matter if much of this either stopped or doubled tomorrow. There are some people working in tobacco control today who will be offended by parts of these chapters. As readers will come to see, I have little patience for tobacco control activities, interventions and programmes that fail to meet the most elementary criterion of potential population-wide public health impact: the ability to reach and influence the large number of people who are or will be affected by tobacco use. Inconsequential interventions keep busy many people working in tobacco control, but their achievements do not translate into anything capable of seriously reducing tobacco use throughout populations, nor the diseases it causes.

There is an eye-moistening parable that I have sometimes heard motivational speakers use in lectures. It describes a man and his son walking on a beach and seeing thousands of fish being washed up on the shoreline by a strong tide. The fish flap helplessly in the sand, with many already dead. The man begins to throw single fish back into the water, liberating them from their fate. The boy questions his father, asking what the point is of saving a few fish when inevitably, for every one saved, hundreds or thousands more will immediately take their place, being washed ashore with each wave. The father replies that while the boy's observation is true, each fish that is saved by his actions will be in no doubt that being helped to live was a good thing.

This parable is usually told as a way of motivating people to understand that their personal acts of generosity and helpfulness can make important differences to others. This is undoubtedly true. Its counterpart in public health is the concept of the "rule of rescue"[15], which sees political and resource allocation priority always given to efforts to save identifiable individuals, rather than unnamed "statistical" individuals whose lives might be saved or quality of life enhanced in years to come by actions taken today. Civilised societies always value individuals.

Rescuing individuals – or for our purposes here, assisting people to stop smoking or from never starting – is nearly always virtuous. People running small interventions in the community such as quit clinics undeniably help many attenders of their clinics to stop smoking. As I will explore in Chapter 5, such interventions can be among the most cost-effective of all procedures in modern medicine[16,17]. But the problem is that not many smokers attend them, and that while such small numbers of "fish" are being thrown back in the sea to be given a second chance, thousands more are being washed ashore by the force of tobacco industry marketing activity and obstruction of effective tobacco control.

The book commences with three preliminary chapters that address key issues that underscore much in the rest of the book. The first re-examines the ethical basis for tobacco control. Many of the most heated debates in contemporary tobacco control practice today reflect ethical conflicts. These debates are between the public health interests and the tobacco industry; with governments about the reasons they offer for not acting; and, sometimes, between participants in tobacco control. Because I will be arguing for and against particular positions throughout the first part of the book, it is important that I should declare the values and ethical principles on which those positions rest. I discuss some of these in Chapter 1.

The second chapter addresses a question I am often asked: "does advocacy work?" Those who ask such a question typically come from fairly narrow scientific disciplines where they are used to exploring research questions in artificially controlled experimental situations. Their narrowness can be frustrating in the face of blindingly obvious changes that have been engineered by advocacy efforts. But the persistence of the question, and the continuing neglect of advocacy as a serious, funded priority even among many public health institutions, requires that it be addressed. Chapter 2 pulls together some previous writing of mine on this topic, trying to explain the futility of trying to "remove the (policy and strategy) eggs from the omelette": of trying to apply overly scientific demands to the project of explaining how policy and public opinion changes. It examines in detail the case of the decades-long advocacy effort to secure comprehensive legislation for smokefree indoor air. It also discusses at length the core advocacy skill of framing, again illustrating this with a case study on the struggle to see bars and pubs go smoke free.

The third chapter argues for the centrality of news-making in ensuring that tobacco control gains public and political support. It argues that the news media are neglected by the public health community in its preoccupation with planning, running and evaluating controlled experimental interventions whose effects can be nailed down by tightly controlled research designs. While the majority of the professional public health community are busy running and studying these typically small-budgeted interventions, the world is full of background "noise" in the form of oceans of news reportage and debate about tobacco control, most of which is highly supportive. This noise is largely neglected as both a vital "intervention" in its own right and as a subject to be analysed for its potential to allow greater and more effective participation by those wanting to progress tobacco control. Much of Part II is a detailed menu of ways to make that happen. Chapter 3 makes the case for its importance.

Agent, host, environment and vector

Part I then moves to explore, in a further four chapters, what I consider the most important topics in tobacco control today if we are to reduce the incidence of diseases caused by tobacco use. This part of the book is not an attempt to review exhaustively the latest and best evidence on each of these topics, but instead to put the case for action or changing emphasis on those issues I consider most critical. These topics can be considered under the time-honoured disease control matrix of agent, host, environment and vector. This matrix has mainly been applied to infectious and vector-borne disease control (e.g. with malaria control, the agent is the malarial parasite; hosts are those who can get malaria after being bitten by a malarial mosquito; environments are the physical environments in which mosquitoes thrive and so need to be monitored and controlled; and the vectors are the mosquitoes that carry the malarial parasite within these environments and bite the hosts who develop malaria.

In trying to understand tobacco-caused disease, the matrix adapts well. In tobacco control the agent is tobacco itself, in all its forms and varieties. The main question here is "can tobacco products themselves be changed so that their continued consumption would significantly reduce health problems caused by their use". Chapter 4 takes up this theme – certainly the most volatile in tobacco control today – and explores at length both the potential and the pitfalls of pursuing harm reduction within a comprehensive approach to tobacco control, including some of the ethical issues arising.

Hosts in tobacco control are those who either use or might one day use tobacco. Here, the main questions are "what are the most efficient ways of motivating and assisting large numbers of smokers to stop their tobacco use?" and "how can we most efficiently prevent non-smokers from starting to smoke?" Chapter 5 considers:

- Why and how most people stop smoking; how we can amplify this; and why we should limit our support for those strategies that have no hope of making a big impact?
- What sort of public awareness campaigns and interventions "work" and which ones merit little effort, in both cessation and prevention?

The "environment" in tobacco control is far more complex than the physical, climatic environment typically considered in the control of infectious diseases. An obvious starting point is to consider the process of how to denormalise further smoking in communities so that smoking becomes exceptional rather than normal. Some big topics emerge here. Chapter 6 considers how we can continue to erode the number of public places where smoking is allowed. It also considers the question of whether employers should be able to refuse to hire (or even fire) smokers when these employees do not smoke at work. I am very much opposed to such a proposition and will argue why such polices should be strongly opposed.

Finally, the "vector" in tobacco control is the tobacco industry and the third parties it increasingly uses to run its arguments in public. Just as malaria control involves studying and seeking to eradicate or biologically control mosquitoes, tobacco control needs to control the tobacco industry's ambitions. Chapter 7 examines how the industry has sought to continue its promotional and advertising activities in environments where "above the line" tobacco advertising is banned, something that will occur in most countries as the global Framework Convention on Tobacco Control is implemented. Australia has advanced experience of this, being one of the earliest nations to ban all advertising and then see the industry seeking to circumvent the spirit and letter of the ban.

Chapter 7 also considers nascent efforts to ban scenes of smoking in films, something I regard as well-meaning but ultimately indefensible in any society that values freedom of expression in the arts and entertainment world.

Chapter 7 also considers how the tobacco industry can be further marginalised in public life as a rogue, "bad apple" industry fully deserving of tough controls and regulation. I will examine its recent efforts at "rebirthing" itself via the global corporate social responsibility movement, and some examples of how these efforts can be derailed. The chapter concludes by considering why the tobacco industry has no place in academic environments, via funding research.

Chapter 8 concludes Part I by asking "how low can we go" in making smoking history. It considers examples that are already occurring of smoking prevalence going below 5% in particular subpopulations, as well as concerns about other subpopulations where smoking remains very prevalent. I speculate in this chapter about the prospect that within perhaps 20 years, smoking might virtually disappear as a major social phenomenon in some nations with advanced tobacco control programs.

An A–Z of advocacy

Part II is a sort of advocacy "cookbook" – a guide to how to promote effective tobacco control. It is a practical, coalface A–Z guide to creating a climate in which tobacco control can become more politically compelling. Many subject headings include examples of the strategy in action.

By the same author

Simon Chapman. *The Lung Goodbye. Tactics for counteracting the tobacco industry in the 1980s*. Sydney: Consumer Interpo, 1983.

Simon Chapman. *Great Expectorations: advertising and the tobacco industry*. London: Comedia, 1986.

Simon Chapman and Wong Wai Leng. *Tobacco Control in the Third World. A Resource Atlas*. Penang: International Organization of Consumers' Unions and the American Cancer Society, 1990.

Simon Chapman and Deborah Lupton. *The Fight for Public Health: principles and practice of public health media advocacy*. London: BMJ Books, 1994.

Simon Chapman and Stephen Leeder (eds). *The Last Right? Australians Take Sides on the Right to Die*. Sydney: Mandarin, 1995.

Simon Chapman. *Over Our Dead Bodies: Port Arthur and Australia's fight for gun control*. Sydney: Pluto, 1998.

Acknowledgements

The University of Sydney supported me with sabbatical leave between April and October 2006 to write the book and I am very thankful to have been hosted by the International Agency for Research on Cancer in Lyon, France, where its director, Peter Boyle, and the tobacco section head, Carolyn Dresler, gave me total freedom to work on the book every day for five months. Annick Rivoire was immensely helpful in helping me settle in. Nigel Gray, who occupied the room next to me, gave constant counsel and acted as a sounding board for my thoughts on harm reduction, as well as being a great friend. Many people have been of enormous influence to me over my career, but here I will reserve my thanks for those who assisted with parts of the book, providing criticism and data: Clive Bates, Gene Borio, Dave Burns, Greg Connolly, Mike Cummings, Rob Cunningham, Mike Daube, Coral Gartner, Jack Henningfield, Ann McNeill, Andrew Penman, Lars Ramström, Yussuf Saloojee, Michelle Scollo, David Sweanor, Ken Warner, Raoul Walsh, Robert West, Shu-Hong Zhu and a BAT scientist who was very generous with his time. Thanks go to David Champion and Katie Bryan-Jones, with whom I wrote two previously published papers that I have blended into Chapter 2, Amanda Dominello for a paper that has in part been included in Chapter 3 and Jonathan Liberman for a shared paper that is reproduced in Chapters 1 and 8. The customary caveat applies here: none of these people necessarily agree with the arguments I develop in this book. I know some of them don't. But they have all given generously of their time.

Then there are those magic people who made my wife Trish's and my time in Lyon one of the best of our lives. Elif Dagli in Istanbul provided us with unforgettable Turkish hospitality on the way over, and our friends and neighbours in Lyon made life in a new city very easy.

Stan Shatenstein has my particular gratitude. Everyone in international tobacco control knows Stan: he seems never to sleep, sending out to the world every day oceans of information that he tracks from newspapers, journals and every obscure source going. Stan and I have struck up a cyber friendship over the years and his polymath interests have alerted me to unimaginably interesting and witty things.

Fiona Byrne has worked with me for five years doing tobacco industry document research. She is a simply remarkable reference detective. I owe her huge thanks for her patience and good humour.

Part I

Major Challenges for Tobacco Control This Century

Chapter 1

Death is Inevitable, So Why Bother With Tobacco Control? Ethical Issues and Tobacco Control[i]

Tobacco control advocates have had the dismal luxury of being able to call on unimaginably "great" statistics to make their case. Globally, an estimated 4.9 million people die each year from tobacco-related illness[18], compared with 3.1 million from AIDS[19], 2.1 million from diarrhoeal diseases[20], 1.6 million from violence[21], nearly 2 million from tuberculosis[22], 1.2 million from road injuries[23] and 1 million from malaria[24]. Among risk factors for disease, only hypertension and undernutrition kill more people than tobacco use[25].

Between 1950 and 2000, it was estimated that smoking caused about 62 million deaths in developed countries (12.5% of all deaths: 20% of male deaths and 4% of female deaths). Currently, smoking is the cause of more than one in three (36%) of all male deaths in middle age, and about one in eight (13%) of female deaths. In the USA, each smoker who dies loses on average 12.7 years of life[26]. By 2020, the World Health Organization estimates that "the burden of disease attributable to tobacco will outweigh that caused by any single disease"[27].

Those are numbers "to die for", but they so often fail to create a sense of urgency in the media, or among policymakers and the public. They are so stratospheric that they have become almost banal. As Joseph Stalin put it: "A single death is a tragedy, a million deaths are a statistic." Tobacco control advocates have long tried to make smoking statistics resonate with a public numbed by endless quantification rhetoric advanced by myriad interest groups. Annual tobacco deaths in different nations have been routinely compared with deaths from so many jumbo jet crashes, the loss of football stadium crowds, and the obliteration of entire medium-sized cities. Conferences and shopping centres display digital death clocks for tobacco where audiences and shoppers are transfixed by the ever-mounting toll[28]. In 2006, when projections of cancer deaths arising from the 1986 Chernobyl nuclear reactor meltdown were published[29] showing that some 16 000 excess cancer deaths were likely to occur until 2065, the International Agency for Research on Cancer, which coordinated the study, stated: "tobacco smoking will cause several thousand times more cancers in the same population"[30]. Few news bulletins picked up on that comparison.

Community concern about health problems can reach its zenith over low-probability threats that sometimes barely rate an asterisk on national cause-of-death tables. Risk communication research shows that exotic, involuntary, catastrophic and sudden risks can strike fear into the hearts of populations and governments far easier than chronic, day-in-day-out dangers like smoking. Conventional wisdom says that a small sum spent on prevention is worth a fortune spent on cures, but cancer charities know which emphasis will see larger banknotes flow into street-corner collection buckets. Governments, with eyes firmly trained on the next electoral cycle, continue to give budgetary priority to acute health problems. Politicians cast themselves in rescue fantasies where grateful patients and their families form the backdrop to photo opportunities of more money being poured into facilities to diagnose and treat the sick. And the news media are generally happy to perpetuate these myopic myths. One person killed after ingesting the contents of a contaminated tin of food can be more newsworthy than 4.9 million dying the world over, each and every year, from consuming tobacco products bought off the very same store shelves.

Smoking kills an obscenely large number of people. But it does so one quiet, private death at a time. A single jumbo jet crash that kills 300 people makes the front pages for days. The collapse of the Twin Towers on 11 September 2001 created a climate of fear that will forever mark the generations who went through it "live" on television. Deaths of tobacco users go relatively unnoticed, except by the smokers' grieving relatives. Hannah Arendt wrote of the banality of evil among the very ordinary men who perpetrated the Nazi atrocities[31]. Tobacco deaths have their own banality in desperate need of redefinition so that communities may become outraged in the face of industry misconduct and government inaction.

Sadly, too many people inhabit the definitions of disease caused by smoking that are promoted by the tobacco industry: that smoking is a decision freely made by sentient adults who are fully apprised of the risks they are taking. They smoke with their eyes fully open to the risks, and are incorrigible in their determination to smoke in the face of this awareness – their perfect right in any society that values the rights of its citizens to make risky decisions on their own behalf. In 35% of press articles reporting on the case of a dying woman who took a tobacco company to court, the notion that she was fully responsible for her own smoking was evident in the reportage[32]. As I will discuss below, such conceptions of being fully informed are highly simplistic, and ignore the implications of nicotine being addictive, that most people take up smoking when children and that the levels of understanding that most smokers have of the risks they are taking are primitive.

In this chapter, I consider the harms that tobacco use causes, arguing that the misery it brings smokers while they are alive is as important but much neglected compared with the sometimes confused preoccupation we have with smoking causing death. I then consider the ethical arguments on which tobacco control rests. Ethical considerations, along with both the quantity and the quality of the evidence on how smoking causes disease, are the twin bedrocks of tobacco control. All arguments about policy and strategy in tobacco control are ultimately about whether the evidence is strong enough to warrant action, and about the values inherent in taking action – or not taking it – where directions for solutions to reduce tobacco's harms are apparent. Each of the sometimes volatile policy debates that I will review in Part I of the book are wringing wet with implied value positions that I believe have not received sufficient critical analysis within the tobacco control community.

During my 30-year career in tobacco control, I have met quite a few people whose motivation for being involved in trying to reduce smoking seemed to me to be primarily moralistic. Whatever they knew about the harms of smoking, this only served as post hoc ammunition for a wider purpose: to try to stop people smoking because smoking was *wrong* before it was harmful. To such people, the origins of its "wrongness" sometimes lay in explicit religious doctrines, but more often lay in some deeply puritanical sense that smoking was a moral vice, redolent with visions of other forms of frightening licentiousness and self-pleasuring.

But the overwhelming majority of people involved in tobacco control do not come to the topic as Calvinistic-like moralists. They come to it as health workers who want to help prevent early death and the attendant misery this can bring to smokers and those close to them. Often they are simply decent citizens with no professional roles in public health, who hope to contribute to the same ends. This of course is unavoidably a moral position too, as history has seen many infamous episodes where life has been devalued. An indicator of these values is the revulsion that many expressed at news of the Philip Morris-sponsored study that advised the Czech Republic's government that early deaths of smokers each saved the government \$1227 on health care, pensions and housing[33].

Tobacco control therefore has a noble purpose, but it is obviously not the only noble pursuit in the world. Occasionally tobacco control activists act as if it were; but it is important that policy debates should be transparent about the implications of overzealous single-mindedness where this discounts other important values cherished by large sections of society. Tobacco control debates are not restricted to circles of people who eat, drink, live and breathe tobacco control. Propositions for the further control of tobacco need to resonate with the values of wider society, and particularly with those held by key political decision-makers.

An articulate 52-year-old woman called me a few years ago. "Give the 'smoking kills' line a rest", she urged. "I've smoked for thirty years. I have emphysema. I am virtually housebound. I get exhausted walking more than a few metres. I have urinary incontinence, and because I can't move quickly to the toilet, I wet myself and smell. I can't bear the embarrassment, so I stay isolated at home. Smoking has ruined my life. You should start telling people about the living hell smoking causes while you're still alive, not just that it kills you."

I took this call shortly after having discovered online, a 23-page document written in 1978 for the British tobacco industry by Campbell Johnson, a public affairs firm. The document seemed to me the very worst I had ever encountered in several years of studying internal industry documents. It read:

> This last point, a brutally realistic one, implies that, with a general lengthening of the expectation of life we really need something for people to die of. In substitution for the effects of war, poverty and starvation, cancer, as the disease of the rich, developed countries may have some predestined part to play. The argument is obviously not one that the tobacco industry could use publicly. But its weight, as a psychological factor in perpetuating people's taste

for smoking as an enjoyable if risky habit, should not be underestimated . . .
In reality, of course, though in its controlled and positive aspects, cancer is
an essential ingredient of life, without which the cells of the human body
would be unable to renew themselves[34].

This second statement was written in 1978, a full 16 years after the Royal College
of Physicians of London published their landmark report on smoking and health
in 1962[35]. This is taken by many to be the date when the first consolidated evidence
condemning smoking as a major preventable cause of disease was considered to
have become established. Here was a public affairs firm setting out the case to its
tobacco client that they should try to make a virtue out of the small "problem"
that smoking kills lots of its users. Moreover, cancer, the most dreaded of all diseases, was to be reconceptualised as "an essential ingredient of life", as important
as food, air, water and shelter. The industry should feel proud that it was just helping nature along. Its "enjoyable" products would go down in history as having taken
their place in this "predestined" theatre of death, as another part in that lay discourse one sometimes hears muttered by people indifferent to the mass death caused
by famines, tsunamis and war that "these things just help trim the population".

We are all going to die

The Campbell Johnson author got one thing right. We *are* all going to die. Death
itself cannot be prevented. Advanced age is easily the strongest predictor of death,
and chronic diseases including most forms of cancer and heart disease become much
more prevalent in later life and are the diseases that will appear on most of our
death certificates. These truisms have acquired profane, almost unutterable status
in contemporary health care debate. Each banal in isolation, they remain banished
from polite discussion as indecent reminders of the pathos of the human dust-to-
dust destiny, occasionally insisting to be heard amid the unbridled optimism of
the scientific legacy. Perhaps the most unabashed manifestation of this denial is the
spamming American Academy of Anti-Aging Medicine, which boasts 11 500 members in 65 nations[36], and unblinkingly speculates about the virtues of people
living to the age of 120 and possibly as long as 170[37]. Whole death-denying and
-defying industries have become established on the back of the age-old human
preoccupation with finding fountains of youth and other promises of eternal life.

Indeed, the dominant medical motto for our age might well be "never say die".
In 2004, following Richard Nixon's declaration of war on cancer in 1971, the
then head of the US National Cancer Institute, Andrew von Eschenbach, caught
the spirit of George W. Bush's all-conquering *zeitgeist* and challenged the USA to
"eliminate suffering and death from cancer" by 2015[38]. In Sweden, it is government policy that the road toll should strive to reach zero, not merely fall[39]. If you
scratch the surface of the Human Genome Project, unstated assumptions about
eternal life are not hard to find in the pitch to the often elderly biotech investors.

Single-issue health organisations, including those in tobacco control, often talk
of research or progress that might one day eliminate their diseases. Lung cancer

was a rare disease before the mass availability of machine-made cigarettes saw its rapid acceleration after 1920 in nations with easy access to cigarettes. It remains uncommon in non-smokers. So if the disease can appear, it can be made to disappear, the thinking correctly goes. The recent development of a vaccine for cervical cancer[40] is self-evidently a wonderful thing. Here is a almost fully translated research advance that promises to end the collected misery and pain that millions of women would otherwise suffer over the years. The eradication of smallpox and the predicted departure of wild polio from the planet are astonishing achievements. So why not conquer everything else? In wealthy nations today there are few causes of death that cannot boast a non-government agency and a research focus dedicated to eradicating the offending disease. Health agencies' mission statements are purged of anything that even hints that a point might be reached when an organisation might be content with a certain incidence of deaths from their cause. Defeat is anathema to medical progress when it comes to death.

Plainly, there is much to admire in all this. If the go-for-gold death eradication scenarios played out for each preventable cause, a huge number of deaths in young and middle age would be prevented. But if no one of any age died from cancer, was ever killed on the roads, or died from any given cause now subject to ever-onward mortality-reduction targets, what would take their place? If the death toll from late-age smoking-related cancer plummeted, if heart disease became something permanently able to be postponed, would this be progress? Which causes of death would increase when others declined? What *would* we die from? And would this be progress?

Isolated from the wider "if not death from X, then what?" question, advances against deaths from particular diseases may be pyrrhic victories if all it means is that cause-of-death deckchairs are being shuffled on life's *Titanic*, only to sink around the same time.

So, because we all have to die of some cause, what's the problem of such deaths being caused by tobacco use? What virtue is there in stopping people from dying at the end of life from diseases caused by their smoking, and instead seeing the same people die from other diseases, probably soon afterwards, not caused by smoking? Plainly, little – if that was all that was at issue. In the eponymous Greek myth, Sisyphus is condemned to an eternity of ceaselessly rolling a rock to the top of a mountain, only to see the stone fall back because of its own weight. Is this not like the ultimate futility of trying to postpone death by defeating each of its possible causes at the end of life? If so, the ethical justification for preventing tobacco-caused deaths needs to move to other considerations. These are not hard to find.

Tobacco causes early death

First, while some people who die of tobacco-caused diseases are very old – and would be likely to die of *something* sooner than later, a massive number of smokers die each year when they are well below average life expectancy. Of people who smoke for many years, about half will die of a disease caused by their smoking and about half of these will die in middle age[41]. Richard Peto and colleagues have calculated that for the year 2000, in industrialised nations alone, 1 945 902 people died of tobacco-caused disease. Of these about half (962 313, or 49.5%) died between the ages of 35 and 69[42]. In less-developed nations for the year 2000, 2.41 million deaths were attributable to smoking[43].

Former Beatle George Harrison was one such person who died early from smoking. His death on 29 November 2001 from smoking-caused lung cancer was noted in some reports as if he had died from any other cause, despite losing more than 20 years of the average life expectancy of a 58-year-old British man. Indeed, the ABC network in the USA went so far as to note that unlike many other rock stars of his generation (Jimi Hendrix, Janis Joplin, Jim Morrison) Harrison had died of "natural causes"[44].

If we assume Harrison took up smoking at the age of 15, and on average smoked 20 cigarettes a day, he therefore smoked for around 43 years, smoking 314 115 cigarettes in that time. Observations of smoking show that a cigarette takes about 5.6 minutes to smoke[45]. We can therefore calculate that Harrison had a cigarette alight for a cumulative total of 1221.6 days, or 3.34 years, of his 58 years. Recalling that he lost about 20 years of normal life expectancy for an Englishman, we can calculate that each of the 314 115 cigarettes he smoked took 33.5 minutes off his life – about six times longer than the time it took him to smoke each one.

Few smokers have any realistic idea of the probability (it is 50%) that their smoking will cause their death, nor of how many years on average they will lose. Since early 2005 my website[46] has hosted a quiz for smokers to assess the extent to which they understand the risks of smoking. One question reads:

On average, how much longer do non-smokers live than people who have smoked for a long time?

- None. On average they will live as long as a non-smoker
- Between 1–2 years
- Between 2–5 years
- Between 6–12 years
- Between 12–20 years
- More than 20 years

As at 26 August 2006, 960 people had attempted the question, and only 297 (30.9%) got the correct answer: "between 6–12 years" ("On average, cigarette smokers die about 10 years younger than non-smokers")[47]. Later in this chapter, I consider the ethical questions arising from smokers' inadequate understandings of the risks they face.

Tobacco can greatly diminish quality of life

So, tobacco kills many people, and it kills many people years earlier than they may have lived had they not smoked. If communities value life and believe that the early, avoidable deaths of many of their citizens are cause for concern, we are then already one large step towards justifying tobacco control. But the *process* of dying from tobacco-caused diseases is also highly relevant. It is here that the wisdom of my 52-year-old caller who pleaded for more attention to the misery that smoking can cause *during* life comes into its own. Tobacco doesn't just kill, and kill many people early, it also seriously erodes the quality of life for millions who live, sometimes for many years, with tobacco-caused diseases before they die.

Most of us have a sense of how we would like to "go" when we die. In the most usual scenario, we see ourselves dying peacefully in our sleep, around normal life expectancy, after having lived our lives free of pain and without major disability, with all of our senses still functioning and being able to continue daily performing most of the activities we enjoy without assistance. We don't want to have to depend on others for basic support in mobility, toileting and eating.

Certainly, there are many lifelong smokers who die this way: who "drop dead" after a decent lifespan, lived largely free of diagnosed disease. Smokers' experience of such people gives rise to the commonly heard self-exempting belief "what about all those people like my Uncle Bob who smoked all his life and died in his sleep at 85?"[48]. But many smokers and former smokers die with significant disability that they may have lived with for years before death. Let us briefly count just some of the ways.

- Smoking is a major cause of cardiac disease, with painful manifestations like angina afflicting millions and greatly reducing sufferers' ability to live a fully participatory life.
- Smoking causes peripheral vascular disease[49], which can cause pain in walking and, in extreme cases, lead to gangrene and amputation of the limbs.
- Smoking is a major causative factor in stroke. Stroke survivors can suffer all manner of mild to severe motor, neurological and sensory problems. People who have had strokes can place huge burdens on their carers for many years.
- Smoking is a major risk factor for blindness resulting from age-related macular degeneration caused by smoking[50].
- Smokers are at greatly increased risk of hearing loss[51].
- Smoking causes periodontal disease, causing teeth loss[52].
- Smoking is a cause of osteoporosis, associated with the risk of bone fractures, immobility and death in older people from pneumonia consequent on that immobility[53].
- Erectile dysfunction. In a recent Australian study of 8367 Australian men aged 16–59 years, men who smoked more than 20 cigarettes a day had a 39% higher probability of having a period of erectile dysfunction that lasted longer than one month[54].
- In 2000, an estimated 8.6 million – 95% confidence interval (CI) = 6.9–10.5 million – persons in the USA had an estimated 12.7 million (95% CI = 10.8–15.0 million) smoking-attributable conditions. For current smokers, chronic bronchitis was the most prevalent condition (49%), followed by emphysema (24%). For former smokers, the three most prevalent conditions were chronic bronchitis (26%), emphysema (24%), and previous heart attack (24%). Lung cancer accounted for 1% of all cigarette smoking-attributable illnesses[55].

One of the most common and chronic diseases caused by smoking is chronic obstructive pulmonary disease (COPD), including emphysema. Emphysema, which is what my caller suffered from, results from destruction of the alveoli (air sacs) in the lung. The effect of this loss of lung tissue on the small peripheral airways is to cause them to collapse when pressure is applied during exhalation or breathing out. When you are with a person with emphysema, you get the impression of it being easy for them to take air in, but not to get it out. In advanced emphysema, which can last many months and sometimes years, the person finds even the simplest energy-requiring tasks hugely exhausting. Walking across a room becomes a major challenge, and climbing even a small set of steps can be nearly impossible. An oxygen cylinder is their constant companion. Speaking more than a few sentences can be energy draining.

People living such lives understandably don't get out and about much, so tend to live the remainder of their lives shut off from the outside world, moving from bed to chair and back again. Understandably, their invisibility to the world means that few people without first-hand experience of a relative or friend living with emphysema have much awareness of the disease. Out of sight is out of mind, which explains in large part why many people find it hard to believe the stratospheric data on the numbers of people killed and affected by smoking. A recent review of global studies of the prevalence of emphysema in different populations concluded that in the population studied the pooled estimated incidence of emphysema was 1.8%, and that 15.4% of smokers had COPD compared with 4.3% of people who had never smoked[56]. Such proportions translate to frighteningly large numbers of seriously debilitated smokers.

In 1980, James Fries first advanced the concept of the compression of morbidity – the notion that the goals of medicine and public health should also importantly involve striving to compress the time in which people experience illness, disability and a significantly reduced quality of life[57]. He argued that a key goal of medicine and public health should be to reduce the number, duration and severity of episodes of illness. A recent systematic review of the *rate* of functional decline in the aged in the USA has shown a significant reduction in this decline in the past three decades, suggesting some success in compressing morbidity (i.e. delaying the onset of illness in elderly people) through both prevention and medical care. However, in many nations the demographic wave of former "baby boomer" generation people now entering late middle and old age will mean that the *number* of people who are disabled, dependent and living with reduced functionality because of multiple chronic conditions will grow to be larger than ever before. Tobacco-caused morbidity will be a significant proportion of these conditions. With this trend compounded by the rapidly growing obesity epidemic, we seem likely to see an unprecedented prevalence of disability in ways that may not have been previously anticipated in disease modelling. Efforts to reduce and compress the incidence of preventable morbidity – such as that caused by tobacco use – will thus become increasingly important as populations age.

Tobacco control needs to pay far more attention to the diseases we get from tobacco use when still alive, particularly those that can affect people in their early middle age. Efforts should be made to empower people living with chronic disease caused by smoking to become more visible and to assist in tobacco control advocacy.

The ethics of tobacco control

To some, it may seem self-evident that with smoking causing so much preventable early death and suffering, that efforts to control tobacco use will always be entirely ethically defensible. But in fact tobacco control policy presents many complex ethical dilemmas that need careful interrogation. Robert Goodin's seminal paper "The ethics of smoking"[58], and his now out-of-print book[59], which expands his arguments, remain for me the most lucid exposition of the ethical issues associated with tobacco control. Starting with the utilitarian philosopher John Stuart Mill's famous essay on liberty[60], Goodin examines both the question of whether smoking ought to be regarded as "a paradigmatically private-regarding vice" that harms only smokers themselves who have chosen, perhaps knowingly, to take their chances. He also considers the extent to which smoking interferes with the liberty of others, and so might be regarded as a legitimate subject of intervention in any civil society.

Mill's key precept states that "the sole end for which mankind are warranted, individually or collectively, in interfering with the liberty of action of any of their number, is self-protection . . . The only purpose for which power can be rightfully exercised over any member of a civilised community . . . is to prevent harm to others"[60].

Broadly, these are the two central questions on which an ethical assessment of the case for tobacco control rests. In the case of the first, the crude argument runs that unless one is an open paternalist who believes it is legitimate to interfere in the liberty of others to protect them from the consequences of their own freely chosen actions, then such interference is ethically unjustified to anyone who subscribes to the ethical force of Mill's core principle. But as I will discuss, such a simplistic assessment is complicated by several key problems: are smokers in fact knowingly taking the risks they "choose" to take? Because nicotine is addictive, what implications are there for the notion that smokers are freely engaging in smoking, particularly because most smokers commence smoking when they are legally children and therefore below the age when informed consent is recognised. And because in welfarist states, the community through taxation provides for the health care of those who are ill, is it reasonable that the state should pay for the costs of caring for sick smokers, who some would argue are "voluntarily" incurring such costs and then expecting the community to pay for them?

In the case of the second major ethical question (does smoking violate the Millean principle of not harming others?), if smoking can also harm people other than the smoker, then a prima facie case exists that smoking in such circumstances should be subjected to ethically legitimate controls. Goodin notes that "there is a world of [ethical] difference between the harms that others inflict upon you and the harms that you inflict upon yourself." The interesting ethical questions arising here concern the levels of exposure at which "harming others" might be reasonably said to commence. And more fundamentally, what is "harm"? As we will consider in Chapter 6, policy debates have emerged about banning smoking in circumstances where the exposure involved and the probability of harm is extremely low.

The ethics of smokers "knowingly" harming themselves

The legal maxim of *volenti non fit injuria* holds that if people voluntarily participate in activities known full well to them as involving risk, then they waive any rights to redress should they then be harmed. They are said to have "brought it on themselves". This is the position taken by tobacco industry defence teams when sick and dying smokers seek to sue the industry for damages arising from the use of tobacco products when consumed according to the manufacturers' instructions.

The key questions arising here concern the proposition that smokers in fact do really "know" the risks to which they are said to be consenting. People can only be said to have consented if we can be assured that they actually knew what it was to which they were supposedly consenting. If smokers falsely believe that their smoking poses no risks to them, or significantly underestimate those risks, then the central premise of the "informed consent" argument justifying allowing smokers to chose to continue knowingly harming themselves is seriously undermined.

Obligations to provide information to consumers about the risks created by products fall mainly upon manufacturers, and the failure to provide information is a common basis of legal liability. This failure may take the form of positively misleading or deceptive conduct or misleading or deceiving through a combination of positive acts and silence, such as where a manufacturer fails to disclose information where a consumer would have a "reasonable expectation" that, if the manufacturer knew some information likely to be seen as important to a consumer, the manufacturer would disclose it.

No person can be reasonably expected to have a full appreciation of all the risks they face in every behaviour or in every circumstance in which they may find themselves. For similarly obvious reasons, the law never requires a manufacturer to disclose *every* conceivable risk that a product might ever create in any circumstance. Generally though, the obligation is to provide "adequate" information or warnings. As often occurs in law, "adequacy" is an imprecise concept that has to be determined in the context of all relevant circumstances. Relevant questions include whether warnings bring clearly and emphatically to the mind of a consumer the risks associated with use; whether they refer to specific risks; and whether they are sufficiently clear or explicit. As a matter of general legal principle, the greater the magnitude of a risk (i.e. the more likely that the adverse outcome will occur), and the more severe the consequences if the risk materialises, the more important is the obligation to disclose.

As stated earlier, globally each year, tobacco products, when used as intended by their manufacturers, cause the death of (currently) some 5 million people[43]. Around half and perhaps up to two-thirds of long-term users of tobacco will die from a tobacco-caused disease[41]. Tobacco thus constitutes a prima facie example of a consumer good for which it is imperative that questions about the communication of risk information be considered.

There is a huge disparity between what is known from epidemiological research about the range, extent and probability of tobacco's harm to users, and both the communication of these harms to consumers and smokers' understandings of these harmful characteristics. The proposition that most smokers are fully or even adequately informed about the risks they take is false, manifestly so in populations with low literacy and education.

Governments regularly impose restrictions and conditions of use on goods and services when unrestricted use or provision may cause unacceptable levels of harm either to users or to those exposed to the use of the product or provision of the service. This is more often the case when the harms caused are imminent ("dangerous") rather than chronic ("unhealthy"), the latter typically requiring many years to be expressed as illness. Restrictions implemented through registration and licensing are imposed on manufacturers of consumer products, motor vehicles and their users, firearms, explosives and the performance of dangerous work. Governments restrict access to or performance of certain occupations (e.g. certification of competence to perform electrical work, building, plumbing, medical, dental and pharmaceutical dispensing) and require formal assessment of medical need for access to products (access to addictive drugs such as morphine derivatives). For a product that causes such immense death and disease, the sale of, and access to, tobacco remains minimally regulated (see Chapter 4).

"Informed" smokers: policy implications

The tobacco industry has long acted to avoid, dilute and delay the introduction of health warnings on packs, particularly when these concern specific diseases[61]. When it was forced by legislation to do so, the cloud had a big silver lining, allowing the global industry to adopt the position that all smokers were henceforth "fully informed". For example, the Tobacco Institute of Australia told the Australian Senate in 1995: "The tobacco industry believes that people who smoke do so fully informed of the reported health risks of smoking . . . If the public is adequately informed then the necessity or logic of further government intervention must be questioned"[62]. However, the core assumption of the industry's position has not been sufficiently interrogated: just what is a "fully or adequately informed smoker?" Moreover, if the concept of the fully informed smoker is seen as critical to policy about the obligations of manufacturers and the responsibilities of government, it follows that we should also ask whether it is, or should be, legal to sell tobacco to an "inadequately informed smoker".

Legal proscriptions on children voting, being conscripted into military service, gambling and entering legal contracts, on selling alcohol and tobacco to children, and allowing them to view explicit sexual and violent films are in part based on the premise that children are too intellectually immature to be able to make informed decisions about matters where they might be exploited or suffer harm. Adulthood, and its legal rights and responsibilities, carries assumptions about individuals being able to reasonably comprehend risks and make informed choices. But such an assumption deserves scrutiny against what is known about smokers' understandings of the risks they face.

There are at least four important consequences for both the tobacco industry and public health policy if the "smokers are fully or adequately informed" argument is accepted uncritically. First, it allows the tobacco industry to resist future reform of pack warnings because it presupposes that all relevant information both known and that might be discovered is already addressed by existing (presumably general) warnings. As Philip Morris' international CEO wrote to an Australian political leader in 1992: "Australians are aware of the warnings against smoking – one would have to be asleep in a cave for 20 years not to be aware – and a change in the existing pack warnings is thus unnecessary."[63]

Second, it allows the tobacco industry to resist other regulatory reforms, such as those dealing with advertising and promotion, product availability (where products can be sold), packaging design or taxation. The Tobacco Institute of Australia's line that "if the public is adequately informed then the necessity or logic of further government intervention must be questioned" can be expected to be deployed in each of these contexts.

Third, the cornerstone of the industry's defence to litigation in most cases brought by dying smokers has been that smokers are aware of the risks they take, through pack warnings and other widely circulated information about smoking and health, and therefore smokers should bear all responsibility for deciding to take these risks. Evidence that the community is "saturated" with information about illnesses said to be caused by smoking and the addictive nature of nicotine (see below) is critical to such a defence. However, the defence remains vulnerable to evidence about the industry's dissembling conduct designed to undermine public confidence in the warnings[64], the reassuring messages it has sent, and continues to send, to smokers and potential smokers through its advertising including alluring pack designs[65], deliberate product manipulation[66] and the significance of addiction.

The fourth area of relevance is concerned with arguments about the costs and benefits of tobacco use to national economies. Industry-commissioned economic reports often assume Viscusi's "rational addiction" precepts[67] about significant awareness of health risks as a basis for arguing that the money outlaid by all smokers should be considered as an economic benefit, thereby allowing the "benefits" side of national cost-benefit ledgers to be artificially boosted significantly.

What is a "fully or adequately informed" smoker?

Four levels of being "informed" about the risks of smoking can be distinguished.

Level 1: having heard that smoking increases health risks. At the most elementary level, one can ask whether an individual has ever heard that smoking is a threat to "health" in its widest sense. Such people might be said to be "aware" that smoking is regarded as harmful. Today, this level of awareness is very high in nearly all nations and subpopulations, and is that to which the tobacco industry invariably refers when it talks about almost saturation-levels of awareness. Evaluation of recent Australian quit campaigns, which highlight the harms of smoking, suggests over 88% awareness of the campaigns[68]. By contrast, in less developed nations, knowledge can be very poor. In China in 1996, 61% of smokers believed smoking caused "little" harm, with 7.5% believing it caused no harm[69].

Level 2: being aware that specific diseases are caused by smoking. Level 1 awareness often involves little understanding of which particular diseases are caused by smoking, while level 2 awareness involves knowing that smoking can cause particular diseases like lung cancer and emphysema. Level 2 awareness in populations is generally much lower than that for level 1. For example, in one Australian study, only 54% of smokers mentioned lung cancer, unprompted, as a smoking-related illness, though the specific warning had already appeared on packs for several years[70]. Although cigarette smoking has been found to increase the risk of developing many different illnesses, most smokers in developed countries with histories of tobacco control can name only a few illnesses when given the opportunity in surveys to name as many diseases caused by smoking as they can, suggesting that many of the health risks are either unknown or not particularly salient.

Here important questions arise as to how many, and which, diseases a person should be aware of before being said to be adequately "aware" of the full range of risks engendered by smoking. In Australia, awareness of pack warnings among smokers remains high[71], yet a 2002 US Surgeon General review and International Agency for Research in Cancer (IARC) declarations about smoking's relationship to disease found 26 other diseases not covered by the six warnings[72]. Informed decision-making and self-regarding behaviour seem impossible without knowledge of many conditions that have not been the subject of health warnings. For example, conditions caused or exacerbated by smoking such as blindness[73], reduced fertility, deafness and impotence substantially affect lifestyle and life decisions. Other conditions, such as bladder cancer and colorectal cancer[74], could potentially be treated if detected early. Here, information may make the difference between survival and death.

Level 3: accurately appreciating the meaning, severity and probabilities of developing tobacco-related diseases. Being aware of claims that smoking causes particular diseases may not involve an individual having even rudimentary awareness or understanding of what these diseases mean. For example, few smokers are likely to actually know what emphysema is, how it destroys lung tissue, and what the quality of day-to-day life of someone living with emphysema is like. Similarly, few would have seen a person (or even a photograph of a person) suffering from gangrene caused by advanced peripheral vascular disease caused by smoking, and so would have a poorly developed sense of the hideous nature of gangrene, including the pain and smell it causes.

Similarly important is an understanding of the severity of smoking-caused disease, the likelihood of surviving 5 years after diagnosis, the probabilities of contracting various diseases, or the relative risk of contracting a smoking-caused disease when compared with other risks of life that people would rank as important. For example, when shown a list of possible causes of death that included car accidents, alcohol, asbestos and poor diet, and asked to indicate the one they were most likely to die from, only one-third of smokers in an Australian study identified smoking[70] despite it being by far the greatest health hazard they faced on the list. A considerable proportion of smokers (28%) thought they were most likely to die from a car accident, and 6% thought they would die from "toxic chemicals". A majority of Australian smokers underestimate the risks of smoking[75], and Weinstein et al.[76] state that "Smokers underestimate their risk of lung cancer both relative to other smokers and to non-smokers and demonstrate other misunderstandings of smoking risks. Smoking cannot be interpreted as a choice made in the presence of full information about the potential harm". A comprehensive list of such studies can be found in the Canadian Cancer Society publication *Controlling the Tobacco Epidemic*[77], commencing at page 231. Such studies indicate that many smokers have a poor understanding of the risks that smoking poses to their health. Additionally, given that most harms from smoking occur later in a smoker's lifetime, becoming manifest often after decades of use, special challenges arise in communicating the lifetime probability of acquiring such diseases.

Level 4: personally accepting that the risks inherent in levels 1–3 apply to one's own risk of contracting such diseases. Individuals may have appreciable levels of awareness as described above, but may nonetheless mediate these through various self-exempting beliefs (e.g. "everything causes cancer these days") that effectively allow for the rationalisation of continued smoking.[48] Level 4 awareness involves smokers agreeing that their smoking poses significant risk to their *own* health. Weinstein's review of international evidence on smokers' recognition of vulnerability to harm concludes that "smokers do acknowledge some risk; nevertheless they minimize the size of that risk and show a clear tendency to believe that the risk applies more to other smokers than themselves . . . People may be quite aware of well-publicised risks and may even overestimate their numerical probability, but they still resist the idea that risks are personally relevant."[78]

In principle, an adequately informed smoker would be one who was able to demonstrate specified levels of awareness and understanding of level 2 and 3 information, and who believed that their own smoking was likely to pose significant risks to their health (level 4). However, settling on what these agreed levels of understanding should be and how we would agree that adequate levels of understanding had been demonstrated presents large challenges (see Chapter 8). Nevertheless, the difficulties presented by meeting these challenges should not preclude their being subjected to serious consideration, drawing on the considerable body of evidence assembled by experts in the visual communication of risk[79] and particularly work undertaken in Canada[77] and Australia[80] in the development of more salient health warnings.

Level 2 awareness would require agreement on which diseases smokers should reasonably be expected to know were increased in risk by smoking. The conclusions of regular reviews by agencies such as the Centers for Disease Control, the US Surgeon General and the International Agency for Research on Cancer could provide a starting point here. Just how this might be operationalised is discussed in Chapter 8.

The tobacco industry's current information inaction

The tobacco industry's past and current practice in communicating with its customers about health risks can be characterised as doing as little as possible, as slowly as possible, in as low a key as possible. As revealed in industry documents, the industry fully appreciates that packs are the premier site for communicating with smokers[65]. Yet the industry has never initiated any form of communication with smokers about health risks via packs. Instead, it defers to government requirements on health warnings, waits for government reforming initiatives and then seeks to delay and dilute the proposed changes[61].

There is much more that the industry could do to inform smokers both through packs and through other means. Rather than wait out the ten-year cycles that have characterised three new generations of health warnings in Australia, the industry could voluntarily add new warnings to packs whenever scientific consensus was declared through major agency reports like those of the IARC. It could run public awareness campaigns citing these new findings (authorised and vetted by health authorities to eliminate characteristic weasel wording) and place website addresses on packs linking to the reports rather than trust smokers to discover these for themselves.

It is not through lack of its own awareness that the industry fails to warn smokers about emerging new risks. Industry documents on the Master Settlement Agreement websites contain many thousands of examples of public domain scientific papers on health effects that have been in the industry's possession often for decades. In any case, even if it did not monitor developing information, lack of awareness ought to be no defence. The manufacturer that buries its head in the sand is hardly less culpable than the manufacturer that deliberately withholds information – the law recognises this through its notion of "wilful blindness". The industry has a continuing responsibility to inform itself, and to act to pass this information to its customers.

In Australia, tobacco companies voluntarily publish additive and emissions data on websites[81], although the ubiquitous use of the nonspecific catch-all term "processing aids" allows them to conceal information about any ingredient they wish not to reveal to consumers[82]. However, because these sites are not publicised by the industry or listed on cigarette packs, very few smokers would be aware of them, or capable of understanding the implications of pyrolysis product inhalation (i.e. the health consequences of repeatedly inhaling, e.g., burnt pesticide residues). Again, the industry could declare *all* the ingredients it uses in manufactured tobacco such as ammonia chemistry and any nicotine analogues[83], explain why it uses them and how they affect addiction, and inform consumers that no information is available about the health effects on humans of inhaling the combusted ingredients it adds to tobacco.

Ethical implications of addiction in tobacco control

All argued so far is greatly complicated by the combined facts of (often rapid) nicotine addiction[84], and that most smokers begin smoking in childhood when they are legally incapable of making informed decisions on important matters. The importance of adequate information presupposes that people are able to make free, self-regarding decisions based on relevant facts. But as the tobacco industry knows, "the entire matter of addiction is the most potent weapon a prosecuting attorney can have in a lung cancer/cigarette case. We can't defend continued smoking as 'free choice' if the person was 'addicted'."[85]

The tobacco industry likes to trivialise the notion that tobacco use is addictive, emphasising that millions of smokers have quit, and that therefore smoking (or nicotine) cannot be addictive. Such rhetoric plays to populist notions that true addiction is wholly involuntary so that the addict, like a sleepwalker, somehow unconsciously goes about procuring and using nicotine, in a zombie-like trance from which they are unable ever to be released once it commences. But such notions are entirely fictitious: narcotics addicts, for example, also often stop using heroin completely[86-88] and few would therefore conclude that heroin is not powerfully addictive. There is almost endless evidence that smoking is powerfully addictive, satisfying all the standard criteria of addiction – except intoxication – that other addictive substances satisfy[89].

I often ask nicotine addiction sceptics to reflect that if nicotine was not addictive, why would hundreds of thousands of smokers every year together shower millions of dollars into pharmaceutical company cash registers? Do they privately like wearing nicotine patches that no one can see? Have they some collectively mistaken notion that drug companies are charities who deserve their support? Or is it more plausible that many are frustrated by sometimes years of failed attempts to quit and have sought pharmacological assistance, at considerable expense?

Few smokers are likely to start smoking believing that there is a strong possibility that they will find it difficult to stop. Indeed, many will be aware that millions of former smokers have successfully stopped smoking, so pack warnings about smoking being addictive are likely to be discounted by many smokers. Much has been written about the notion of voluntarily assuming the risks of addiction[90], that is, assuming the risks of becoming addicted before one is addicted. The notion of voluntarily assuming the risks of having one's capacity for future voluntary activity impaired is highly problematic. John Stuart Mill argued that we would not respect a person's voluntary choice to sell themselves into slavery, and Goodin argues that "acquiring a lethal and hard-to-break addiction is much more like a slavery contract than it is like an ordinary commercial commitment" (such as a legal contract)[58].

Further, because relevant information on the risks of smoking is forever evolving, much relevant information can only be learned once one is already addicted.

If agreement could be reached on what constituted being adequately informed about the risks of smoking, it could only be a level applicable at a particular point in time. Being "adequately informed" is not a static "once in a lifetime" state. New information emerging 10 years after a person commences smoking today comes after they are already addicted (and their capacity for voluntary activity has been impaired). But how can one *voluntarily* assume the risks to which the new information relates once one is already addicted?

Anglo–Australian common law contains a deep-rooted doctrine of "voluntary assumption of risk" (*volenti non fit injuria*). Under this doctrine, defendants have a complete defence to negligence actions if they can show that a plaintiff voluntarily assumed the risk that later materialised into injury.

The test of voluntary assumption of risk is not an easy one to meet. The person who tries to use it has to show that the plaintiff perceived the existence of the danger; *fully* appreciated it; and *voluntarily* accepted it[91]. The strictness of the test, and the rationale for the strictness, were well encapsulated by Lord Justice Scott in 1944, when he wrote:

> That general maxim has to be applied with especially careful regard to the varying facts of human affairs and human nature in any particular case just because it is concerned with the intangible factors of mind and will. For the purpose of the rule, if it be a rule, a man cannot be said to be truly "willing" unless he is in a position to choose freely, and freedom of choice predicates, not only full knowledge of the circumstances on which the exercise of choice is conditioned, so that he may be able to choose wisely, but the absence from his mind of any feeling of constraint so that nothing shall interfere with the freedom of his will[92].

Goodin concludes his analysis of the ethical implications of whether addiction undermines free will by saying "the issue is not one of impossibility [of quitting] but rather of how hard people should have to try before their will is said to be sufficiently impaired that their agreement does not count as genuine consent. The evidence suggests that nicotine addicts have to try very hard indeed"[58].

When smoking harms others

It is an elementary tenet of civil society that the exercise of freedom should not involve harming others. The evidence that began to emerge in the early 1970s with epidemiological reports showing that infant respiratory problems were associated with parental indoor smoking rapidly came to revolutionise the ethical basis for tobacco control. My smoking was no longer simply bad for *my* health, it was now also bad for *your* health too. Essentially paternalistic precepts about protecting one's own health were joined by imperatives not to endanger other's health. Smoking was suddenly not merely a personally risky action, it was also a public menace requiring the same sort of protections that other forms of public harm attract. In perhaps the most quoted statement of the era on the topic, the Roper market research organisation advised the tobacco industry in 1978: "What the smoker does to himself may be his business, but what the smoker does to the non-smoker is quite a different matter." Passive smoking was "the most dangerous development to the viability of the tobacco industry that has yet occurred."[93]

It is now history that secondhand smoke emerged at the beginning of the 1980s as the unstoppable Trojan horse of tobacco control[94] that has caused nothing less than a revolution in the way smoking is treated in public policy. While controls were introduced to protect non-smokers from involuntary exposure, the bigger public health impact has been on active smokers. When you can't smoke at work, on public transport, in cinemas and increasingly in restaurants, bars and even private homes, smoking opportunities are radically reduced and your consumption across 24 hours falls significantly[95]. Many smokers also quit when they cannot smoke at work, many being grateful for the imposition.

The ethics of tobacco control when it seeks to prevent harm to others are therefore very much more straightforward than those urging paternalistic interference in the freedoms of smokers to harm themselves. In 2006, public debate about the rights and wrongs of restricting where smokers can smoke has all but abandoned reference to the bedrock rationale for the restrictions: the health impact on non-smokers. In a study of several years of reportage about advocacy and counter-advocacy to ban smoking in Australian bars, the hotel industry (which opposes the bans) rarely ever mentioned or engaged with health issues, seeking instead to define the debate as being about economic and ideological concerns[96]. Seeking to argue that smokers have a right to risk the health of others is indefensible, so those wanting to defend public smoking have been forced to frame their arguments with other values.

The principal ethical issues remaining about reducing non-smokers' exposure to secondhand smoke relate to questions of when such exposure should be regarded as sufficient to warrant restrictions. In various places in the world, proposals are being advocated for smoking to be banned in outdoor settings such as streets, beaches and parks. Some have even argued that smokers should be banned from working with others even when they do not smoke at work, because even the smell of a smoker is "harmful". I will consider these arguments in detail in Chapter 6.

Ethical aspects of the social costs of smoking

Finally, it is often argued that governments have a legitimate interest in controlling smoking because the social and economic costs of smoking far outweigh the benefits. Governments, having an interest in the relationship of health to economic development, will want to reduce smoking to reduce the costs of smoking. Against this, the tobacco industry has sometimes argued that smokers "pay their way" by having contributed a lifetime of tobacco tax (which non-smokers do not pay) to the government. Should they need to call on the public purse for the costs of caring for them while they are sick from a smoking-caused disease, the argument runs that smokers' tobacco tax contributions should be seen as the equivalent of a sort of "insurance" payment towards such costs if and when they arise.

In Australia, for example, in 1998–99, government expenditure on the hospital costs of treating tobacco-caused disease was estimated at $A718.4 million[97], whereas tobacco excise was approximately $A5 billion. The authors of the report noted "tobacco tax revenue does in fact exceed by a considerable margin the tobacco-attributable costs borne by the government sector".[97]

However, as the authors of the above report went on to explain, government-borne costs are only a fraction of the total economic costs of tobacco use, which include large items such as the benefits foregone to the economy by smokers dying early who would have otherwise contributed to the economy through their labour, investment and expenditure. Items like production losses in the workforce, a reduced workforce size, absenteeism costs, the cost of smokers' breaks and welfare costs for disabled smokers and the welfare support costs of non-working dependants of smokers who have died need to be factored in.

There is also an ill-considered but often repeated folk wisdom about how much governments love smoking because it is a goose that lays a very fat, reliable and easily collected golden tax egg each year. A corollary of the reasoning here is that people who do not smoke somehow take the money that they would otherwise spend on tobacco each day and put it into a box under their bed, never spending it and benefiting neither the government through tax nor the economy through expenditure benefits. This is pure nonsense, of course. Non-smokers spend their money on other goods and services, which in many countries attract a value-added expenditure tax.

However, tobacco products typically attract a double taxation: sales tax and tobacco excise. Most other goods only attract sales tax. All nations place a tax on cigarettes (mostly per stick) and on loose tobacco (by weight), which is paid by tobacco manufacturers directly to government. The manufacturers recoup this cost from retailers, who in turn pass it on to smokers. So smokers do pay extra (often considerable) tobacco taxes that people who do not smoke do not pay. But importantly, tax is not strictly an economic benefit. It is simply a transfer payment – a way that governments arrange for money to be channelled to them.

By arguing this way, tobacco companies are in effect arguing that it is acceptable for tobacco to cause disease, so long as the public cost of treating that disease does not exceed tobacco tax revenue. This is in key respects little different to the ethical foundations of the Nazi death camps, where inmates were killed when their value to the "economy" of the camps fell to an unacceptable level through the decline in their health. In both philosophies, all that matters is the health of the economic balance sheet: let smoking kill people early, as long as the net value to the economy is in the black.

Tobacco tax paid by smokers (not by the tobacco companies) cannot be considered as an insurance policy for the tobacco industry against government intervention to reduce tobacco use. If cigarettes were a consumer good that did not cause disease, then governments could both avoid expenditure on tobacco-caused illnesses and collect revenue that could be used for the benefit of all taxpayers.

The companies argue that smokers pay their way. What they fail to say, however, is that tobacco companies do not. While most costs associated with smoking are borne by smokers and their families who suffer the tragedy of premature death and disablement, we would all be significantly better off if smokers spent their money on other products and services that required more labour input and were therefore more employment generating than tobacco[98,99].

Conclusions

There is a strong, ethically coherent case for tobacco control. This case rests on the way that addiction, typically effected when smokers are below the age of legal consent, reduces the autonomy of individuals to act in their own interests. The consequences of the world's most common addiction are a global toll of premature, often painful death, preceded by sometimes years of chronic disability. The moral squalor of the tobacco industry's case against effective tobacco control is compounded by its decades of contempt for its best customers, manifested in a global programme of "smoker reassurance"[100], lying about addiction[101,102], and undermining (which continues today) of every policy or programme that might reduce tobacco use and the harms it causes.

Note

i   Sections of Chapter 1 have been previously published as Shatenstein S, Chapman S. The banality of tobacco deaths. *Tob Control* 2002;**11**:1–2; Chapman S, Liberman J. Ensuring smokers are adequately informed: reflections on consumer rights, manufacturer responsibilities and policy implications. *Tob Control* 2005;**14**(Suppl. II):ii8–ii13; and Chapman S. Never say die? *Med J Aust* 2005;**183**(11–12):622–624 (© Copyright 2005 *The Medical Journal of Australia*, reproduced with permission).

Chapter 2

The Place of Advocacy in Tobacco Control[i]

In 1991, a prominent Australian heart transplant surgeon, Dr Victor Chang, was murdered on the way to work in a bungled extortion attempt. For weeks afterwards, the Australian media were dominated by news accounts of his death and efforts to find his killers. Dozens of eulogies were written and a research foundation established in his memory. Why was the story so huge? When you deconstructed these reports for their common subtexts and news values, most told the story of Chang as a quietly achieving, unassuming and highly skilled surgeon whose talent allowed everyone from nameless, statistical patients to named, very public citizens to be "born again". In effect, Chang was being framed as a secular Christ-like figure who could almost raise the dead[103].

Let us imagine for a moment that instead of a transplant surgeon being murdered, that a policy analyst from a highway authority was killed that day. Or someone who had worked tirelessly for 20 years to build an injury surveillance system. Or the architect of a successful national smoking cessation campaign. It's almost inconceivable that a nation would similarly mourn the death of a bureaucrat, a policy analyst, an epidemiologist or what the press like to call a "crusader" for some public health issue. Yet the public health impact of a transplant surgeon's work and those of public health workers working to collect evidence, set up early warning systems, or successfully advocate for laws and standards are simply incomparable.

The first heart transplant was performed in 1967. Globally, by 2003, some 62 800 heart and heart/lung transplants had been performed[104], an almost indescribably tiny fraction of the number of people with heart disease in the world during those 36 years. Because of the skills and costs involved, heart transplantation will always have an utterly insignificant role in any public health response to heart disease. But it looms large in the public imagination as part of the arsenal of solutions to heart disease that deserves charitable and government support. Far more people have won lotteries than have had a heart transplant since the operation was first performed. Its relevance to the lives of ordinary people in the vast populations of developing nations like China and India could not be more remote. Far more years of life are saved and disabilities avoided each year by prevention workers than by the cutting-edge efforts of surgeons or the work of oncologists treating those already suffering from cancer. As a review in the *New England Journal of Medicine* concluded about progress against cancer: "The most promising approach to the control of cancer is a national commitment to prevention, with a concomitant rebalancing of the focus and funding of research."[105]

Prevention has produced spectacular public health outcomes in diverse fields of public health, from immunisation, to HIV control in nations that have embraced a harm reduction philosophy, to road injury reduction. In a Scottish study comparing the contributions of cardiology treatments to lifestyle changes (smoking, cholesterol, blood pressure) the latter accounted for some 35 991 life years gained (with reductions in smoking accounting for over 50% of this) whereas pharmacological treatments gained 12 025 life years, almost three times fewer[106].

In 2006, the chief epidemiologist at the American Cancer Society, Michael Thun, examined the contribution of falling smoking rates in the USA to the falls in incidence rates of all cancers. He concluded: "Even our most conservative estimate indicates that reductions in lung cancer, resulting from reductions in tobacco smoking over the last half century, account for about 40% of the decrease in overall male cancer death rates and have prevented at least 146 000 lung cancer deaths in men during the period 1991 to 2003. A more realistic straight line projection of what lung cancer rates might have become suggests that, *without reductions in smoking, there would have been virtually no reduction in overall cancer mortality in either men or women since the early 1990s.* [my emphasis] The payoff from past investments in tobacco control has only just begun."[107]

Whenever success stories are being gathered to demonstrate the importance and potential of prevention, tobacco control is seldom far from the top of anyone's list. Despite this, the proportion of government health care expenditure devoted to preventive efforts is typically derisory[108]. In Australia, for example, the Federal government today receives about $A5.5 billion each year in tobacco excise tax, often declares tobacco control to be a leading public health priority, and yet currently allocates about $A6 million annually to tobacco control. Plainly, there remains much to be done to effect a rebalancing of resource allocation to give greater prominence to prevention.

The paradox of successful prevention[109] is that it works when *nothing* happens. People who *don't* get lung cancer at 50 don't tend to walk around saying "thank heavens for the Cancer Society". Few of us when turning the car safely into our driveways each night bless those who've advocated for random breath testing or traffic calming measures. There are no "waiting lists" or queues for prevention. I've never heard callers to radio attacking government over delays in implementing a Pap smear reminder system. Accordingly, there is a widespread sense in politics that while the community think prevention is very worthy and will be all approving when asked to complete opinion polls, few people would consider it a top-of-mind vote-deciding issue. But political red-alert hospital "facility plight" stories are legion because of the power of the "rule of rescue"[15].

Policy wish lists

Every field of public health practice has its "wish lists" of upstream policies, programmes and levels of funding that its practitioners dream of securing so that progress can be accelerated to reduce the diseases or injuries being caused. But in all fields of public health, there remain yawning gaps between what is being implemented to effect change and what those working in those fields know would make a difference.

Public health advocacy is the broad process that seeks to bridge these gaps, by placing and maintaining issues like tobacco control prominently on public and political agendas, eroding barriers to the adoption and implementation of policies and the adequate funding for programmes, and counteracting the efforts of interest groups who stand to lose from the implementation of good public health policy. In the overall project of public health, it is the discipline that can mean the difference between emerging knowledge of how to prevent disease sitting largely unread in an obscure specialised research journal, and the importance of that research being recognised in the introduction of a new law, regulation, funding for further research or intervention programmes.

It is critical that advocacy is understood to be a *strategy*, and not as an end in itself. As such, advocates should always be able to point immediately to the public health objectives that any given episode of advocacy is trying to address. These objectives can include:

- New laws and regulations.
- Enforcement of existing laws and regulations, including stronger penalties.
- More funding for programmes.
- Tax rises or reductions on products to depress or increase demand.
- Changing clinical or institutional practices.
- Having other sectors direct energy at health issues.

Explicit objectives can also be set for the process of advocacy itself. These can include:

- Ensuring that an issue is discussed publicly and politically where it is being suboptimally discussed (framing issues to make them more compelling to the media and decision-makers).
- Having an issue discussed *differently* in ways that are more conducive to the advance of policy and funding ("reframing" issues that are being discussed, but in ways that are helpful to public health).
- Discrediting the opponents of public health objectives.
- Bringing important, different voices into debates.
- Introducing new key facts and perspectives calculated to change the focus of a debate.

Since comprehensive tobacco control policy blueprints were first articulated in the 1970s by agencies such as the World Health Organization[110] and the International Union Against Cancer[111] five stock platforms have characterised comprehensive tobacco control policy:

- A ban on all forms of tobacco advertising and promotion.
- Health warnings on packs.

- Mass-reach public awareness campaigns that highlight the harms of tobacco use, promote prevention and encourage cessation.
- Controls on smoking in enclosed public spaces.
- The progressive taxation of tobacco products to reduce demand.

Thanks to sometimes decades-long advocacy efforts, today many nations have gone a considerable way to implementing this orthodoxy, and the historic Framework Convention on Tobacco Control (FCTC)[112] now guarantees that each of these are backed by internationally enforceable treaty obligations. However, the widespread optional rather than obligatory language throughout the FCTC seems likely to neuter many of its key clauses, leaving it up to countries how to interpret language such as "sovereignty", "appropriate", "latitude", "individual", "flexibility" and "may" that is strewn throughout the FCTC[113]. I would argue that nations friendly to the tobacco industry, like Germany and Japan (which have ratified the FCTC), would never have signed anything that threatened seriously to hamstring the tobacco industry. The USA may never sign it.

Despite the progress that has been made, even in nations with the most advanced tobacco control programmes, a smoking prevalence of under 20% of the adult population remains uncommon. This has stimulated the development of what might be called a second wave of arguably more radical proposals. Some of these remain highly controversial within the field, as were proposals to ban advertising and prevent smoking in workplaces, restaurants and bars when these were first proposed decades ago. Items in a "wish list" for tobacco control in the twenty-first century that have been called for by various agencies and advocates are outlined below.

Agent controls

These are controls on tobacco itself:

- Full regulation of tobacco products so that all ingredients would need approval and full consumer disclosure (such as maximum carcinogen levels, bans on flavouring agents designed to make tobacco more palatable).
- A ban on all misleading product descriptors such as "light" and "mild".
- A ban on filter ventilation holes[114].
- Mandatory international reduced ignition propensity ("RIP") standards for cigarettes[115].
- Progressive increases in the retail price of cigarettes to the point that they become "special occasion" commodities rather than hour-by-hour consumables.

Host-directed factors

These are efforts to reduce demand for tobacco:

- Determination of tobacco industry earnings from under-age sales and requirement that all these earnings be fully repatriated to an independent trust dedicated to reducing youth smoking.

- Commit governments to allocate all tobacco tax earnings from youth sales to the same independent trust, to run world's best practice youth prevention campaigns.
- Establishment of independently audited youth smoking reduction targets and associated punitive taxes on the tobacco industry if target reductions are not met.
- Requirment of all smokers to pass a test demonstrating their adequate knowledge of the harms of smoking (as in driving knowledge exams), and to obtain a smoker's "informed consent to smoke" licence[116] (see Chapter 8).

Vector controls

These are controls on the tobacco industry:

- Legislation to recover costs from the tobacco industry of treating tobacco-caused illness.
- Legislation to oblige tobacco companies to pay for costs of smoking cessation in anyone wanting to quit and choosing to use professional help or pharmacotherapy.
- Licensing of all tobacco retailers and removal of licence to sell on any conviction of selling to minors.

Environmental controls

These are controls on where tobacco can be smoked, and on how it is promoted:

- Full implementation of smoking bans inside all places of employment, including bars and casinos (this remains far from comprehensive in all but a handful of nations).
- Introduction of generic plain packaging to eliminate promotion via packaging and branding[117].
- Further implementation of graphic pack warnings[118].
- "Mopping up" bans on all remaining and future instances of tobacco promotions (see Chapter 7).
- Banning tobacco product displays in shops (i.e. under the counter storage)[119].
- Banning mail-order sales of tobacco (via internet marketing)[120].
- Banning smoking in cars when children are inside.

Advocacy: the neglected sibling of public health

Despite its undeniable track record of achievement and the implied application end point of all public health and medical research (to improve health and well-being), advocacy remains a marginal activity in the broad field of public health. Most public health researchers aspire to have their work published in high-impact journals, reasoning that this is a key measure of their work's importance and influence. Publication in these journals accords peer recognition, enhances promotion prospects and can attract media[121] and hopefully public and political attention[122] to research and its implications for public health. Currently, the epidemiology journal with the highest impact factor is the *American Journal of Epidemiology* with 5.068. In wider public health, the peak journal is the *Annual Review of Public Health* with 4.293. Forty-eight percent of the journals indexed by the Institute of Scientific Information have impact factors <1.000[ii], meaning that in these the average paper is cited less than once in the 2 years after publication[iii].

These numbers that define high impact in public health research are depressingly modest, as are the global circulations of the journals themselves (*Tobacco Control*, the international journal I edit, has about 1200 paid subscribers). Moreover, the audience that might hear a paper at a main session of the world's largest public health conference (the American Public Health Association) is relatively tiny. Add to this library shelf-use studies indicating that 20% of journals are responsible for 80% of borrowings, with many bound volumes of scholarly journals never being opened in a survey year[123], and it all makes a salutary contrast with the audience size of even low-rating late evening national news programmes or the readerships of even provincial newspapers. While epidemiological research should provide the foundation for public health advocacy, only a tiny fraction of often high-quality research ever percolates out of academic circles to inform advocacy efforts or be brought to public attention.

In most research environments it is *de rigueur* to rehearse a conference presentation that might be heard by 30 people at a specialised session. Yet a radio or television interview heard by millions including key decision-makers is often undertaken with a casualness that contrasts with the unparalleled opportunities it presents to influence change. If a public health research report is selected as newsworthy by international news syndicates, its salient features in the eyes of journalists will be broadcast to hundreds of millions, and occasionally billions of people. People repeatedly nominate news media as their leading source of information on health issues, and there are few examples of major legislative or funding reforms in public health that have not been preceded by protracted periods of news coverage involving advocacy by those both promoting and opposing change. Chapter 3 considers the critical role of the news media in advocacy for tobacco control.

I assume tobacco control workers aspiring to be influential understand that the goals of epidemiology and public health lie well beyond the pursuit of growing scientific publications that will be read by few and cited by even fewer. They want their research to influence political or institutional policy and practice, or the personal agendas of large numbers of people, and so hope that there can be a continuum or partnership between epidemiological research and advocacy. They will often find the journalistic compression of their often voluminous research reports into two hundred words or a popularised radio sound bite to be a traumatic experience that tramples on most of the heavily qualified conventions of scientific writing. Yet they will recognise that without such attention to their work, it may never influence any policy or practice.

However, few postgraduate courses in public health place anything but passing attention on how to advance or advocate the policy implications of research. Public health advocacy remains barely a subdiscipline within public health. Unlike medical psychology, education, sociology, anthropology, economics, biostatistics or epidemiology, advocacy has no journals dedicated to critical analysis of its methods, wins and losses. It has few textbooks[1,124–127] and even fewer recognised training programmes, although in recent years an impressive body of scholarship has been published[iv]. Against the time and attention devoted to planning, implementing, and writing up research, the relative neglect of both the skills and analysis of advocacy is remarkable, given its achievements.

Every branch of public health can point to the critical role of advocacy in translating research into policy, practice and sea changes in supportive public opinion. So why does the study and teaching of advocacy remain so neglected? Having worked in public health advocacy for nearly 30 years, I have come to see this as a reflection of advocacy's perceived incompatibility with the reductionist epistemology that underscores most public health enterprise. Academic public health has been most comfortable with those branches that most closely satisfy the criteria of a science. While there are aspects of the advocacy process that are emerging as almost fail-safe ingredients in predicting the course of campaigns, much in the day-to-day practice of advocacy draws more on the less replicable truths of political science, and particularly on framing strategy[128]. Epidemiology, with its aspirations to define immutable notions of reality, demands precision in its specification of agent, host and environmental factors to satisfy these ambitions. Advocacy, by contrast, recognises the dynamic interplay of a myriad of actors and influences that often lie well beyond the reach of the evaluator's desire for control. I continue this theme later in the chapter.

Advocacy is contested

Many epidemiological findings with potential to improve health are welcomed by the public and decision-makers alike. To generalise, in cases where there are no vested interest groups who stand to lose by policy or legislative changes; where these changes require little resource investment; where they might be commodified into profit-making solutions; or where there is already overwhelming community support for implementing change, publicity rather than advocacy may be all that is required. Our emerging understanding of risk reduction in sudden infant death syndrome[129]; of iodising salt to reduce mental retardation[130]; and of supplementing diets with folate to prevent neural tube defects[131] are good examples of red carpet receptions being given to epidemiology.

But advocacy is typically met with a hostile reception from some quarters. Advocacy shares strategies with public relations, but differs in that it invariably involves *contested* definitions of what is at issue. Advocates therefore often find themselves engaged in public conflict with sometimes powerful interest groups or governments determined to resist the changes being advocated. This has always been the case with tobacco control, where the tobacco industry, other affiliated industries profiting from tobacco use and sponsorship, research agencies assisting the industry, and political parties grateful for campaign donations have each resisted tobacco control. For the faint-hearted, advocacy can take on the spectre of a fraught, highly politicised activity, threatening to make enemies particularly of retributive government figures and litigious industries. This can seem a far cry from the mannered and often inconsequential exchanges in letters pages of journals where scientific disputes occur.

In this chapter, I will examine two recurrent concerns about public health advocacy that seem to inhibit greater engagement by those in public health and epidemiology. The first problem is summed up in a question I am often asked by an uncomfortable person in an otherwise supportive audience: "Do you believe that with advocacy it's a case of 'anything goes' . . . that the end justifies the means?" This question goes to the heart of the motivated intent of advocacy and its core strategies: of the way that advocacy sets out to be effective and the extent to which this can sometimes generate controversy about the ethical boundaries between information and persuasion. The core issue here concerns the ways in which problems are defined or framed and the naivety of assumptions that there is some "correct" way of defining a problem.

All tobacco control debates should eventually be concerned with reducing the health problems caused by tobacco use, but as we will see, opponents of tobacco control often seek to try to redefine an issue under debate as being more fundamentally about other values they judge to be more important. While the *goal* of tobacco control advocacy might be to refocus political attention onto the importance of reducing the health impact of tobacco use, the *means* by which this will be achieved will often see various other considerations let off the leash to invigorate debate. Successful advocacy may see a whole host of considerations other than health issues being aired, all in the interests of growing support for values that are compatible with the tobacco control goals being sought. Successful advocacy occurs when advocates' definitions of what is at issue come to dominate public and political debates.

Multiple definitions of the same events

Successful advocates cannot avoid engaging in politics and the core problem of politics has been described as the struggle for ascendancy between multiple definitions of the same events[132]. Multiple definitions of the same events abound in tobacco control. To the tobacco industry, a tobacco advertisement might be defended as a legitimate means of a legal industry to inform its customers about its products. To someone trying to have tobacco advertising banned, the same advertisement is merely another effort by modern day Pied Pipers to beguile adolescents with benign images of an addictive, carcinogenic product. The interest group that succeeds in having its definition of these same events or issues adopted by those able to implement legislative or policy changes will generally be the group that gains ascendency.

The second concern I'll discuss is typically expressed through the question "what evidence have you that advocacy actually *works*?" The attribution of effects to interventions in public health is subject to hierarchical models with the double-blind randomised controlled trial enthroned as the emperor of evidence. By contrast, efforts to attribute causal effects from advocacy processes to their outcome objectives are fraught with problems, and therefore implicitly denigrated as soft or weak. This tends to mean that the most robust "truths" about public health interventions tend to cluster around highly defined and controllable interventions such as the efficacy of therapeutics and vaccines. Efforts to influence political decision-making over years or even decades – the typical time frames in advocacy – are about as far as one can get from such circumscribed, highly controlled interventions. Unless one takes the rather dismal view that in public health the only things that count should be those that can be comprehensively and unambiguously counted, many case histories of important public health successes would be relegated to the dustbin of inconsequentiality.

Does the end justify the means?

When public health advocates articulate their goals, they seldom attract dissent: few decent people are willing to publicly disagree that deaths from heroin over-dose are tragic, that work environments should be safe, or that it would be good if fewer people were killed on the roads. Where advocacy becomes contentious is when it spells out its strategies for achieving these ends, and where these strategies conflict with others' agendas. Safe injecting rooms and heroin prescription trials for illicit drug users[133], smoking bans in pubs[96] and restaurants, and further restrictions on the liberties of motorists[134], for example, all attract protracted, emotional debate.

In disputes about these, all analyses of both advocates' and opponents' positions inescapably reflect the values that inform these. An assessment of the "facts" is rarely the sole decisive feature of political decision-making in public health. When tobacco control advocates emphasise health problems caused to bar staff by second-hand smoke, and pub owners emphasise their concerns about loss of profit, both are talking about the same phenomenon – banning pub smoking – but both are reflecting very different "realities". An intervention will be deemed justifiable or not depending on the way these values are assessed by participants and observers to these disputes.

Advocacy is always unashamedly purposive in its intent

The objectives of advocacy participants are not merely to place their concerns on the public table, retreat and wait patiently to hear if the ensuing community or political debate and the decisions reached are favourable. Once committed to an objective, advocates set out to maximise support for it by strategic planning of the ways they will argue their case, including special attention to counteracting or refram-ing any rhetorical strengths in their opponents' arguments. Discourse in academic public health circles is disciplined by principles of evidence and critical appraisal. By contrast, the currency of advocacy is metaphor, analogy, symbol and efforts to present data in ways that are resonant and memorable to often inexpert target audi-ences. The apposite soundbite that "a non-smoking section of a restaurant is about as useless as a non-urinating section of a swimming pool" contains no data, but conveys more to the average person than the earnest pronouncements of hundreds of scientists at indoor-air-quality conferences could ever hope to achieve with the same broad communicative purpose. Above all, debate in advocacy needs to invoke subtexts or value bases that have widespread support ("this issue is like that issue") so that the solutions proposed to problems are seen as consonant with solutions demanded for problems with parallel value issues underlying them.

The motivated intent of advocacy gives rise to some interesting debates about whether there are meaningful ethical distinctions to be drawn between information and persuasion. I have often noticed criticism of advocacy efforts that imply that there are fairly narrow established or acceptable ways of talking about problems, and in my opening remarks in this chapter noted the concern that is sometimes expressed that "anything goes" in advocacy.

Accuracy is cardinal

Obviously advocacy that is ethical must never utilise claims that are known to be incorrect. The quickest way for an advocacy campaign to fail is for its core scientific foundations to be rapidly gutted by opponents pointing out that one's case is based on fallacious information. The scientific foundations for tobacco control are immense. As US Surgeon General Dr Antonia Novello said in the preface to the 1990 Surgeon General's report on tobacco: "It is safe to say that smoking represents the most extensively documented cause of disease ever investigated in the history of biomedical research."

Tobacco control advocates who try to exaggerate or misrepresent evidence debase these respected foundations, and risk undermining their credibility more widely: people have long memories for those shown to be loose with the truth. The tobacco industry's almost congenital reliability for lying and dissembling is one reason why its credibility and trustworthiness is held in such low esteem by the community[11,135]. Its recognition that the evidence-based bedrock to tobacco control is so powerful is why the tobacco industry has devoted so much effort over the years to trying to undermine these foundations via hired scientists[136–138] who were, in the words of the industry, "prepared to do the kinds of things they were recruited to do"[139]. Incidents of advocates fabricating data or otherwise poisoning the waters of scientific integrity are thankfully uncommon. Disputes about evidence within the tobacco control field are little different to those in epidemiology generally, reflecting the continually evolving status of scientific knowledge, and varying consensus about when collected evidence is robust enough to move to higher status as accepted understanding.

More commonly, though, concerns are expressed about the introduction of argument into advocacy discourse that is held to be irrelevant or "emotional". Public health traditionalists seem to believe that the only acceptable way to present a case about a public health problem is to let the evidence "speak for itself". By this they typically mean a rather narrowly defined range of evidence dominated by biological, toxicological, environmental and economic data. But all public health issues, including tobacco control, have a range of alternative realities to these narrowly prescribed dimensions, which can be very legitimately invoked in public discourse.

Communication always involves choices about how we select, assemble and express the information that we deem relevant to others' reception of what we are wanting to say. Every time we express ourselves publicly, we decide that fact X is relevant, but that fact Y is not, and in doing so begin to frame a definition or closure around what we are claiming to be at issue so that a "preferred" meaning is framed for those we hope are hearing us. If it is inevitable that we steer others' considerations by this unavoidable process of selection, then it is self-delusional to pretend that we are not nearly always hoping that when we give people information they will find it motivating in the ways we had planned. If advocates find that the ways their target audiences receive this information are unmotivating, they try to present it differently in the hope that another way works better. To pretend that there is some neutral, value-free way of presenting information is naïve – the process is inevitably governed by communicative expectations and intentions on the part of the sender[140].

If, as I have argued in Chapter 1, what is ultimately being debated in public health disputes is the primacy of certain values over others, then it is wholly appropriate that the rhetoric of advocacy should seek to highlight those values. This means that it will often need to remind its audiences of what is fundamentally at stake in a debate. What an epidemiologist deems fundamental and relevant may well underscore why an issue is the subject of advocacy in the first place. Epidemiologists' currency in debate is probabilistic data on risk, but this is not how communities define problems, nor why they can become outraged about low-risk issues, remain indifferent to some high-risk exposures or support some policy responses and not others. While the drama of public advocacy played out on television news regularly features venerable scientists in laboratory settings or filmed against the cinematic cliché of a wall of books, news genres in public health also routinely feature distraught victims personifying injustices, corporate villains defending venality over community health, formerly faceless bureaucrats and politicians smarting under the arc lights of public scrutiny and whistleblowers speaking out at risk to their careers.

All these news conventions work to frame the meaning of public health issues, and advocates wishing to have journalists pay attention to their issue need to have an instinctive understanding of the popular subtexts of their issues, as much as the factual dimensions of the debates in which they engage. Many health issues where advocacy debates occur involve consequences that *are* highly emotional. An infant burned in a house fire caused by a discarded cigarette *is* tragic, and any advocate who communicates that they have little emotional rapport with such tragedy effectively disqualifies themselves from being a potent advocate.

The attribution problem in advocacy

The persistent bugbear for sceptics about advocacy is their need for reassurance that it "works". Forgetting that Australia has seen a cultural and legislative revolution in which all tobacco advertising has been banned in the past 20 years; has some of the world's toughest pack warnings; has more than halved the proportion of men who smoke since the 1960s (and reduced the proportion of women by about one-third over the same period); and has had a continuing fall in male lung cancer rates since the early 1980s; sceptics often say to me "advocacy is very interesting, but can you prove to me that it actually works?" There are two major challenges inherent here. The first involves problems in specifying exactly what advocacy *is*, and the second concerns the development of meaningful ways of measuring its influence. Interventions in clinical trials of drugs are discrete and designed to be wholly replicable. Everything possible is done to remove or account for confounders so that those assessing the drugs can be confident that any observed changes are due to the action of the drug. By contrast, advocacy never operates in such pristine environments, but seeks to penetrate and repeatedly respond to decision-making environments that can literally change by the hour during periods of intense campaigning. While the appellation "opportunist" is generally pejorative, in advocacy it is high praise and an essential quality in responding to the many twists and turns that arise in every extended effort to promote change. Whenever necessary, advocates don't hesitate to introduce new strategies not initially planned out of some reverence for the inviolate sanctity of the independent variable or "black box". Such indiscipline in epidemiology would border on profanity. For advocates, public health evaluators often seem to be preoccupied by relatively trivial interventions selected because of funder interest ("did our household brochure change behaviour?") or the ease of bolting on evaluation instruments.

Unravelling gossamer with boxing gloves

In 1993 I published a commentary in the *British Medical Journal*[141] on the problem of how, in tobacco control − or indeed in any complex area of public health − we can be sure we know what impact policies and programmes have on the outcomes we are seeking, such as the quit rate in a community. Over the years, many public health teachers and students have told me that they found it very useful. I have updated it in the next few pages.

Consider a recent day in the life of an Australian smoker, John. As he wakes, John listens to a news item on his clock radio that the present Formula 1 Grand Prix will be the last to have tobacco advertising in Australia. In his half awake state, he reflects that since the mid-1970s he has woken to many similar announcements concerning various forms of tobacco advertising. These have occasioned discussions at his office and in social gatherings, where smoking has become a common and sometimes highly charged topic of conversation. Newspapers have also been thick with news about smoking. In 1988, for example, he might have read up to 1600 separate items in newspapers alone, of which only 17% would have delivered even a vaguely comforting message[142]. Not a day passes without him reading something in a newspaper, or hearing something on radio or television about smoking and how it harms you in dozens of different ways, or how governments are doing something to make it less appealing.

As John smoked at the breakfast table, his two children playfully chorused their latest anti-smoking slogans, "Smokers suck! But we get half the muck!" It seemed there had been dozens of these taunts over the years. Undoubtedly they had picked them up from school, where he knew that they regularly were given lessons about the health consequences of smoking. His wife, who didn't smoke had, like a lot of people, slowly turned into someone who actively disliked smoking. She had recently begun seriously talking to him about whether he might go outside when he wanted to smoke. In making this request, it seemed to John that she was not really being overzealous: most people he visited these days didn't seem to want you to smoke inside their house[143].

On the way to the train station he stopped to buy a new pack. Proffering $A9.50 for his usual pack, the shop assistant reminded him that they had now gone up by 20c a pack in the latest Federal budget. John had calculated that by smoking a pack a day, he was spending $A3540 a year on cigarettes – the price, with lots of spending money leftover, of a ten-day holiday in a luxury hotel in Bali. He also noticed that the pack he had been given had one of the newly introduced picture warnings on it. His had a photo of a foot with gangrene. He'd never seen *that* before.

Boarding the train, he pondered that here was yet another place he couldn't smoke. Public transport had gone smoke-free in 1976, joined later by all planes. You hadn't been able to smoke inside an Australian air terminal in years, unless you wanted to join a sad-looking bunch inside one of those awful "smoking rooms". And just before the 2000 Sydney Olympics, the government had banned smoking in restaurants. You just never saw anyone smoking in a restaurant anymore[144].

As he read the morning newspaper, he was confronted by a full-page advertisement from a life insurance company offering substantially reduced rates for non-smokers[145]. "I guess they would know all about the business sense in that" he was forced to reflect. He also noticed how many of the "share accommodation" classified advertisements specified that only non-smokers need apply. Of 335 advertisements that day, 42% specified this requirement[146] – a higher rate than any other quality sought by advertisers. He also noticed that every government job advertisement and a not inconsiderable number of private sector ads stated that "a smoke-free workplace was company policy". Out of curiosity, he had once spent a wet afternoon browsing an internet dating site and was struck by how many of these people sought a date who was a non-smoker[147].

Arriving at work, John stubbed out what would be his last cigarette until lunch time. He'd raced his way through three between getting off the train and walking into his building[45]. He was sometimes disconcerted to feel like a bit of an addict doing this – not a good feeling. Way back in 1988, his office had introduced a total smoking ban. Since then there had been a virtual stampede throughout the Australian business world to do the same. The ban at work had certainly forced down his own consumption. He'd read that the average smoking office worker had reduced daily consumption by around 20% because of these bans[95]. He'd also heard some of his colleagues say that they were going to quit[148], because "it's as if you can't smoke *anywhere* these days . . . and that makes the decision to quit a lot easier."

At lunch time, John went with some colleagues to a nearby Pizza Hut restaurant. The entire chain had gone smoke-free many years ago. On the way he then passed a street sign warning him that he could be fined for discarding his cigarette butt in the street – the non-biodegradability of butts made them a major pollution problem, especially in a city where stormwater ran into the picturesque harbour around which the city was built. Being environmentally conscious, he felt awkward about his usual throwaway method of disposing of butts. But what were you supposed to do with a dead butt?

Home that evening, John relaxed in front of TV where on the news he heard a report linking smoking with yet another dreaded disease – this time they were saying that parental smoking was linked with childhood leukaemia[149]. "Was there *anything* that smoking didn't cause?" he thought to himself, reflecting on all the news reports he had heard about the subject over the years. Being a sports fan, he zapped his TV between channels showing the national soccer and basketball competitions. And there it was again: anti-smoking sponsorship messages on the sidelines and even on the players' clothing. And then to put the icing on the cake, a gruesome government advertisement showing how much black tar a smoker would inhale in a year was shown several times during commercial breaks.

The next day, John decided – again – that he would finally quit. He'd made many unsuccessful attempts before[150]. Over the next 12 months he made another three or four unsuccessful attempts, one inspired by a brief warning given to him by his doctor, and another being a period where he used nicotine gum after his pharmacist had suggested it. Eighteen months after his initial decision, he smoked what would be his last cigarette. In doing so, he joined approximately 4.14 million Australian adults who today identify themselves as former smokers.

Shortly after he finally stopped smoking, he was phoned by a researcher working on the evaluation of the current government media quit smoking campaign. John joined respondents who had seen the campaign; who strongly agreed that the campaign made them think about quitting; and who responded (unprompted) that health reasons, cost and social unacceptability were the three main reasons they stopped smoking[151].

The researchers subsequently wrote a scientific paper where they claimed that their statewide media campaign was probably the factor responsible for a quit rate within the state that was higher than that found in other states. This claim was based on extrapolations made from the sample of aggregated recent quitters like John.

So how do we explain John's decision to quit? What do we make of a community cessation rate extrapolated from data including John's responses and its partial *attribution* to the government campaign? And what should we make of John's *own* account of *why* he quit? In the research literature of tobacco control, such questions are seldom asked and even more seldom thoroughly investigated. Where questions of attribution are assessed, it is usual that the influence of a particular variable such as advertising or a health education campaign is examined using standard pre-post or intervention-control group designs. Occasionally, a limited number of potential confounders like price changes are incorporated into such studies. Control areas are seldom if ever matched with intervention areas for anything remotely like the range of variables described in the above scenario. Essentially qualitative variables such as tobacco advertising are conveniently homogenised into measurable units such as cost, as if all advertising campaigns were of equal impact[152]. This would be news indeed to many in the advertising industry who know too well how many of their efforts seem to make little difference to brand sales.

Yet from the foregoing scenario it is obvious that in the life of every smoker there are a plethora of interventions, campaigns and influences to which they are exposed over many years. From John's perspective, these did not pass by him in any neat, sequential order nor in any way that would allow him to reliably quantify their respective influence on his gradually changing perception of his own smoking and the evolution of his decision to quit. At many times in his recent smoking history, it would have been quite impossible to isolate and quantify the effects of any one of up to a dozen concurrent variables. Quantitative evaluative research processes avoid the methodological imbroglios that are inherent in accepting the reality of the dynamic interplay of the sort of factors described above. There are at least four outstanding explanations for this. Together, these work to grossly oversimplify our understanding of both the dynamic interplay of factors that actually work to precipitate quitting, and our understanding of how advocacy works to ensure that many of these influential "hares" are set running in smoker's minds.

1. Reductionist epistemology

Evaluative research in tobacco control is located almost entirely within the scientific tradition. This tradition assumes a reductionist epistemology whereby the task of science is to discover and quantify the exact relationship between variables. Any difficulties in assessing these relationships are assumed to lie with the imprecision of the methods used to assess them, and not with the very conception of the nature of how it is that a complex behaviour like smoking changes throughout a population or an individual's lifetime. The ambition to quantify exactly the assumed relationship is seen as a task worthy of pursuit, whereas consideration of the *gestalt* of how various cultural, economic, organisational and educational factors actually combine to influence smoking behaviour is viewed as messy and unscientific. The only manageable truths in this tradition are those that are simple and uncomplicated: advertising bans and price rises reduce aggregate demand, education programmes decrease the incidence of uptake, and so on. The messy *gestalt* is entangled in the explanatory gossamer of a myriad of experiences, conversations, memories and exposures to interventions, but researchers bearing reductionist precepts and methods wear the equivalent of boxing gloves in their attempt to unravel these delicate threads. Disentangling the precise effect of just one variable of interest is like trying to retrieve eggs from an omelette.

2. The explanatory privileging of recent factors

It is not just *single* factors, but also *recent* factors that are privileged by reductionist explanations. The view seems to be that the effects of recent interventions and policy changes could be expected to be less confounded by the intrusion of other influences than policies and events enacted further in the past. This assumption is fuelled by attributions often given by individuals when they nominate specific events (e.g. a quit campaign, recent illness or symptoms, death of a relative, an intense period of haranguing from their children, a straw-that-broke-the-camel's-back price rise) as "why" they quit. Such explanations may well represent accurate and heart-felt perceptions of the *precipitating* or proximal factors that prompted quitting, but reveal little of the complex historical distal precursors that may have been neces-sary to predispose individuals to quit when finally subject to the precipitating event. For example, it may be the case that demand sensitivity to price rises is dependent on a widespread acceptance of the tobacco–disease nexus. Respect for the importance of such plausible predisposing factors is rare in evaluative studies about smoking control.

3. Concern for policy tractable factors

Concern is often expressed that research should concentrate on better understanding of how to influence so-called "policy tractable" factors that influence smoking. These are factors that are amenable to manipulation by government policies such as price, advertising, packaging and smokefree laws. They stand in contrast to factors said to be also relevant to smoking, which include age, sex, cultural proscriptions on smoking, social class, occupation, income, school performance, and parental, peer, sibling and workmate smoking. All of these are not as directly or even at all amenable to influence through government policy.

Pragmatic considerations of "what can we *directly* influence?", have directed research attention onto the role of precise factors like price or large public information campaigns. Again, the problems arising from the reductionism involved here tend to be overlooked in the fervour to produce action-oriented research that can be fed into policy and political processes.

4. Relationship of evaluation to funding

Health promotion campaigns that involve relatively large sums of money are gen-erally subject to intensive scrutiny bred from the competitive funding climates in which they operate. Unlike "passive" preventive strategies such as price controls and advertising restrictions, which require little or no money to implement, health promotion campaigners are continually asked to justify their funding. Evaluation of the effects of health education campaigns against smoking are thus partly inspired by a concern to be able to show that an intervention is effective, or better, cost-effective. Such considerations produce a highly selective orientation to evaluation driven by a priori concerns to assess interventions deemed worthy of evaluation, rather than an attitude towards explanation of the quitting process that is open to the possibility of a thoroughly "messy" account like the scenario above.

Confounding run amok

Individual platforms of comprehensive tobacco control policy are seldom implemented by governments in isolation from others. When a government is committed enough to introduce bans on smoking in restaurants, it will have done this in a spirit of wanting to reduce the burden of death and illness caused by tobacco and accordingly will be predisposed to introducing other policies with similar intent. In practice this has meant that nearly all countries where evaluation studies of tobacco control policies and programmes have been undertaken have been characterised by the coalescence of a multitude of these factors, much in the manner described in the scenario.

Advocacy for smokefree bars, as described later in this chapter, was not orchestrated by any central public health group who, driven by evaluation imperatives, marshalled the firing of orchestrated salvos into the media or the mailbags of politicians. For each of the memorable milestones there were literally countless instances of long-forgotten letters written to editors, people calling up discussion programmes on radio, minor news items in newspapers and radio, and casual conversations about passive smoking being unpleasant and unhealthy, carried out in innumerable settings. Each and every advocacy foray into the mass media was not recorded, quantified or evaluated, although content analysis of news reportage on smoking shows passive smoking to be the single most reported issue in tobacco control[142,153]. Tobacco control advocates were frequent participants in all of these and often acted as catalysts or spark plugs for a flurry of activity.

Many of these factors are introduced in an ad hoc, opportunistic way rather than any way remotely analogous to the timed and controlled drip-feeding of therapeutics in laboratory or clinical trials. Politicians and tobacco control advocates understandably have little or no regard for the violation of the sanctity of control groups, areas or periods so coveted by researchers hoping to conduct a neat study unconfounded by unexpected influences. Instead, they will have their noses constantly in the political wind for opportunities to engage in media advocacy, to lobby for tax rises, further restrictions on advertising and so on. In large countries like Canada and the USA, where federal, state, provincial and local governments have jurisdiction over different elements of tobacco control policy, it is often the case that at any given time quite complex different configurations of tobacco control activity will be playing out in different parts of the country. Some of these events will be newsworthy and picked up by national media networks, which will amplify a local issue into a national concern, thus further corrupting pristine research designs. Most evaluative studies simply pretend that all this does not occur and that the independent variables (policies and interventions) they are evaluating constitute the only players in the landscape.

Conclusions

What does this analysis suggest for the future of evaluation of tobacco control policies and programmes? The sort of methodological problems discussed above should not induce an evaluative paralysis in tobacco control researchers. They should not inspire any abandonment of the evaluation of outcomes in tobacco control nor any shying away from the challenges of the attribution problem. Continuing debate about ways of sampling and controlling for differing "microclimates" of influence and intervention between areas, states and nations will be very welcome. Also, though, a more open recognition of the limitations of reductionist thinking in considering the causes of declining tobacco use throughout populations could redirect researchers into considering the potential of qualitative methods as important adjuncts in the explanatory process.

Mark Twain wrote that if your only tool is a hammer, then all your problems come to look like nails. And so it has largely been with the dominant explanatory paradigms in tobacco control research. Social scientists have long argued for multiple methods or *triangulation* in studying complex human phenomena. Triangulated research can involve use of different investigators, theories and methods to study the one phenomenon with the assumption that the weaknesses in each single method will be compensated by the counterbalancing strengths of another. This is not to argue that triangulation can ever produce a single "true" reality beyond the frameworks and interpretations provided by each research approach. Data collection methods and interpretive approaches drawn from ethnomethodology, oral history and discourse analysis hold promise as ways of rendering complex social processes like the natural history of smoking cessation more transparent.

The degree of analytic sophistication possessed by most politicians and funding bureaucrats will rarely require any venturing into the complexities of the attribution problem. Such people invariably want two-paragraph answers to questions like "Do these school programmes work?" or "Will banning advertising reduce demand?". They are slaves to entrenched, simplified decision-making processes that conspire against answers predicated on any honest admission of the highly intertwined nature of the relationships involved.

International tobacco control agencies and expert groups have long called for *comprehensive* policies to turn the public tide against tobacco. They have also been dismissive of efforts by the tobacco industry to attribute population-wide trends in tobacco consumption to the presence or absence of single variables. The rationale for comprehensive policies lies not in any belief that the individual platforms of such policy simply have incremental, additive effects on demand. Rather, it lies in the recognition that each of these platforms is nurtured by the others, creating a synergy that produces the sorts of slide in prevalence seen in many countries today.

Banning smoking in workplaces

In an attempt to draw together much of the preceding discussion and show the complexity of the advocacy process in action, I will now consider in detail the evolution of smoking bans in Australian workplaces, with particular focus on the "endgame" still being played out today in Australia: the banning of smoking in bars and casinos. I will draw on material I wrote with two Masters students at the University of Sydney, David Champion and Katie Bryan-Jones, in two papers where we examined, respectively, the news discourse on advocacy for smokefree bars, and how key political decision-makers in the state of New South Wales (NSW) see the politics underlying the incrementalist history of the erosion of smoking in enclosed public spaces.

Today in Australia, all indoor workers except bar and casino workers work in smokefree environments. Smoking is banned by law on all public transport, in all cinemas and public halls, and in all indoor eating areas of restaurants – the latter since 2000[144]. From July 2007, all but one Australian state (the Northern Territory) will ban smoking inside pubs and bars.

About 70% of Australian homes discourage visitors from smoking indoors[154]. Cigarettes foregone due to workplace bans were estimated to have reduced overall consumption in the community by 12.7% between 1988 and 1994[95]. The tobacco industry's own internal estimates are consonant with this[155], and a recent report[156] suggests that workplace restrictions on smoking have done more to reduce tobacco consumption in the USA than any other strategy. The virulence and endurance of tobacco industry efforts to discredit the science of environmental tobacco smoke risk[138,157,158] suggest this assessment is almost certainly accurate (see 'Scream test' in Part II).

Early epidemiological reports on the elevated health risks faced by non-smokers living with smokers[159,160] added a public health dimension to a growing community discourse that cigarette smoking smells unpleasant[161] and that non-smokers' amenity was being unfairly affected by laissez faire smoking policies. During the 1980s and 1990s, several milestones put extra pressure on employers who were reluctant to introduce workplace smoking bans. These included publicity surrounding expert reports[162,163], successful litigation by workers over adverse health effects from passive smoking[164,165], publicity given to vanguard bans by the civil service dating from December 1986, a major legal case where the tobacco industry was found guilty of having misled the public on passive smoking[166,167] and repeated polls showing large majorities of workers supporting smokefree workplaces, including in bars[168].

Since at least 2001, NSW senior politicians have been quoted as saying that smoking bans in all workplaces are "inevitable"[169]. However, unlike the responses of the Irish, Norwegian, British, Italian and New Zealand governments to ban smoking in all public places, the NSW government did not respond to this "inevitability" with timely and comprehensive legislation; it instead continued effectively to exempt bars and clubs from a total ban. In early 2005, a final date for a complete indoor smoking ban in bars and licensed clubs was set for adoption in July 2007, although intense lobbying from the hospitality industry resulted in the government adopting a definition of an "enclosed space" that will allow smoking in areas that are up to 75% enclosed.

Bars as the last bastion

The pattern of bars being the "last bastion" to be addressed in smokefree air legislation appears to have no exceptions anywhere in the world where smokefree legislation has been introduced. The protracted paradox of those most exposed being the least protected, together with interest in how the hospitality industry – often with backing from the tobacco industry[170] – has succeeded in resisting smoke bans in spite of the risks posed particularly to its staff, makes this a compelling subject for study.

With each year that bars avoid smokefree legislation, further evidence accumulates about indoor air quality in bars[171], bar workers' secondhand smoke (SHS) exposure[172,173] and their improved respiratory health when their workplaces go smokefree[174]. Similarly, as the community's experience of smokefree workplaces, restaurants and public transport becomes ever more routine, public support for smoking bans to be extended to bars also increases[168]. A large body of research has also accumulated showing either positive or negligible economic impacts on bar earnings following bans[175].

In Australia, the tobacco industry has a long history of attempting to discredit studies showing the harms of SHS[176] or to circumvent smoking bans[177]. The Australian Hotels Association (AHA) and Clubs NSW have now replaced the tobacco industry as the dominant public voice opposing smoking bans in Australia[96]. Having acknowledged direct support from the tobacco industry[170], the AHA's opposition to bans is a classic example of the tobacco industry's "third party strategy" in action[178].

David Champion and I gathered all press articles published in capital city Australian newspapers between 25 March 1996 and 3 March 2003, dealing with proposals to ban smoking in bars, clubs and pubs. We were interested to see the ways in which parties to the debate sought to define what was at issue. A description of our sampling and approach to analysing the content of the news coverage can be found in the original paper[96].

All direct quotes or journalistic summaries of statements attributed to named individuals in each article we found were coded into five themes: Health, Economic, Cultural/Ideological, Practical and General, which we defined as follows:

- **Health:** statements about health issues and SHS exposure regarding patrons or staff, including statements both asserting and denying or playing down the connection between exposure and health risks.
- **Economic:** statements about the economic consequences of introducing smokefree hospitality venues, suggesting positive, negative or neutral consequences.
- **Cultural/Ideological:** statements about public support or opposition to smokefree bars; non-smokers' and smokers' "rights"; neglect of bar workers' occupational health status; that bans are "un-Australian"; that bans constitute "prohibition" or overly bureaucratic interference in the conduct of business; that the issue is "political"; that policy should be left to individual venue management through self-regulation; and statements about legal liability and discrimination.

- **Practical:** statements about the practicalities of implementing smokefree bars; the futility of arbitrary smoking and non-smoking zones; comments about the adequacy or inadequacy of ventilation solutions; and matters regarding the timing of bans.
- **General:** statements containing no value-laden comments of support or opposition to smokefree bars were coded "general". Examples included an AHA statement that they were "surprised to hear [the government] was flagging wider bans" and statements from health advocates clarifying how, when or where smoking legislation would be implemented.

From 1996 to 1999, there was an average of 21 articles published every year. By 2001 and 2002 this had increased more than threefold to 73 per year. Those attributed to AHA spokespeople grew continuously from 1998, with sharp growth from 2000 onwards, following the "fall" of restaurants to smokefree status that gained momentum from 2000 with the announcement of a ban in NSW. When restaurants went smokefree, the debate predictably shifted entirely onto hotels and clubs, where the AHA had an obvious vested interest. By 2002, the AHA was being quoted at twice the rate of tobacco control advocates, suggesting aggressive advocacy by the AHA. In May 2001, there was intense press coverage of the Marlene Sharp legal case in Australia, in which a court found that a non-smoking, near-teetotal bar worker's throat cancer was caused by exposure to SHS[179].

Despite the preponderance of AHA quotes, across the full sample period there were more than three times as many *articles* reporting on the issue of tobacco control positively ($n = 171$) than negatively ($n = 48$). These positively slanted articles highlighted the merits of tougher smoking bans, efforts to include gaming areas in smoking bans and reports on studies showing that smoking bans did not harm business. Negatively slanted articles tended to highlight claims that smoking bans would destroy a bar tradition, cut earnings, cause job losses and presented a spectre of unfairly besieged hotels fighting back.

Table 2.1 shows the distribution of statements made by AHA and tobacco control spokespeople. The AHA consistently emphasised economic issues (40% of all their attributed quotes) and cultural/ideological frames (36.3%), while tobacco control interests emphasised health concerns (32.4% of all their quotes, while virtually absent from AHA statements – only 10/413 statements) as well as cultural/ideological frames (42.1%). Practical concerns were expressed three times more often by the AHA than by tobacco control groups, but much less than the dominant economic and cultural/ideological discourses favoured by the AHA. Each of the four main themes (health, economic, cultural/ideological and practical) will now be explored in greater detail.

Health framing

Statements on health came overwhelmingly (nine to one) from health groups, with the AHA remaining largely silent on health issues, being quoted only ten times. The right of hospitality staff to work in a smokefree environment, irrespective of

Table 2.1 Frequency of frames used by tobacco control (TC) groups and the Australian Hotels Association (AHA).

	Number of quotes (%)		
	TC	**AHA**	**Total**
Health	97 (32.4)	10 (2.4)	107 (15.0)
Economic	47 (15.7)	165 (40.0)	212 (29.8)
Practical	21 (7.0)	64 (9.0)	85 (11.9)
Cultural/ideological/legal	126 (42.1)	150 (36.3)	276 (38.8)
Miscellaneous/general	8 (2.7)	24 (3.4)	32 (4.5)
Total	299	413	712

the willingness of some to work in smoky environments, and the unacceptable "exceptionalism" that gave protection to all workers except bar staff was the core frame used by health groups. Health groups and labour unions representing hospitality workers appropriated the "last bastion" debating frame first used by opponents of bans, and argued that "the hospitality industry is the last bastion where workers have to suffer someone else's smoke", that "all other workers are being protected at their place of work", and that "no employee should be forced to work in conditions where they are in constant contact with a known carcinogen". Health groups highlighted research showing hospitality workers were the group most exposed to environmental tobacco smoke.

On the few occasions the AHA was quoted on health it mainly denied the risks involved saying it had made use of "specialist medical advice, giving the all-clear for adults exposed at work" and that "evidence in relation to passive smoking and adverse health effects remained weak and inconclusive".

By 2000 the AHA began to acknowledge the risks associated with SHS and stated that they "had always taken its health responsibilities to staff and patrons extremely seriously" but defended their position by claiming that they make "all employees aware of the risks in their initial orientation", and that hotels were now making every effort in "educating staff about the risk". Some hoteliers reported that they had made it a "condition of employment for non-smoking staff to sign a waiver acknowledging they understood and accepted the risks of passive smoking", a strategy that would have been legally vulnerable if challenged in court. The waiver, they reported "was protection against legal action".

Economic framing

The second most frequent framing used in the debate was economic, with the AHA making economic statements 3.5 times more often than health groups. The AHA consistently warned of "horrendous ramifications" and "certain bankruptcy" for many small pubs, particularly in country towns, which "could not afford to install the necessary ventilation equipment". Ventilation solutions were never part of what was being proposed by health groups, so the AHA tactic here was to both propose an alternative (bogus) solution while emphatically claiming it would be financially ruinous for many hotels. The AHA constantly promoted the spectre that "business will decrease". Smoking bans had "the potential to kill off a number of small country pubs which rely purely on their bar sales" and that smoke bans would be "devastating for hotels" because "if you took the smoking out then you'd be closing the door". There were numerous predictions of "catastrophic consequences" and that "the cost to society would be immense". This apocalypse would cause "major flow-on effects including higher land taxes and increases in car regos [registration]", which would reduce the ability of the government to provide police and health education programmes.

In particular the AHA warned of the loss of "thousands of jobs" and referred to domestic and international experience to support their claims: "in Boston they laid off three people in every bar and café" and "in California about one in five surveyed respondents said they had laid off staff". It claimed that 13% of Californian bar jobs disappeared after anti-smoking laws were introduced and that similar employment repercussions would happen in Australia. The AHA "said the revenue decline would cost up to 3000 full-time jobs" and that in casinos, smoking restrictions had already "been blamed for the shock axing of more than 100 jobs". The bans would "be a blow to the tourist trade" and "if you're going to introduce cultural change, you have to be a little bit sensitive to that other very important culture we like – jobs".

Health groups countered these arguments by claiming US evidence showed smoking bans could improve patronage. They noted that the AHA was using similar predictions of disaster that it "had used for more than 20 years" that random breath testing would also empty hotels and cause job loses. They argued that the AHA was only interested in money, claiming that the economic arguments were "like the scene in *Jaws* when people are saying 'you've got to close the beach' and they won't because it's tourist time and people are making money".

Cultural/ideological/legal framing

From the entire sample of quotes, core cultural or ideological statements were the most frequent (39%). The AHA consistently maintained that smoking was a core part of Australian culture and almost a historical birthright: "going to the bar and having a beer and a smoke is part of our culture", "people have been smoking in Australia since they [Captain James Cook] landed here at Botany Bay"; "any type of ban affects our culture" and that further bans would discriminate against individuals' rights. They maintained that while it was "fashionable to be against smokers" a "complete ban on smoking in bars was taking things too far, we would be turning smokers into lepers". Health groups and politicians were engaging in "cultural engineering" and "while statistics showed only 20.3% of Australian adults smoked, a total ban on smoking was discriminatory and un-Australian" and that "smoking in the pub is the Australian way" because "people can't enjoy a beer if they don't have a smoke".

The AHA questioned the need to legislate against smoking, arguing that self-regulation had been working. "Under self-regulation, hoteliers were attending seminars and installing air filters." This, the AHA argued, "was a much more sensible means of handling smoking". "Many hotels also introduced smoking and non-smoking areas many years ago and to introduce an outright ban now will alienate people."

The AHA argued that tobacco is a legal product and so we cannot alienate those who choose to use it because "the majority of smokers are very considerate". If it was legal to buy cigarettes in hotels it should be legal to smoke them inside hotels.

Finally, the AHA invoked populist antipathy for prohibition, arguing that "it is merely prohibition and history tells us prohibition doesn't work". They argued bans were no more than "red tape which pacifies the crusaders but achieves little else".

Health groups mixed health framings with ideological angles, maintaining that while patrons choose whether to go to smoke-filled pubs, the argument that bar staff have the same choice was "redolent of Dickensian mine owners asserting that they didn't force 10-year-olds down mines: they could always get another job". They also highlighted the threat of the legal consequences if smoking were allowed to continue. They argued that "employers knew the risks to patrons and employees" and that the AHA was "leaving themselves open to potentially huge legal claims" that would result in "huge ramifications" for the hospitality industry. Tobacco control groups argued that the AHA was under a legal responsibility to protect workers: "we've clearly warned employers that they're accruing a legal liability for those who will inevitably suffer illness or death from unsafe work environments". They argued that insurance companies will inevitably say that "if you want workers' compensation insurance, then make your establishment smoke-free". Health groups compared passive smoke to asbestos, suggesting "where the danger is known, it's quite clear that employers can be in breach of legal obligations where they've failed to act" and "if they want to lift the threat of legal liability which hangs over their heads [pubs and clubs] will need to go totally smoke-free".

Some health groups claimed that the government "showed a lack of political courage" and that the "onus was on governments to protect workers, as the hotel industry has been blocking smoking bans and lobbying governments to delay actions for nearly a decade". Politicians were seldom quoted but also acknowledged that more restrictions in pubs and clubs were inevitable. Other politicians downplayed the issue saying "a total ban was an option, albeit an unlikely one, but that the Government wanted feedback from pubs and clubs before making any decision". They signalled there could be "further advances in legislation but said the Government would not react in a knee-jerk way", while other Government ministers were quoted as saying they "remained committed to achieving smoking bans in hotels in the future".

Practical framing

In 1996 the AHA argued that dispersing smoke with fans, exhaust systems, open windows and air grilles was the practical solution to heightened public concern about secondhand smoke. Further legislation would now be impractical as the hotel industry "was aware of the passive smoking issues and could do numerous things to improve air circulation to reduce the problem". The AHA claimed it was now "policy to encourage hotel owners to install state-of-the-art ventilation systems".

Health groups countered the ventilation solution by arguing that "even the best ventilation systems do not clear the air completely" and that "they do not protect workers from the health problem and do not protect hotels and restaurants from being sued by workers or patrons". The Australian Medical Association wrote that it "had received scientific advice that to remove cancer-causing particles from the air that the air-conditioning would have to be so powerful it would suck the beer out of your glass". Health groups argued that sections divided by an arbitrary line was analogous to having a urinating and non-urinating section in a swimming pool.

Discussion

Public health advocates campaign about SHS because it is a preventable health issue that can readily be addressed through legislation. The hospitality industry has campaigned against these efforts because it claims smoking restrictions will deter patrons and because of a myopic belief that part of the atmosphere of bars is that unhindered smoking is a "natural" companion to drinking. The endgame of the history of restricting public smoking is essentially a struggle for ascendancy between these two fundamentally different conceptions about what is at issue in the contested debate about bar smoking.

Now that health groups' concerns have prevailed, with all but one Australian state governments banning smoking inside bars from July 2007, it is reasonable to reflect both on why the debate took as long as it did to reach its conclusion, and why the health-led argument eventually triumphed. This discussion must be unavoidably speculative because there is no "official" or definitive answer to either question, no person or group of people whose judgment on these questions could be considered inviolable, and no moment when the decision was made, referenced against a particular incident or other critical event. As we will see shortly, Katie Bryan-Jones and I have explored the political dynamics of the evolution of laws against public smoking in the state of NSW and our findings support this complexity.

The dominant patterns of news discourse mapped in this study suggest three fundamental oppositions that jousted for ascendancy. First, the health of workers and the public was pitted against the commercialism of the hotel industry. Second, two radically different appropriations of what it allegedly meant to be "Australian" became contested. Third, debate about practical matters pitted those who worked in bars every day with those who could be painted as having little credibility when it came to the practical administration of a hotel or pub.

Health vs commercialism

Health advocates were most often quoted on comments about the health problems of passive smoking, while the AHA almost totally avoided any engagement with health matters. As authorities and advocates on health matters, health groups are contacted by journalists as sources that are expected to provide a health perspective. While the tobacco industry has a long history of attacking the evidence about the harms caused by secondhand smoke, it also recognised that "The tobacco industry is still attempting to win an unwinnable argument . . . namely that there is a valid scientific controversy concerning smoking and health issues"[180]. It thus enlisted third parties such as hospitality associations to fight smoking restrictions[181].

The AHA largely kept away from the health agenda and sought to frame what was at issue by means of other agendas. This absence gave health groups years of almost uncontested opportunities to raise the core health issues. As new research continued to be published and publicised, the absence of government response to ever-growing evidence of harm became less and less politically sustainable, and the word "inevitable" began to be used by politicians to refer to bans. Either explicitly or by implication, the health perspective remained the core, unavoidable starting point of every media report about SHS.

Ways to be "un-Australian"

As we saw, the AHA dug deep into a store of references about cultural heritage in the attempt to frame smoking bans as antithetical to quintessentially Australian tableaux about authentic day-to-day life. Here, references to country town pubs and men who would be denied being allowed to smoke with their beer after a hard day's work. One taunted smoking ban advocates to go to the "Royal Hotel in Coonabarabran [a quintessential country town in NSW] in the middle of a drought, bushfires and hardship, and tell the old man at the bar he's not allowed to smoke with his beer. I'm not going to do it. They've been doing this for years". Those proposing bans were by implication people who were out of touch with ordinary Australian values, who were employed in occupations that were not really "proper" jobs, and so whose advocacy needed to be placed in those perspectives and seen as a minority opinion seeking to be imposed on the community. If there was a weakness in this powerful set of interlinked frames, it was that the references and word pictures invoked in its support were decidedly backward-looking and relatively easily dismissed as being out-of-touch with world views held by many people in contemporary Australia. Restaurants had gone smokefree in 2000 to widespread acclaim and with few if any major problems[144], and with public opinion overwhelmingly in favour of smokefree pubs[168], it is likely that many exposed to the AHA framing here would have found it out of date.

By contrast, health groups' take on being "un-Australian" was to bracket their health messages with ideological statements about fairness and it being manifestly inequitable and indefensible to deny the most occupationally exposed group the same protection that all other workers enjoyed under law. Being "un-Australian" is common parlance for behaviour or policies that are not egalitarian. Health groups reframed the AHA's "last bastion" status of hotels and bars as a neo-Dickensian irrational application of public health policy and were never directly challenged.

Practical matters

Because it represented the owners and managers of pubs, it might be expected that the AHA would have a decided advantage over health advocates when it came to public argument about the practicalities of implementing smoking bans. They worked in these environments every day, whereas health group spokespeople could be readily painted as people who rarely ventured into pubs and so whose idealism and impracticality could be emphasised. The AHA rapidly moved to embrace separate accommodation (sometimes defined by farcical "magic line" rules) and ventilation – especially air-conditioning – as their solutions of choice.

However, both of these solutions were very vulnerable to ridicule and imagery about high-powered, uncomfortable and expensive air-conditioning systems that would be financially beyond the reach of small bars and evoked scenes of draughty, uncomfortable environments.

Our findings were consistent with those of Magzamen et al.[182] who concluded that the tobacco industry in the USA created an effective central message that has been used consistently over time. They showed that by consistently delivering well-thought-out framing strategies, public health groups can also be effective in getting adequate attention for their arguments in the media, which were able to help them in maintaining smokefree environments in California's bars. Australia's recent success in securing dates for the implementation of smokefree pubs is similarly likely to have owed much to the enduring media advocacy by health groups.

Political insights into advocacy for smokefree bars

In a complementary study[183] to the one just described, interviews were conducted with 21 key stakeholders in the state of NSW, including politicians, their advisors, health officials and tobacco control advocates, on the dynamics surrounding the debates and outcomes of legislative attempts to control secondhand smoke and about how to progress SHS legislation. Key findings, showing direct statements from those interviewed, were as described below.

Inevitability and incremental advances

> I think most analysts would see that it's almost inevitable that it will finally happen, but the intriguing question is, what are the forces that are making it happen so slowly?
>
> Health advocate

Interestingly, despite suggestions that SHS was "relatively unimportant" [bureaucrat] and had "never been a big issue" [politician] on any government's political agenda, a political advisor reflected that there were few issues that sparked as much political, media and community interest as the debate over smoking. Nearly every participant agreed that the "writing is on the wall" [political advisor] for bars and clubs to go smokefree. However, the consensus among supporters of smokefree legislation was that "nobody [in government] is prepared to take the plunge" [union representative], for reasons outlined below.

Tobacco control supporters recognised that "as with a lot of progress in tobacco control, it rarely happens suddenly; in fact, it never happens suddenly" [advocate], and acknowledged that incremental changes were important first steps in the early days of SHS advocacy. However, with bar and club workers remaining exposed to SHS, advocates were frustrated that "the timeframe that [the government] out-line[s] is less ambitious than any of us ever contemplated back in 2000. We thought that maybe it would be a few years at most" [advocate].

A ministerial advisor acknowledged advocates' frustration, but explained that other government priorities make "things move more slowly than you'd like them to". Another advisor admitted that it was no longer a question of *if* smoking should be banned in pubs and clubs via legislation, but rather a question of *when* and *how* the government would act. However, this advisor suggested that, while it was clear that removing smoke from workplaces was the right health decision, SHS was a politically challenging issue that would not be fixed quickly. Instead, politicians and advisors indicated that incremental advances and compromises between vari-ous stakeholders are "the only way government can work" [political advisor] because of the government's need to take into account a variety of stakeholders. These interviewees also suggested that incremental change is "not unreasonable" [politi-cian] because it "allows the community to go with you" [politician].

Because of the government's desire to balance various issues and stakeholders, politicians and advisors suggested that health advocates who are open to compromise and incremental progress will more likely be heard and received by the govern-ment. However, advocates felt challenged by this position because "if you just sit back and are nice to politicians all the time, does that really get you anywhere? . . . Somehow you've got to tell them that 'more needs to be done and that what they've legislated hasn't gone far enough'" [advocate] in protecting the public from SHS.

Advocates cautioned that incremental steps can slow progress towards compre-hensive bans and contribute to the sense that an issue has been taken care of and, as a result, take some pressure off politicians to act more strongly. For example, several informants felt that compromises for smokefree zones (such as no smok-ing within one metre of the drink service area) in bars and clubs were ways for the government to deal with the issue "politically" rather than "fundamentally" [advocate], by compromising health standards.

Competition for the agenda with immediate issues

> I think that deep down they know it's the right thing to do, but that there are more immediate concerns, and I think that probably is what weighs more heavily on their minds.
>
>   Advocate

When attempting to explain the reasons why SHS legislation has failed to attract political urgency, most informants agreed that acute health issues, such as hos-pital bed shortages, unavoidably take precedence on the political agenda. Because political terms are only four years long, some bureaucrats suggested there is not much political investment in preventive health measures, such as smoking restrictions, because health improvements may not be evident for many years. A former health minister explained that "you cannot escape today by focusing on tomorrow". While championing tobacco control "was seen to be providing leadership and bringing some vision to the portfolio, from the negative view, it could be seen as taking time away from . . . [more] pressing issues".

Advocates suggested that one difficulty in raising the profile of SHS has been that "the idea of chronic exposure . . . is a difficult concept for people to take on board" [advocate]. While interviewees across the political spectrum acknowledged that the evidence shows SHS is a health risk, tobacco control proponents indicated that they must still battle "an underlying sense of disbelief that [SHS] couldn't be as dangerous as everyone is saying" [advocate]. Because people do not often immediately become ill from SHS, advocates have found the dangers of SHS "a very difficult story to sell" [advocate] to both the public and politicians. Another advocate suggested that smoking was banned in workplaces and airplanes because people viewed involuntary exposure in a small environment as unacceptable; however, with bars there is a sense that people choose to go to bars and, thus, are voluntarily exposed.

Issue wear-out and sense that tobacco control has been "done"

> To use a transport analogy, it's a bit like putting a road through the mountains, and now we're down to curbing and guttering the highway. But putting the road through is the important thing.
>
> Politician

Interviewees across the political spectrum also agreed that issue wear-out was inhibiting the attention given to SHS as a relevant and urgent issue. One advocate suggested that the biggest threat to advocates' success of achieving smoking bans in pubs and clubs was "a strong sense . . . that tobacco has been 'done'" by both members of the political and public health communities. Most informants indicated that politicians probably feel that they have already addressed the issue adequately, because most workers are now protected, and that they are content that "there are a few things to tidy up, but there are more important issues to worry about at the moment" [politician].

Tobacco control advocates also commented that issue wear-out has made it difficult to be heard by politicians or political advisors because the arguments and stakeholders surrounding the issue on both sides have remained the same. One advocate proposed that "unless you've got something new to say, [politicians] are not that interested". However, the challenge recognised by many interviewees, regardless of their affiliation, was that there was not much new to say on either side of the argument: health advocates cite the health evidence showing the harms of SHS, the economic studies from other jurisdictions show that businesses are not harmed by bans and increasing public support, whereas as we saw previously, the industry attempts to keep SHS issues framed around economic losses and ideological arguments.

Power of industry opposition

> I just think there was a lot of political lack of will because the tobacco industry was still very active in its misinformation campaign, [and] that the hotels and others just kept saying "look, we'll go broke".
>
> Advocate

Most interviewees acknowledged that the hospitality industry has played a significant role in inhibiting the passage of comprehensive legislation. Supporters of SHS bans, including a representative from a restaurant industry association, expressed frustration with the level of influence that pubs and clubs have been able to wield in policy negotiations. These informants proposed that clubs and hotels have successfully avoided complete bans because they are "highly regarded" [politician] organisations that are "fairly important in the Australian context" [union representative]. Many important local identities tend to be hotel or club owners or associates, and "that web of influence can be very important to politicians" [advocate]. A bureaucrat noted that because of this influence "there is a deeply entrenched view in government that there are no wins, and a lot of potential to lose, by tackling the bar situation."

Most participants, including many of the politicians interviewed, also held the belief that the bar and club industries' political power was a reflection of financial donations to political parties. In contrast, political advisors were adamant that political donations played "zero" or "less of a role" than some advocates imagined. Instead, political advisors suggested that these industries' influence with government is through the currency of job loss arguments – however spurious – because "if you make decisions that cost jobs, that's a very serious political issue" [political advisor].

Interviewees also suggested that the hotel and club industries have successfully promoted a pervasive sense in the community and among influential politicians that bars are somehow inherently "different" to other workplaces. Informants noted that bars are seen as a reasonable "last bastion" of smoking by many people, and that smoking in bars is "somehow emblematic of some form of Australian life that needed to be protected" [advocate]. Health bureaucrats, discouraged that their health-based policy advice is often ignored by politicians, believed that because of industry lobbying, the government was often more interested in a "comfort standard" [bureaucrat], such as ventilation systems and no-smoking zones that have been scientifically shown to be ineffective in reducing the health risk of tobacco smoke.[184]

Evidence is outweighed by economic, ideological and anecdotal arguments

> It's not that they're not persuaded by the evidence, it's just that those other forces outweigh what they're trying to do.
>
> Bureaucrat

Although all interviewees recognised SHS as a health risk and noted that governments would not act without a scientific and economic evidence base, they held different views regarding the extent to which evidence can influence political decisions. Advocates stressed that "you need to have your solid evidence – that's the foundation of your advocacy". However, politicians and political advisors indicated that evidence has limited power in governmental deliberations and noted that governments "can't make decisions based on the science alone" [advisor]. One political advisor went as far as to say that "evidence" presented by any lobbyist is often viewed with circumspection because lobbyists tend to "spin" findings to suit their position.

As suggested by some interviewees, if evidence was the only factor in political decisions, the government would not have supported the partial restrictions supported by industry groups or have delayed comprehensive legislation for decades. Several interviewees proposed that the value of economic studies and scientific reports supporting smoking bans is diminished in political debates when countered by anecdotal economic and job loss arguments. A political advisor commented that it was one thing to talk to an industry lobbyist about projected economic losses, but it was "a very different thing to talk about a family member who has his entire business attached to a pub". A politician suggested that anecdotes and "folklore" stories of economic ruin have always carried more weight in political conversations than scientific studies and other forms of independent evidence. Many interviewees also indicated that international evidence does not hold as much weight in political decision-making, as opponents can counter that Australia is "different", and highlighted the need for more Australian-specific studies to be conducted.

The gambling factor

Participants also described how in recent years, the club and pub industries have framed their arguments around the threatened loss of gambling profit if smoking were banned in clubs and pubs (which have gaming machines), as gamblers tend often to be heavy smokers. Because of the "mutually beneficial income" [advocate] both the government and clubs get from gaming, some interviewees suggested that emphasising possible gambling profit loss might be "a convenient [argument] to distract attention away from the real issues – protecting people's health" [bureaucrat]. Several interviewees suggested that a problem facing advocates today is that there are no solid independent local studies relating to the impact of smoking bans specifically on gambling revenues in Australia. For example, because hotel-based gambling is not legal or widespread in most international jurisdictions that have already banned smoking in bars and clubs, the economic studies on which advocates have relied have never included the impact of smoking bans on gambling venues in pubs or hotels. Opposition groups, such as the AHA, have exploited this Australian "difference" and have argued that foreign studies of public support and positive economic impact are therefore irrelevant.

What does the public believe?

> There isn't a visible constituency . . . that [resonates] with politicians, that gives them the impression, the belief, that there are real numbers attached to this issue for them electorally.
>
> Advocate

Nearly all interviewees agreed that public opinion is an influential factor in political decisions; however, what was considered to constitute evidence of public opinion differed between interviewees. Supporters of smoking bans have "always been heartened by the results of public opinion polls" [advocate] that show majority popular support for bans, and expressed frustration that these appeared to have little impact on politicians. In contrast, politicians and advisors explained that political assessment of public sentiment is often "more of a gut feeling" [advisor]. One advisor considered that people who go to pubs and clubs in rural areas are a different constituency than in the city, and suggested that this electorate was not ready for smoking bans.

Despite documented public support for smoking bans, interviewees noted that policymakers appear to believe that those in favour of bans are not as passionate about their preferences as those opposed to bans, and that the intensity of the public's support in regard to bans in pubs and clubs remains in doubt. One advocate suggested that the only times politicians hear of smoking bans are from the "usual suspects": the same predictable handful of tobacco control advocates. Many informants reported that the public seldom vocalises its support to parliamentary representatives. In the face of industry lobbying, an advocate suggested that if politicians believe that smoking bans are not a pressing issue for their constituents, they think "why should we incur all this angst from the AHA?"

Interestingly, despite smokefree venues becoming the norm and politicians claiming that smoking bans are not an important issue for their constituents, informants hinted that policymakers still fear that there could be political "backlash" from select segments of the population. Some Labor Party members indicated that their members have a strong sense of "camaraderie with blokes in this country" [politician] who want to smoke in their "traditional" local pub, and that the government believes rural constituents are less likely to be supportive of smoking bans than city-dwellers [political advisor].

While a former health minister acknowledged that in hindsight there was no political fallout from banning smoking in workplaces and restaurants, he indicated that past reluctance on the part of both major parties to pass legislation in the early and mid-1990s was due in large part to its sense that "there was political concern and fear that there could be a voter backlash in the event of the restriction of smoking" because many people smoked. However, previous concerns of voter backlash regarding workplaces, public transport and restaurants have proven to be unfounded, with the public supporting the restrictions, as evidenced by high compliance rates and increasing public support.

What will overcome the inertia of incrementalism?

> The law of inertia, isn't that what's going on? You need something more powerful in order to change the direction. The inertia right now is to do nothing.
>
> Union representative

Similar to analyses of other tobacco control policy attempts,[185–188] nearly all informants in this study believed that the challenge rests with advocates in NSW to "find a pathway . . . to make it politically advantageous" [advocate] for politicians to take action. Advocates and bureaucrats both acknowledged that the Health Department representatives had "laid everything on the table . . . [but] they can't influence the political process" [advocate] to move the issue forward on the political agenda. Similarly, while minor party politicians and independent members of parliament had successfully pushed SHS onto the political agenda in the past by introducing bills and debate in parliament, there was general agreement that only a bill introduced by the government would be accepted at this stage.

A political advisor stressed that although advocates may feel like they are "knocking their heads against a brick wall", they should "keep knocking because someone's [eventually] going to let you in". Advocates indicated that "the single most important thing . . . [is] that we remain committed and persistent" [advocate].

Although participants were unable to state conclusively what they believed would be the "smoking gun" [union representative] that would overcome the inertia of incremental compromises regarding pubs and clubs, they had a variety of suggestions of what tactics advocates should take to win the final endgame.

Keep the issue focused on workers' rights and health and discredit industry arguments

Tobacco control supporters stressed the importance of keeping the issue of smoking bans centred on the concept of workers' rights and health protection. They suggested that the best way to counter the promotion of the "Australian narrative" [advocate] that smoking and drinking go together, is to frame smoking bans around the idea that "there is something fundamentally un-Australian about exposing workers to risks that we protect other workers from in every other situation" [advocate]. By highlighting SHS as a health inequity and making "the connection between the unpleasant experience" and the proven danger of SHS resonate with both the public and politicians [advocate], advocates may better influence community support and counter industry arguments about revenue loss.[188,189]

Mobilise a visible constituency

Most interviewees felt the most powerful force that would convince politicians finally to act would be the mobilisation of a visible and diverse constituency demanding smoking bans in pubs and clubs. However, tobacco control supporters were sceptical about their ability to get the public impassioned about the issue because "we've reached a stalemate where places the empowered middle classes go are largely smokefree" [politician]. A union representative cautioned that "we're not going to necessarily get the public's perception to move all that much more than it already is" because "to the extent to which you remove the problem for the majority" there remain fewer people who will view the issue as a problem.

Use the media strategically

Nearly every participant commented that the media have "enormous power" [politician] in influencing both the public and political views about SHS. Media were seen as the "predominant" method to educate the public [advocate], to "push politicians' buttons" [bureaucrat], and to contribute to changing social norms and expectations regarding the acceptability of passive smoking.

Advocates and other lobbyists indicated that they needed strategically to utilise the media by being available for public comment, calling into talkback radio programmes, writing letters to the editor, capitalising on new evidence or events, and putting forward a vocal tobacco control position to counterbalance industry comments.

Partnerships with other groups

Another strategy suggested by some informants to increase health advocates' profile with the public and gain more access to inside policy discussions, was partnerships with organisations, such as the labour unions, which the government sees as an important constituency. Advocates and the labour union representative noted that the formation of the Smokefree Australia campaign, comprising health charities, health advocacy groups and labour unions, broadened advocates' advocacy opportunities and access to politicians. For example, one advocate described how different organisations and individuals can play complementary "good cop/ bad cop" roles, with one organisation complimenting the government on its progress, and the other taking a harder, more critical stance in the media. Although some advocates cautioned that it can be challenging to present a united lobbying front and find agreement on issues, they believed a more cohesive strategy and acknowledgement of diverse allies could assist in advancing SHS on the political agenda.

Demonstrations and grassroots campaigns

Interviewees described demonstrations and grassroots campaigns as another potentially influential strategy to put external pressure on the government. However, many participants said that the success of such strategies was dependent on the groups and individuals participating in the campaign, highlighting the importance of recognising each advocacy group's strengths and weaknesses in contributing to the SHS campaign. For example, some interviewees described how a hospitality labour union had effectively utilised grassroots lobbying to promote smokefree places – and had succeeded in influencing the Health Minister to include a ban on smoking at casino tables as part of the Smokefree Environment Act 2000. In contrast, while a community non-smokers advocacy group indicated that its rallies and letter-writing campaigns had given visibility to SHS issues, other advocates cautioned that the group is perceived as "killjoys" [advocate] that lack credibility with policymakers and the community.

More court cases needed

> If you get a couple of [litigation] cases where major pubs or clubs go down, and you'll have the government . . . falling over themselves to introduce urgent legislation if necessary in Parliament.
>
> Politician

Additional cases of litigation was another frequent suggestion about what would increase momentum on passive smoking legislation. Most participants said that previous court cases[165] had stimulated public debate, provided advocates with an opportunity to increase media advocacy, and allowed for tobacco control lobbying to be more favourably received by some politicians. Fear of litigation was viewed as a reason more clubs and pubs have voluntarily gone smokefree [union representative], and the reason why the government went ahead with earlier SHS legislation [political advisor].

The power of litigation to influence policy outcomes is supported by tobacco industry documents that show that the tobacco industry and its allies perceived early court cases as major setbacks[176]. However, one advocate commented that at this stage court cases may not be "as threatening as they used to". For example, the most recent case in 2001 in which the NSW Supreme Court awarded damages to a non-smoking bar attendant who had developed throat cancer[179], did not "achieve the outcomes we were all hoping for" [advocate]. Although the case established a legal precedent and prompted supportive media articles that bars and clubs can be responsible for workplace-caused tobacco-related disease, it did not result in additional political action.

Competition with other states

Many bureaucrats and politicians noted that NSW prides itself on leading other Australian states in government initiatives, and suggested that "one-upmanship" with other states might provide the stimulus for the NSW government to move faster [bureaucrat]. One politician noted that Australian states are like "dominoes" and when one state takes the first step, the others will likely follow shortly after. For example, all Australian states followed the lead of the Australian Capital Territory (ACT) and then NSW by banning smoking in restaurants, and others have introduced laws to varying levels of comprehensiveness.

Find champions in government

> You've either got to have a lot of constituents knocking on the door saying I want something done, or you've got to have a politician with a fire in the belly who takes this problem and says we bloody need to deal with it.
>
> Politician

In addition to putting external pressure on policymakers through the outside advocacy strategies described above, interviewees suggested that advocates must find a champion in government and convince him or her that supporting smoking bans is a good political decision. In the past, legislative attempts have only been successful when championed by a senior government politician. Several interviewees suggested that if the Premier or another high-ranking politician had the courage to stand up to critics and back the issue, legislation to ban smoking in pubs and clubs could happen without much resistance.

Discussion

In the past 20 years, the tobacco control movement in NSW has advocated successfully for considerable SHS legislation and regulation, and non-smoking indoor areas are now the public norm, enjoying wide support. Yet the bar, club and casino industries continue to avoid total bans in their environments. In the 3 years since the interviews for this study were conducted, an agreement for comprehensive SHS legislation that includes bars has yet to be reached in NSW, with the government having again made concessions to industry, this time in the form of a definition of "enclosed spaces" that will allow smoking in areas that are substantially enclosed. Other Australian states (Tasmania and Queensland), Ireland, Norway, New Zealand, England and Scotland, and several state governments in the USA and Canada either implemented total indoor smoking bans, or legislated for their introduction.

The factors inhibiting the adoption of comprehensive restrictions, as described in this study, appear not to have dissipated. Interviewees' comments show that SHS restrictions in NSW have been contested and never been defined solely as being about achieving health outcomes, but have been delayed by several broad factors including: issue wear-out; the continued influence of industry groups who have successfully opposed regulation; and political perceptions that there is not a salient constituency demanding smoking be banned in bars and clubs.

Industry influence

A major challenge for proponents of SHS regulation, as with most tobacco control endeavours, lies in the public benefits of regulation being perceived as diffuse, while the potential costs of regulation are concentrated on a vocal single-interest group – the clubs and hotel industry. In September 2004, in anticipation of the announcement that NSW would end smoking in pubs, the AHA sent its members a fax claiming their businesses would be "destroyed", that there would be "20% job loss" and that "61% of bars in Dublin will not survive much longer"[190], despite reports from Norway, New Zealand and New York showing the recent adoption of bans in these venues had minimal impact on business.[191–193] Although economic and ideological arguments against SHS legislation would appear to be both wrong and outdated, industry groups have succeeded in promoting a politically potent combination of these to the heart of NSW politics.

Issue wear-out

Advocates operating in incrementalist political environments face the challenge that they may achieve only some of their goals before their issue is "worn out" and perceived to be "done" by politicians. Consonant with Nielsen's[189] observation of tobacco control in the USA, windows of opportunity[194] for creating tobacco control legislation may be closing in Australia as well. Issue wear-out and a sense that tobacco has been "done" may explain why other more immediate political concerns continually take precedence over SHS on the political agenda, why the public does not appear impassioned about the issue, and why SHS does not appear to politicians as a politically urgent problem that must be addressed.[195]

No visible constituency

Although strong and unambiguous public opinion can be a powerful motivator to persuade government to act[187,188,196], interviewees did not believe that politicians feel that the public demands legislative action in the way that often characterises other health issues that receive urgent political attention. As long as politicians do not perceive that a significant number of their constituents support smokefree laws as a significant problem that needs urgent attention, they will not feel the need to progress towards complete bans any faster[194,195,197,198].

As advocates suggested, because most politicians often only hear from the "usual suspects" on this issue, advocates would be advised to mobilise other constituencies to vocalise support of smoking bans in bars and clubs. These new voices might include constituents in marginal political seats, bar workers, doctors and other health workers, whose voices might resonate with politicians and provide personal stories to counter the anecdotes about falling custom presented by opposition groups. If advocates are able to demonstrate overwhelming public support that spans the spectrum of constituents, politicians and their advisors will have to defend publicly their continuing refusal to ban smoking in all workplaces and will be less able to dismiss public opinion surveys as unrepresentative of the NSW population.

Lessons for the endgame

Although advocates believed that past advancements towards smokefree areas were accomplished primarily through their groundwork strategies that would eventually be realised in the form of policies and laws, the support of a key legislator[188] was imperative in putting SHS on the political agenda both in 2000 (with restaurants and other public places) and in 2005 (with the latest bars and clubs). No informant interviewed claimed to have precise knowledge about what influenced the Premier's apparently personal decision to ban smoking in restaurants in 2000, alluding to his decision as a more or less inevitable response to the growing anti-smoking social environment in which he felt politically comfortable to act. Similarly, the entrance into politics of another champion in 2005 in the form of the newly appointed Minister for Cancer was undoubtedly crucial to again pushing bans in bars and clubs onto the political agenda[199,200]. As noted, the resulting legislation has been compromised in the face of industry lobbying, but the new law, which will be implemented in July 2007, will see all fully enclosed rooms smokefree – another increment towards the final comprehensive total indoor smoking ban.

With the NSW government still making concessions to industry demands, the strategies outlined by the participants in this study still have relevance to tobacco control advocates faced with similar incremental approaches. As with other studies, it appears that in NSW advocates have been the most successful when they utilise strategies that place outside pressure on policymakers, rather than trying to lobby from inside the political sphere, in which the industry excels[186,187,201].

In the past years, local advocates have capitalised on some of the tactics described in this study. An outstanding example was a 2005 media campaign in which an Irish bar patron mocks the NSW government for believing its residents are not ready for comprehensive bans when the Irish have been able to do it. This appropriated Australia's concern to not "lag behind" other countries. By continuing to utilise their partnerships with groups that have visibility with the government and working on advancing smoking bans through the use of outside strategies – particularly media advocacy and the mobilisation of additional voices – advocates can continue to create visible demand for smoking bans in bars and clubs and hold politicians accountable for the inequity of their exceptionalist policy of protecting all workers other than bar staff.

Conclusions

Governments in the end stage of policy controls of SHS are often attracted to continuing drawn-out incremental policy advances rather than risk confrontation with hospitality and tobacco interests. Advocates concerned to shorten the duration of this endgame must continue to insist that governments address the issue "fundamentally" rather than "politically". Efforts are needed to both broaden and amplify community voices calling on governments to "finish the job". Publicity featuring the growing number of state and national governments that have successfully implemented total bans over the past decade, as well as continued public support is likely to make incrementalism an increasingly unattractive political option.

Notes

i   Parts of this chapter are drawn from revised and edited versions of Chapman S. Unravelling gossamer with boxing gloves: problems in explaining the decline in smoking. *BMJ* 1993;**307**:429–32; Chapman S, Wakefield M. Tobacco control advocacy in Australia: reflections on 30 years of progress. *Health Educ Behav* 2001;**29**:274–289; Chapman S. Advocacy in public health: roles and challenges. *Int J Epidemiol* 2001;**30**:1226–32; Champion D, Chapman S. Framing pub smoking bans: An analysis of Australian print news media coverage, March 1996–March 2003. *J Epidemiol Commun H* 2005;**59**:679–84; and Bryan-Jones K, Chapman S. Political dynamics promoting the incremental regulation of secondhand smoke: a case study of New South Wales, Australia. *BMC Public Health* 2006,**6**:192 (http://www.biomedcentral.com/content/pdf/1471-2458-6-192.pdf).

ii   http://www.cncsis.ro/PDF/IF_2004.pdf

iii Institute for Scientific Information (http://www.biotechmedia.com/y2005-Impact-Factor-Def.html).

iv   See http://www.health.usyd.edu.au/current/coursework/media.php

Chapter 3

The News on Smoking[i]

The first rule of politics and the first principle of advocacy is simply to "be there". If the only people who know and care about your issue are like-minded colleagues, your issue will not be considered mainstream, but confined to the margins in key arenas where legislation, policy and funding decisions are made. Mae West once said "It's better to be looked over, than overlooked". Getting looked over requires advocacy for tobacco control to be taken seriously by those in positions to unlock the barriers to reforms. In today's society there is no more reliable way of "being there" than for your issue to be considered newsworthy.

Like everyone else, a health minister wakes each morning to the sound of a clock radio, from which news bulletins and commentary flow. The preferred morning newspaper is read at the breakfast table. The drive to work will see the car radio tuned to the most important news station or hopping between several. One of the first people to deliver a briefing on arrival at the office will be the press secretary, who will highlight any opportunities and threats that have already arisen that morning. The minister may have already received and made calls from and to radio stations about some of these issues. If there has been anything big happening that is perceived as needing follow-up media work, fact-finding or other investigation, the minister's schedule might be changed to accommodate the new priorities.

This sort of respect for the importance of news media is uncommon in public health, and almost rare in research circles. I earn my living as an academic. Each year, I apply for research grants, and if I'm lucky, after applying at the beginning of one year, I get the grant at the beginning of the next. During the next few years I undertake the research and perhaps 18 months after that – often several years from when the need to do the research was first conceived – I might hope to publish a paper in a prestigious journal with several thousand subscribers worldwide, of whom maybe only 10% might actually read the paper. Over the next couple of years, a well-received paper might be cited in 50 other research papers, although many research papers are never cited at all. If it was a very important paper, more than 100 others might cite it in its lifetime. On its strength, I might get invited to a prestigious international conference where, again if I'm *really* lucky, maybe 3000 people might applaud at the end of my speech. Repeated cycles of this scenario lead to academic progression and the idea that such a researcher is productive.

But supposing I was to then give an interview to a TV news programme, or participate in a current affairs debate on the topic of my research. Literally millions of people will then be exposed to the key findings and implications of my work. If it is picked up by international news agencies, it might be run in hundreds or even thousands of newspapers, radio and TV stations and news websites. Numbered among these audiences will be many politicians and decision-makers who will have direct responsibility for some of the policies on which my research might have bearing. And this exposure is noted very keenly by politicians. As a veteran reporter of 40 years experience with the *Wall Street Journal* said:

> Well done investigative reporting produces public outrage (or policy maker outrage) that forces new regulations and laws or tougher enforcement of exist-ing ones. Ten-thousand-watt klieg lights turned on a situation focuses the minds of policy makers very fast.[122]

And just as importantly, there will be the hundreds of thousands or sometimes millions of ordinary citizens whose interest I might ignite and whose attitudes I might hope to condition through not just the research itself, but through the way I and the journalists frame the story. Some of these will be smokers who will reflect on the implications for their own smoking of what they heard. Others will be people who share the concerns I have expressed and might repeat these to others in conversation. A small number may be people so incensed about the problem described that they might take some action such as writing a letter to a news-paper or a local politician. In these small ways, the tobacco control message per-colates through communities literally every day, so common is tobacco-related news.

While the public health community is too often absent from public discourse about its work, the tobacco industry understands the process very well, investing in efforts that include commissioning columnists, using industry-friendly scientists and organisations[137,177,202], and utilising public relations agencies to spread material in its interests. For example, a 1997 Philip Morris internal memo recorded:

> We have seen tangible and immediate results where we have been able to dis-seminate materials for local placement in newspapers and magazines. The media is obviously easier to persuade in some countries than in others, but in those places, such as the Philippines, where the press tends to be more receptive, our local colleagues have managed to get published the articles we send on a whole variety of issues[203].

In this chapter I will first review the importance of the news media in advocacy for tobacco control. I'll then describe a simple way that any agency can generate significant increases in media coverage. Part II of the book contains many strat-egies for generating news on tobacco control.

Impacts of the media

Against a background of declining tobacco use and generally positive changes in other heart disease risk factors, a systematic review of 14 multiple risk factor intervention trials for preventing coronary heart disease[204] concluded that reductions in mortality in the intervention groups were insignificant and changes in risk factors only modest, when compared with the reductions also seen in control groups. The Minnesota Heart Health Program reported similar outcomes[205] and the major multi-community smoking cessation trial, COMMIT[206,207], had a similar modest effect on reducing smoking. In such trials, risk factors like smoking typically head south in the planned directions – but not much further than those in the control groups not subject to the interventions. Compared with typical community health promotion initiatives, which operate on token budgets, all of these interventions were large scale, although still funded with petty cash when compared with the promotional budgets used by the tobacco industry.

Favourable improvements in the secular trend for risk factors such as smoking, and programme contamination of control groups have generally been cited as putative explanations of the lack of difference between intervention and control groups, with media leakage – the most uncontrollable factor – deemed mainly responsible[208]. Doubtless, some of this leakage involved news coverage of specific interventions intended only for the eyes and ears of the experimental populations. However, it is highly myopic to assume that it is only discrete interventions orchestrated by health agencies leaking into control areas that, in aggregate, constitute the possible forces generating positive downward secular trends in the wider population.

Melanie Wakefield and Frank Chaloupka[209] have called for more attention to the description and quantification of tobacco control "inputs": the range of variables that might singly or synergistically influence an outcome like cessation. They noted that the preoccupation with outcomes in evaluation research is often accompanied by overly casual accounts of the policy and intervention variables that are assumed to be the causative factors potentially producing change. They argued for the further development of a range of indices to measure the comprehensiveness of tobacco control policies and programmes. For our purpose here, they also noted the importance of quantifying and accounting for "environmental" issues such as unpaid news media coverage of tobacco issues.

This importance cannot be over-emphasised: were it possible to quantify all media coverage of tobacco in societies with 24-hour access to a multitude of radio, television, internet and print media, such coverage would routinely eclipse even the most intensive coverage gained through discrete formal public health "campaigns". Along with bioterrorism and abortion clinic violence, tobacco was one of the top three health issues to draw public attention between 1992 and 2002, with over 55% of the public reporting that they closely follow news on tobacco[210].

And it is not only news that holds potential to reach, engage and influence millions of people against smoking. For example, the movie *The Insider* (the dramatisation of the Jeffrey Wigand story) grossed $58.7 million in cinemas worldwide. The movie of John Grisham's book *The Runaway Jury*, grossed $49 440 996 in the USA alone. The film of the satirical novel by William Buckley, *Thank you for Smoking*, grossed $4 491 102 in the USA in its first week of screening in 2006[211]. Together, these "moral tales" about the tobacco industry have been seen by many millions of people globally, including many who see them on video or DVD after movie release. The producers of such films have no interest in not polluting research designs by keeping their movies out of control population study areas. The news and debate about tobacco is unstoppable and is everywhere.

Much of this massive reportage is not easily dismissed as inconsequential ephemera: some of the most potent and recalled episodes in the history of tobacco control have been powerful prime-time television documentaries, prolonged news episodes such as US presidential candidate Bob Dole's foot-in-mouth saga over tobacco policy[212], the coverage of legal cases against the tobacco industry and the early deaths of celebrities from tobacco-caused disease (e.g. Yul Brynner, ABC newsreader Peter Jennings and many other examples listed at the WhyQuit.Com website http://whyquit.com/whyquit/notables.html).

Tobacco control has long been highly newsworthy[142,213]. In one year, 38% of all front pages of the *Sydney Morning Herald* carried at least one health story[214]. Of these, tobacco stories ranked second after those about health services. A US report examining print and broadcast media coverage from 1995 to 2003 showed tobacco and weight loss news received comparable coverage[215]. From a journalist's perspective, tobacco control offers rich pickings that are likely often to conform to editors' notions of newsworthiness (see "Discussion" under "Criteria for newsworthiness" below). Tobacco control is resplendent with stories of conflict, corruption, moral rectitude and venality. To the endless fascination of the media, practically every organ of the body can be afflicted by tobacco use and tobacco's stratospheric toll on health lends itself to numerous excursions into quantification rhetoric[216]. Celebrities' efforts to quit[217] or criticism directed at the influence of their smoking on young people are now routine news events[218,219].

As the tobacco industry is fond of noting with its unique brand of cynicism, the tobacco epidemic has generated an epidemic of research, much of which is covered by the news media. The media's appetite for villains finds bountiful sustenance in the form of the tobacco industry, which has entered journalistic lexicons as an index case shorthand device for referencing ethical low life in the business community[220]. Two quick examples: "They behave like the tobacco companies" says one critic of the giant American and European pharmaceutical companies"[221], and the headline: "Gas heater firms 'like tobacco companies'"[222]. Repeated, commonplace framing of the tobacco industry in such an unfavourable light seems likely to be associated with the community's ranking of tobacco industry representatives' trustworthiness as lower than that of used car salesmen, traditionally the populist low-water mark in expressions of ethical behaviour[11,135]. This in turn may be a critical factor in generating political antipathy towards the tobacco industry in some political circles – as John Seffrin, president of the American Cancer Society, noted: "Most politicians know that you don't stand too close to a pariah in the next photo op." The importance of denormalisation and of vector control is considered in greater detail in Chapters 6 and 7, respectively.

News coverage of tobacco issues can have important consequences. There is some salutary historical evidence that coverage of smoking in the news media can be influential in promoting smoking cessation. For example, Warner's (1977) analysis of the impact of publicity flowing from the release of the 1964 Surgeon General's report suggests that the report's release (and subsequent news coverage) caused immediate (though transitory) decreases of 4–5% in annual per capita tobacco consumption[223]. Similarly, Reid et al.[224] identified unpaid media publicity as the main cause of the 30% decline in smoking prevalence among British males in the 20 years after the publication of the first report on smoking and health by the Royal College of Physicians of London in 1962. During this time in the USA and the UK, anti-smoking information and publicity was almost wholly disseminated via news reportage and commentary, with major government health promotion campaigns not starting until the 1970s, particularly in the USA. Other than news coverage and the first bland, nonspecific pack warning introduced in the mid-1960s, there were no other obvious variables that could explain why smoking began and continued its downward descent.

Pierce and Gilpin analysed coverage of tobacco issues in the most popular US magazines from 1950 to 1990, and related patterns of news coverage to tobacco use cessation and initiation data from the National Health Interview Surveys (1965– 1992). They found that for approximately 30 years, "the annual incidence of cessation in the USA mirrored the pattern of news media coverage of smoking and health"[225]. In New Zealand, Laugesen and Meads[226] showed that consumption, measured by weekly purchases of tobacco from a selected number of tobacco outlets, was significantly related to the weekly number of news stories about tobacco, although the effect was short-lived. They estimated that news coverage had approximately the same impact as a 10% increase in price. On a smaller scale, an US evaluation of a week-long local newspaper series on smoking cessation, which caused around 4% of readers to quit for at least one week, was calculated as having an impact equivalent to that resulting from the establishment of 380 dedicated cessation clinics[227].

Because of space and time constraints, news media gatekeepers (journalists and subeditors) must, of necessity, be highly selective in what they decide will constitute the day's news. All potential issues of interest "compete" with one another for news attention, with only a fraction being selected to fill a bulletin or news section. Agenda-setting theory posits that the degree of emphasis placed on an issue by the mass media is influential in determining the priority accorded to such an issue by the public[228]. News sets the public agenda, influencing ordinary people's conversations at home, at work and socially about what is happening in the world and stimulating discussions about the moral and ethical subtexts that are implicit in many stories.

Because of this process of selection, news does not merely mirror what is "out there", but instead authorises and legitimises a limited range of topics and the ways in which they are publicly talked about as being more worthy of public attention than others. Tuchman argued that "The mass media limit the frames within which public issues are debated, and so narrow the available public alternatives".[229] The news media have the ability to choose, create, sustain and shape an issue for public consumption, thus influencing how issues are presented or framed for consideration both by the general public and by decision-makers[230].

Shanto Iyengar[231] demonstrated that news discourses often implicitly pose questions of responsibility for problems and their solutions, so that audiences are simultaneously presented with an account of a problem and directions for think-ing about who is responsible for it and its solution. For example, when news covers a research report on children's recall of tobacco advertising, journalists would start coverage of the story by using the study to define the problem. They would then typically seek to spotlight a tobacco company spokesperson as an exemplar of those responsible for it, and then cut to someone such as a politician with responsibil-ities for addressing tobacco use by children. Repeated episodes of similar stories come to be interpreted as a chronic problem that is not being addressed. Such sagas can gradually transform into stories about irresponsible or neglectful government, and become emblematic of wider discourses about government's performance.

Framing

Advocates need to have advanced understanding not only of *what* issues are being considered, but *how* they are being defined and shaped for public consumption. News texts such as press articles and television bulletin items are constructed in such a way as to guide how those who receive the messages should interpret and make sense of events, as well as how they should incorporate this knowledge into their general understanding of the social world. By referring to certain discourses and narratives, news producers attempt to provide signposts that indicate how they prefer audiences to understand a text. As David Morley explains, "while the mess-age is not an object with one real meaning, there are within it signifying mechan-isms which promote certain meanings, even one privileged meaning, and suppress others: these are the directive closures encoded in the message". Media analysts refer to this construction as the preferred or dominant meaning of a media text[232].

Similarly, news can be thought of as episodes of mini-social dramas, populated by news actors. As such, it can be subjected to dramaturgical analysis[233] of the roles in which each person is "cast" by news directors in stories. Tobacco stories can have victims, villains, whistle-blowers, "crusaders", puritans and "nannies", depending on how a story is framed. Stories on tobacco and its control abound in such dominant meanings: before it ran for public cover to escape what was becom-ing torrential negative framing in the news, the tobacco industry used to appear routinely cast as corporate Pied Pipers, dissemblers, shadowy figures in the back-ground of politics, indifferent merchants of death, and bottom feeders in the world of corporate ethical sludge. As Thomas Sandefur, then chief of the Brown and Williamson tobacco company, told the US Congress in 1994: "Congressman, it's hard for me to envision becoming more of an outcast than I am."[234]

In analysing news coverage, researchers have long considered the process of framing, a key concept in political science. A "frame" implies the structure through which something is viewed, as with photo or window frames. The frame chosen proposes a way of seeing the issue. To frame in news discourse is to "select some aspects of a perceived reality and make them more salient . . . in such a way as to promote a particular problem definition, causal interpretation, moral evaluation and/or treatment recommendation."[235] News coverage unavoidably "frames" an issue for consumers through the language used, the sources consulted and the opinions cited. Efforts to reframe are necessary when the dominant way of seeing an issue is problematic for public health. Table 3.1 lists examples of characteristic ways in which the tobacco industry and tobacco control advocates talk about particular topics or phenomena.

The brevity of news reporting requires that those seeking media coverage must frame their issue so that it resonates for journalists in the typically short window of opportunity that opens for each issue when a journalist opens a press release or receives a phone call pitching a news story. Those seeking to have their issue rise above others and capture the interest of journalists in highly competitive news environments must learn which news frames are deemed newsworthy by journalists and strive to position their proposed news offerings optimally within such frames. Equally, those working in tobacco control need to become students of how interest groups opposed to tobacco control successfully frame their arguments in ways designed to capture news attention and the dominant meaning of particular policies.

Descriptive analyses of the framing of tobacco within news are important because they can improve understanding of both the successes and limitations of public health efforts and campaigns in relation to tobacco. An appreciation of which particular tobacco issues receive news media attention helps to provide context to an understanding of changes in public attitudes and behaviour, as well as the success or failure of policy initiatives. Research in this area has focused not only on what the volume of tobacco coverage can reveal, but also what we might learn from the analogies, metaphors and historical comparisons used in framing news stories.

Kennedy and Bero document the emerging reportage of passive smoking in the US press over 14 years[236]. Part of their interest lay in examining the process of patronage of industry consultants through which passive smoking continues to be reported as "controversial" – an appellation now seldom used to describe the relationship of active smoking and illness outcomes. Lima and Siegel's study of the coverage by the *Washington Post* of the American tobacco settlement[237] used frame analysis to consider the dominant ways in which the reportage effected closures around what was thereby defined to be *at issue* in the debate surrounding the settlement. Both papers not only quantify one dimension of the "grey", largely unresearched "inputs" that characterise modern cultural discourse on smoking, but also offer strategic insights for tobacco control advocates seeking to become more active participants in such discourse.

Criteria for newsworthiness

Below are some commonly ascribed criteria for newsworthiness, with examples of tobacco news stories.

- **Audience:** Journalists ask "Will the people who listen to this radio station/read this magazine be interested in this story?" Targeting the right media outlets will therefore be a key consideration if your story is not of national significance.

Table 3.1 Ways in which the tobacco industry and advocates for tobacco control talk about certain topics.

Issue or event	Industry framings	Tobacco control framings
Tobacco	A natural agricultural product, redolent with wholesome associations of honest farmers tilling the soil and campfire yarns	A highly genetically engineered crop, pickled in chemicals at all stages from field to factory, responsible for unparalleled global death
Tobacco additives	Unremarkable, harmless compounds to be found in many foodstuffs	Secret lab-made chemicals, with totally unknown health impacts when the burnt particles and residues are inhaled in smoke; a "spoonful of sugar" that helps the "medicine" go down
Cigarette packs	Highly valued trademarks that require many months to be altered should health bureaucrats require this	Highly market-researched components of a total marketing programme designed to make cigarettes seem like designer objects and fashion accessories
Pack warnings	Responsible information provided to adult consumers who are already fully aware of the risks they take. Graphic warnings unnecessarily disturb sensitive people and may make them blasé about other risks	Liberated information previously kept from smokers by the industry's refusal to provide readily understandable and memorable information about how smoking is likely to harm its users
Tobacco sponsorship of sport	Generous corporate support of adult-oriented sports that never caused anyone to ever take up smoking	Pernicious association of smoking with healthy, exciting, mass-appeal sport, including millions of children
Tobacco advertising	Product information for adult smokers	Information-free efforts designed to distract from concern about smoking harms and forge associations between all manner of desirable qualities and smoking
Smoking in movies	Artistic licence, totally uninfluenced by tobacco industry	Product placement secured via devious third-party subterfuge
Smoking in bars	Tolerant, courteous accommodation of both smokers and non-smokers	Shredding of the occupational health rights of bar staff in ways unacceptable in every other occupational setting
Smoking caused fire deaths	Tragic, rare events caused by typically intoxicated persons unamenable to education about correct disposal of completed cigarettes. Reduced Fire Risk ("RFR") cigarettes have unknown potential to prevent fires in "real-life" settings	All-too-common deaths, many caused by on-going refusal of industry to voluntarily introduce reduced ignition propensity ("RIP") cigarettes because of fears of consumer distaste for cigarettes that tend to go out
Cigarette litter reduction campaigns	Responsible efforts by a responsible industry to educate forgetful smokers about the importance of a clean environment	Cynical public relations efforts to distract from the industry's overall contribution to death and disease and to define litter reduction as having nothing to do with reducing the source of litter

A story about a newly discovered risk to the fetus from smoking might be better sent to a women's magazine than to a newspaper, where it might risk being spiked as "more of the same" old stuff about smoking being harmful.

- **Timeliness:** Does your story feed into something that is happening now or soon? A critical article about tobacco sponsorship and Formula 1 will attract much more interest around the time of your country's F1 race than months away from it.
- **Impact:** Has this story got strong visuals? For television this will give it huge advantage.
- **Prominence:** People die of smoking every minute of every hour. A smoking death in itself is not news. But if a prominent smoker dies, that's news.
- **Conflict:** Are people having an argument about this? Are they different people from those who we all know are always arguing about this issue? Is there a new (preferably prominent) community identity weighing into the tobacco industry or government inaction?
- **Uniqueness:** Is your news something genuinely fresh and new? Will people reading it for the first time react "how interesting – I never knew *that!*" Smoking causes blindness too? Amazing!
- **Proximity:** Is this story about something in your city? Local outlets can be depressingly parochial, but that's the reality.
- **Myth debunking:** Does this story turn a common way of thinking about something on its head? A myth-that-will-not-die in Australian tobacco control is that women smoke more than men: they never have, but the story persists in the imaginations of journalists and many of the public.
- **Danger in the familiar:** Is your story about something very ordinary and familiar that is now revealed by research as being harmful? In large part, this has been the essence of why secondhand smoke continues to be such a strong story.
- **Moral tales:** Is this story essentially the retelling of an age-old "moral tale" about good and evil? Is someone trying to cover up their association with the tobacco industry?

Making news on tobacco control

News does not magically appear in the news media. Instead, much of what appears as news is a product of deliberate organised activity on the part of those hoping to shape coverage. Among the most common sources of stories are tip-offs from sources known and trusted by journalists as reliable and knowledgeable. Part II of the book provides many ways of doing this. One easy way is for tobacco control agencies to see a core part of their work as trying to provide journalists with access to newsworthy research published in sometimes obscure research journals or websites. Stories about new research discoveries are legion in the media. Below is a description of a pilot study I conducted in 2000, to test the feasibility of such an idea.

Tobacco issues judged both as potentially newsworthy and likely to contribute to current tobacco control advocacy objectives were located using two methods. First, for each of the five weeks of the study *Current Contents* was searched using the search terms "tobacco OR smoking". This provided dozens of research reports and author contact details from the weekly updates published in over 7500 research journals. From these, candidate reports judged as likely to be newsworthy were shortlisted. Next, the worldwide web was searched for news of reports and events on smoking that might be newsworthy. From this process, reports judged likely to both attract news attention and to advance an explicit tobacco control policy objective were selected to be fashioned into news releases.

Copies of the research papers were obtained from their authors, who were contacted by email for permission for us to publicise their paper's findings. Email addresses of the authors were located by searching websites of the author's employing institution for a staff list. Google is the easiest way of doing this.

A media release was drafted and a comment on the significance of the report was sought from the lead author and/or a local expert. This comment and contact details were provided on the release. Media releases were sent to the newsrooms of the major metropolitan newspaper, radio and television stations in New South Wales on midweek days. A total of six media releases were distributed in this pilot study.

Press, radio and television reportage of tobacco and health issues was obtained from a commercial media monitoring service so that the "strike rate" for attracting reportage of our releases could be compared against the total of all reportage on smoking and health issues in the week following each release (see Table 3.2).

Table 3.2 News releases and number of news "strikes" following media releases (total coverage of tobacco control issues during the week in brackets).

Media release	Newspaper articles	Radio news spots	Television news spots	Total coverage and percent of coverage given to releases
1. Smoking ban in Californian bars does not reduce custom	0 (15)	7 (20)	0 (2)	7 (37) 18.9%
2. Smoking fathers increase cancer risk in offspring	1 (8)	2 (9)	1 (5)	4 (22) 18.2%
3. Smoking may increase prostate cancer death	0 (28)	0 (50)	0 (7)	0 (85) 0
4. Call for government action on tobacco pesticides	0 (28)	7 (50)	0 (7)	7 (85) 8.2%
5. Major passive smoking review	0 (23)	1 (38)	0 (6)	1 (67) 1.5%
6. Smokers outside buildings smoking "harder"	7 (26)	29 (37)	3 (9)	39 (72) 54.2%
Total	8 (100) 8%	46 (154) 30%	4 (29) 13.8%	58 (283) 20.5%

Table 3.2 summarises the number of occasions that news coverage precipitated by each release was published or broadcast, expressed against the denominator of the total number of items about tobacco control broadcast or published in each week of the release. Below, each release itemised in Table 3.2 is discussed in turn.

Release 1: Smoking ban in Californian bars[238]

Tobacco control objective: To increase public and political support for smokefree indoor hospitality venues.

Media advocacy objective: To introduce information into public debate showing that bars would not lose customers if they went smokefree, thus eroding a key barrier to political support for smokefree bars.

Perceived newsworthiness: In Australia, as elsewhere, policy debates about banning smoking in indoor hospitality venues such as bars and restaurants were being hotly contested. A key platform of opposition to such proposals was that such venues would lose smoking customers. The tobacco and hospitality industries have actively promoted this notion, which has proved pivotal in several policy debates. A key finding of this study[238] was that a hard-drinking Californian "sports" tavern did not lose any trade after a local ban on smoking was introduced. We considered this report would prove newsworthy in that it provided a body blow to the local tobacco and hotel industries' repeated forecasts of economic catastrophe should a ban be introduced in Australia. Traditionally framed as being at the cutting-edge of modernity, California had banned smoking in the last bastion of smoking: the male-dominated sports bar.

Results: The item was reported seven times on radio, representing just less than one in five reports on tobacco across all three media in that week.

Release 2: Smoking fathers increase cancer risk in offspring[239]

Tobacco control objective: To encourage more men to quit smoking, particularly when contemplating fatherhood.

Media advocacy objective: To introduce a new piece of information about yet another danger posed by smoking.

Perceived newsworthiness: There has been a long history of news interest in the harms that smoking mothers can cause their babies *in utero*, with the subtext often focusing on notions of bad mothering and selfishness. We considered this report to be potentially newsworthy in that it promised an intriguing new twist on the harms wrought by smoking. The findings reported from this Chinese case-control study described increased childhood cancer rates in the offspring of smoking fathers. With relatively few Chinese women smoking, and sperm damage from tobacco use being already reported, the results were biologically plausible. We sensed that the newsworthy aspects of the report would lie in it "turning the tables" on the traditional "blaming" of mothers for risking harm to their babies through their smoking. It promised to open up a whole new discourse about paternal preconception responsibilities, perhaps attracting the attention of some journalists who might be attracted to the idea that men should share responsibility for quitting with their female partners.

Results: Again, just under one in five of all reports on smoking that week were generated by our release.

Release 3: Smoking may increase prostate cancer death[240]

Tobacco control objective: To encourage more men to quit smoking.

Media advocacy objective: To publicise the relationship between smoking and a hitherto unreported adverse health outcome predicted to be of great concern to many men.

Perceived newsworthiness: This study reported a fatal prostate cancer rate ratio for current smokers of 1.34 (i.e. a 34% increase compared with non-smokers). We judged that this story had potential to "piggy back" on the growing media interest in prostate cancer, the second leading cause of cancer death in Australian males, and a cancer that has been largely devoid of preventable risk factors.

Results: Despite recruiting a prominent local professor who often appeared in the media and had recently written a book on prostate cancer, this release was not picked up by any news medium. It may have been that journalists considered the low relative risk reported to be insufficiently dramatic, or that prostate cancer has not yet acquired invincible newsworthy status.

Release 4: Call for government action on tobacco pesticides

Tobacco control objective: To add momentum to calls for more comprehensive labelling of cigarette packs and to add another dimension of concern to smokers' apprehensiveness about their tobacco use.

Media advocacy objective: To frame tobacco as anything but a "natural" product, but as one that was polluted with pesticides that smokers were not being told about.

Perceived newsworthiness: Pesticide residue in food is known to be of greater concern to consumers than nutritional issues like fat and fibre[241,242]. Pesticides, being "unnatural" and produced by industrial corporations, satisfy most of the criteria for predicting community outrage about risk[243]. On locating a large website devoted to pesticides in tobacco, we judged that themes about non-disclosure to consumers, and lack of standards and routine testing would prove newsworthy.

Results: Only seven radio reports resulted, in a week that featured many press reports about passive smoking.

Release 5: Major passive smoking review reinforces call for bans[244]

Tobacco control objective: To build public and political support for a legislated ban on smoking in enclosed areas.

Media advocacy objective: To publicise that – yet again – another major scientific review had declared passive smoking to be harmful.

Perceived newsworthiness: The release on the worldwide web of the report on passive smoking of the Californian Environmental Protection Agency coincided with a spate of news coverage about passive smoking in Australia arising from efforts by the local tobacco industry to suppress a government expert report[245]. We anticipated that alerting the Australian media to a major overseas report would most likely attract interest with reasoning like "the American public have been allowed to see a major government report on passive smoking . . . why can't the Australian public see a local version?"

Results: Our judgment proved overly ambitious, with only one report resulting.

Release 6: Smokers outside buildings smoking 'harder', study finds[45]

Tobacco control objective: To reinforce community understanding of smoking as a form of drug dependence and thereby to contribute to the debate on regulation of cigarette ingredients such as nicotine.

Media advocacy objective: To provide research information on a commonplace sight (smokers outside buildings).

Perceived newsworthiness: The study showed that office smokers smoking outside buildings – a common sight in Australian cities for the past decade – were smoking "harder" than people smoking outside in more leisurely settings. Three aspects of the study seemed likely to be newsworthy:

- The study provided evidence that far from being cool and sociable office "rebels" taking advantage of their status as smokers to allow them to take time off work, many smokers were desperate addicts fleeing from offices to engage in near-frenzied smoking behaviour to satisfy their cravings
- Were policies that drove smokers out of buildings inadvertently harming smokers by causing them to smoke "harder" as observed? That is, had tobacco control policies blundered?
- How much time were smokers spending outside buildings, and was this fair to non-smokers who had no need to take repeated "time-out" episodes from work?

Results: This release attracted 39 news reports, making it nearly twice more reported than all the other releases combined.

Discussion

In the 5 weeks during which the six news releases were issued, more than one in five of all monitored news reports on smoking issues were generated by the releases issued in this pilot study. These findings are consistent with studies of the origins of reportage, which have shown that much contemporary journalism is stimulated by receipt of media releases and other efforts to get into the news. Our "hit rate" in major metropolitan media, with their greater access to electronic news gathering, was considerably lower than the 78% reported by Mindell in regional newspapers in the UK for a similar exercise[246]. However, provincial newspapers have a reputation as being relatively easy targets for news generated locally as such stories do not have to compete for editorial attention with national and international news.

Media releases 3, 4 and 5 were distributed during a time when there was high media coverage of passive smoking and the potential effects of smokefree public place legislation in New South Wales (NSW). This high background level of reportage (mean = 76 over these 2 weeks) was 52% higher than the average reportage rates for the 5 weeks. This may have jeopardised further coverage of smoking in our releases, with editors and journalists perhaps judging "we've had enough smoking stories this week". Public health advocates cannot always predict when competing stories will relegate their own to the editorial "spike".

Radio covered our stories more than newspapers or television news. This probably reflects the greater number of news bulletins on radio compared with television, and the smaller number of newspapers ($n = 3$) in our study sample than radio stations ($n = 10$).

Locating the newsworthy stories and research papers involved weekly computer searching sessions, each taking less than 15 minutes, particularly once the search parameters had been bookmarked. All lead authors of the scientific papers granted permission to distribute the media release. The most time-consuming aspect of the process was our attempts to persuade local Australian experts to comment on local implications of international research papers. Four such people refused, suggesting the low priority that some researchers give to contributing to public dissemination of research[247].

Some stories that were identified as potentially newsworthy were reported in the media before a media release could be generated. Journalists, especially with the advent of the internet, are increasingly able quickly to locate interesting journal articles/news stories without assistance from outside groups, especially when they are reported in widely read journals such as the *Lancet* and *British Medical Journal* (*BMJ*)[248]. However, there are a great many newsworthy reports published in specialised journals that do not have their own publicity divisions, and so seldom if ever come to public attention.

The process of locating newsworthy stories and issuing media releases is an extremely cost-effective way of generating selected reportage that can expose hundreds of thousands, if not millions of people to information about public health issues. Public health advocates have the ability to assist researchers, who often give low priority to publicity, in disseminating significant findings through unpaid publicity. This has the potential to influence knowledge levels, public opinion and policy change.

Note

i   Material in this chapter has been drawn from Chapman S. The news on tobacco control: time to bring the background into the foreground. *Tob Control* 1999;**8**:237–9; Chapman S, Dominello A. A strategy for increasing news media coverage of tobacco and health in Australia. *Health Promotion Int* 2001;**16**: 137–43.

Chapter 4

Dead Customers are Unprofitable Customers: Potential and Pitfalls in Harm Reduction and Product Regulation

In late 1984, freshly graduated with my PhD, I arrived in Adelaide for my first senior public health appointment as director of health promotion for the South Australian Health Commission. Within days, I lunched with the Health Minister, John Cornwall, a pugnacious Labor Party minister who will be recorded in Australian public health history as the politician who introduced the first successful comprehensive tobacco control act into an Australian parliament. We went to a Thai restaurant and he explained that politically, because of the unconditional support for tobacco control of a minor party, the Australian Democrats, he was able "to pursue a relatively aggressive [tobacco control] agenda despite a marked lack of enthusiasm among my parliamentary colleagues", as he later recorded[249].

He said he wanted to introduce the world's best tobacco control programme and asked what this should look like. We unfolded paper napkins, and on these over a couple of hours, sketched out the ingredients of what would become the South Australian Tobacco Products Control Act, 1986[250]. Some months before the Act was passed, I proposed another item: banning smokeless tobacco. Greg Connolly, a Boston dentist with an interest in tobacco control, had sent me his review in the *New England Journal of Medicine*[251], which described a worrying incidence of oral cancer in parts of the USA caused by the use of oral moist snuff. We don't want that stuff in Australia, I thought. John Cornwall agreed.

Unlike parts of the USA, Scandinavia, South-East Asia, the Middle East, North Africa and the Indian subcontinent, Australia has no widespread tradition of oral tobacco use. Its use was then and continues today to be confined to a relatively small number of immigrants from northern Europe and the Indian subcontinent, the latter buying illegal sachets of gutka and pan masala from specialist tobacconists and South Asian grocery shops[252], typically stored under the counter. We reasoned that Australia was in a perfect situation to prevent the uptake of smokeless tobacco. Provision was made for the current small number of users to import enough for personal use. It is often said "if cigarettes were invented today, with all that is known about them now, no government would allow them to be manufactured or sold". So, there we were in South Australia in 1986, armed with the Connolly group's review, about to ban a "new" tobacco product before it could take root in an environment where tobacco advertising and promotion might have helped it flourish. It seemed eminently sensible at the time.

The US Tobacco Company had been showing great interest in Australia as a potential new market and when South Australia banned smokeless tobacco in 1986, other Australian states followed quickly, with the federal government placing a permanent ban on the commercial supply of chewing tobacco and oral snuff on 17 April 1991[253]. New Zealand also banned smokeless tobacco around the same time, and using the same reasoning, the European Parliament has refused to allow smokeless tobacco products to be sold in Europe[254,255] outside of Sweden where its availability has always been legal.

For many years, I counted my role in the ban as one of my most tangible achievements in public health. But today, in 2006, I ask myself whether I was wrong and another unwitting victim of the Law of Unintended Consequences. I will never know the answer to that question, but the most contentious, complicated and divisive debate in tobacco control today is without doubt that surrounding harm reduction through tobacco product modification: the idea that in addition to encouraging prevention and cessation of use, policy should encourage the development and use of tobacco products that might result in fewer deaths in continuing tobacco users.

As a concept, harm reduction has a long history in public health. Industries such as the automobile industry, where users take risks with every use of the product, have long sought to design and engineer ways of making cars safer in both preventing crashes and minimising harm when they occur. The concept has gained huge credibility in the areas of HIV/AIDS control and the illicit drug abuse fields[256], boasting a global society (the International Harm Reduction Association), although in those fields its precepts remain heresy for those wedded to absolutist abstinence values, such as the Bush administration in the USA.

Moral and political conservatives typically don't see tobacco use as morally problematic in the same way that they see "sinful" licentiousness like sex outside marriage and illicit drug use. With these, fornicators and drug users are seen effectively to "deserve" any harm they bring on themselves[133,257] and policies that could soften the harm they might cause themselves are seen as "sending the wrong signal" to the community[133], as the Australian Prime Minister, John Howard would put it.

However, in the tobacco control field, political conservatives see tobacco as simply another consumer choice. If harm reduction claims could be shown to be truthful, then those opposing harm reduction effectively inhabit the same ethical space as those moral conservatives who oppose harm reduction in the HIV/AIDS and narcotics fields: they believe smokers should either quit or "face the consequences". Tobacco harm reduction advocates argue that it is vital that we support the development and then the carefully regulated availability of tobacco products that, while not being 100% "safe" (a nonsensical notion, as nothing is completely safe), might be far less harmful to users than conventional tobacco products. Numbered among these people are several of the finest analytical minds and experienced industry watchers in contemporary tobacco control. While it is possible they are all on a fool's errand and risk a repetition of the dangerous false reassurances that the "light and mild" saga provided to smokers for over 30 years[258], such a hypothesis would require an almost conspiracy theory-style account of why so many intelligent and committed people have wandered so far off the orthodox tobacco control rails.

Harm reduction circumspection

Harm reduction detractors come in several stripes. The most easily dismissed are those absolutists who are gut-level tobacco prohibitionists. Such people don't believe that any form of tobacco product could ever have an acceptable level of risk. *Any* level of risk in *any* tobacco product is unacceptable to them. Expert panels have estimated that total mortality risks of low-nitrosamine smokeless tobacco (LNST) such as Swedish snus (to be discussed below) are of the order of 90–95% lower than that for smoked tobacco[259]. The US Institute of Medicine report concluded that "The overall risk [for smokeless tobacco products] is lower than for cigarette smoking, and some products, such as Swedish snus, may have no increased risk"[258]. Absolutists would immediately point to the 5–10% residual risk and the "may" and declare that to be entirely unacceptable. The 90–95% potential improvement, with all the lives that might be saved, would not be important.

However, every participant in this debate chooses to take "acceptable" risks with their and others' health and safety every day. We drive cars; we expose ourselves to solar radiation at the beach and in parks. We expose ourselves to diagnostic radiation at the hands of dentists and doctors. Some are content to be obese and sedentary. In each of these contexts we develop mental heuristics involving costs and benefits that assist us to make our choices. But for tobacco prohibitionists, tobacco use is *absolutely* unacceptable with only zero risk being acceptable when it comes to considering harm reduction.

Then there are some who, while not necessarily taking issue with the claims about reduced risk, object to allowing any form of nicotine to be made available to those who might want to use it. Basically, they object to the idea of people being addicted, regardless of the risk reduction that this might bring. Some see important ethical issues arising from a policy that would facilitate millions becoming addicted to a product that will cause many of them to pay for decades of nicotine use, even if the health risks were demonstrably lower. They are uncomfortable with nicotine replacement therapy for the same reasons: using nicotine is "wrong" before questions of harm even arise. They would be adamant in their opposition to allowing onto the market nicotine delivery devices with higher or faster-acting dosage than the current generation of nicotine replacement therapies. This is essentially a moralistic position, more than a position anchored to public health considerations.

A third group are those who agree that low-nitrosamine smokeless tobacco (LNST) could have a key role in harm reduction but that its potential benefits and risks depend upon how its availability and marketing is regulated and monitored to detect unintended consequences so that policy changes could be then rapidly implemented. This group are not mesmerised by the Swedish snus experience to be discussed below, and question the transferability of the possible positive aspects of that experience to other countries and cultures[258,260]. This group are also hardened realists, experienced in watching industry tactics and understandably suspicious of the embrace of product regulation that some transnational tobacco companies now routinely give. These same companies, such critics note, also advocate programmes that purportedly discourage tobacco use by youth – who represent the economic future for the companies. They also both openly and covertly oppose all forms of effective tobacco control. With good reason we don't trust them on these issues, so why should we trust them on harm reduction . . . yet again? These critics argue that the companies are "giving an inch to gain a decade" on supporting product regulation, and cleverly playing to the theoretical, seductive appeals of reduced harm which, as we will see, will not be ultimately testable for several decades, if ever. They would point to the tobacco industry's well-documented game plan to divide and conquer the tobacco control movement[261], and see harm reduction as one of the industry's chosen vehicles to do this. These cynics would assess the entire momentum for harm reduction as the latest chapter in an industry strategy to fill the tobacco use "downtime" caused by widespread smoking restrictions[262]. You can keep smoking and use a smokeless product at times when you can't smoke. Such a pattern of use, critics argue, would in fact be unequivocally a harm *increasing* development, as many smokers are stimulated to quit when they cannot smoke at work and other places.

A variation on this argument comes from those who don't engage with the data on reduced risk, but who see the key point of tobacco control being whether tobacco companies gain financially, not that tobacco-caused disease should drop. As one writer to Globalink, the listserver of the international tobacco control community, put it: "I would consider it a tragedy if individuals identifying themselves as representing the tobacco control community either wittingly or unwittingly lent support to the venal objectives of any tobacco company."

The tobacco control community is much divided about harm reduction. In one recent study of US expert opinion, there was widespread agreement about the "theoretical plausibility" of harm reduction; that characteristics of "good" and "bad" harm-reduced products could be identified; and that government regulation is essential but unlikely in the foreseeable future. But beyond these generalities, there was no consensus on key aspects such as preferred regulatory strategies[263]. Debates about harm reduction regularly break out into lengthy and often acrimonious slanging matches. Clive Bates, former director of UK Action on Smoking and Health, and one of the most astute minds I've encountered in tobacco control, was one of the first to refer memorably to harm reduction opponents as "quit or die" advocates: people who effectively say to smokers "either quit smoking, or die from it: we will not countenance you getting access to a tobacco product which might *reduce* your chances of dying."

Others, myself included, while intrigued by the Swedish experience, wonder how much the accelerating harm reduction debate risks distracting from more concerted action in the main, tried and tested strategies for reducing tobacco-caused disease: strategies that today see more ex-smokers than smokers in some nations in the vanguard of tobacco control, and subpopulations with reported smoking prevalence at 10% or even less (see Chapter 8). I look at such nations that now have reported 20% or less adult smoking prevalence, with an apparently brakeless downward trajectory, and I wonder about questions of proportional effort: in an overview of the most important "bangs for the buck" in tobacco control, harm reduction will probably rank low in such nations.

But I also look at the great majority of the world's nations where tobacco control is anything but successful. China, for example, has an estimated 350 million smokers – mainly men – and shows few signs of the declines in smoking that characterise nations with robust tobacco control programmes. I am writing this book in France where, despite some advanced tobacco control policy, smoking levels remind me of those I saw in Australia 30 years ago. In such countries, hundreds of millions of people in successive generations of smokers are likely to continue to smoke for decades to come, with half of long-term users dying from their smoking[47]. If the average toxicity of the tobacco products they use could be substantially reduced, this might lead to significant reductions in death and disease. Those who are indifferent to the possibility of reducing even fractionally such preventable carnage through harm reduction need to be very sure that their alternatives will do the same thing faster.

Lars Ramström from Sweden has in recent years been a leading advocate for snus as a harm-reduced tobacco product. In 2006, one of the leading opponents of harm reduction via smokeless tobacco cited a paper published by Ramström 16 years previously where he had written "taking up snuff must be seen as an introduction to the tobacco habit and possibly a first step towards taking up cigarettes"[264]. Ramström changed his mind about snus[265,266], when data emerged that changed his view. The economist John Maynard Keynes, who had a reputation for often changing his views, once replied to an accusation of inconsistency: "When the facts change, I change my mind. What do you do, sir?" The tobacco control movement has been wedded to the abstinence goal. Have the facts changed enough to make us change our minds too?

Overview

In this chapter, I will try to cut through the thicket of arguments about product modification and harm reduction to try to assess its likely contribution to our ultimate goal in tobacco control: reducing death and disease from tobacco use. I will start with a brief overview of the history of tobacco harm reduction, from its earliest hopes and manifestations to the form and preoccupations of the debate today. In particular, I will summarise current thinking about the Swedish LNST product, snus, which appears to be a genuine reduced-harm product. I will consider why pharmaceutical companies that market nicotine-replacement smoking-cessation products have hesitated to modify these products so that they provide smokers with nicotine "spikes" similar to those obtained by smoking, which would be more satisfying and offer greater competition to cigarettes as nicotine delivery systems.

I will then examine the harm reduction argument as it applies to combustible forms of tobacco, which overwhelmingly dominate global tobacco consumption today. I will review the current thinking among senior tobacco control analysts about the challenge posed by the fundamentally unacceptable proposition that tobacco products should remain unregulated: that unlike foods, beverages and pharmaceuticals, tobacco products should not be required to conform to any product "safety" specifications. Finally, I will summarise my personal conclusions about the future and realistic potential of harm reduction, arguing that tobacco control advocates should lobby strongly for the establishment of internationally networked regulatory authorities for tobacco and nicotine delivery systems, whose main goals would be to regulate all aspects of tobacco and alternative nicotine delivery devices, using harm reduction principles.

Product regulation

No discussion of harm reduction can avoid a parallel engagement with the topic of tobacco product regulation. If we were to agree that harm-reduced products could be produced and marketed, immediate questions arise about the standards – and their enforcement – that would need to apply to any product claiming to be a reduced-risk product. More fundamentally, questions arise about whether and how the tobacco industry should be able to make any claims to consumers about such products. The anarchic alternative to product regulation is to allow the status quo to continue where, alone among all products that are taken into or applied onto the body (foods, drinks, pharmaceuticals, cosmetics), tobacco products may be modified by almost any non-prohibited substance[i] (see "Ingredients" below), and the industry may withhold any aspect of this information from government and consumers and be accountable to no one for its decisions. The standard concept of product safety criteria in consumer safety is an oxymoron when it comes to tobacco, with the result that the only serious attempt to have the government regulate tobacco foundered on the contradictory implications of this conclusion[267]. The cartoonist Tom Toles captured this dilemma beautifully when, in 2000, the US Supreme Court ruled that the Food and Drug Administration could not regulate cigarettes because they were too dangerous to regulate (Fig. 4.1).

At the conclusion of the chapter, I will therefore also consider the regulatory challenges that arise in the harm reduction debate. I know of no serious-minded person working in tobacco control who believes the tobacco industry should not be heavily regulated. This is very easily said, and Philip Morris today says it with consummate ease: "That's why we support strong and effective regulation for both our products and our industry, and we are committed to working with governments and the public health community towards that goal"[268]. But the devil, as always, lies very much in the detail. Philip Morris's fiduciary duty to its shareholders would preclude it from ever supporting any policy that threatened to reduce the company's profitability. The question for public health is whether the existence of companies profiting from nicotine addiction can ever be compatible with the pursuit of public health goals.

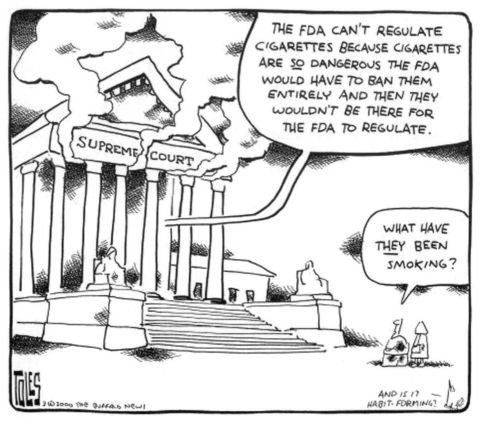

Fig. 4.1 TOLES © (2000) *The Buffalo News*. Reprinted with permission of Universal Press Syndicate. All rights reserved.

Everything old is new again?

Innocents might think of tobacco products as simply dried tobacco, and in the case of cigarettes, dried tobacco rolled in paper, generally with a filter at one end. Nothing could miss the point more. The modern cigarette is a highly chemically engineered drug delivery device primarily designed to deliver the drug nicotine, and possibly other undeclared nicotine-like analogues[83], to the user in doses that will cause rapid addiction, and in a manner that will cause the addicted user to repeatedly dose themselves about ten times per cigarette, hundreds of puffs a day, week after week, year after year[269]. Fortunately for the industry, the formula often works rapidly. DiFranza and colleagues have shown that among teenage smokers, 40% report standard symptoms of nicotine dependency[270].

Ways to engineer tobacco products

Tobacco chemists have a cornucopia of variables to play with in their goal (as one memorable tobacco industry document succinctly put it) of making it "harder for existing smokers to leave the product"[66]. Plant geneticists have provided the ability to grow genetically modified high-nicotine-yielding tobacco. Tobacco chemists and designers are also able to manipulate virtually any component of tobacco and any other ingredient they might wish to add for purposes that include:

- Making the product easier and less unpleasant to smoke, particularly for young starters[271], women and African-Americans[272], who often dislike the harshness of tobacco smoke. Menthol smokers, for example, have a significantly shorter time to the first cigarette of the day compared with non-menthol smokers (smoking within the first 5 minutes of the day: 45% vs 29%, respectively)[273], with some authors suggesting that menthol may both enhance addiction and cause changes in inhalation that may pose greater risks to health[274,275]. Significantly, various sugars are often added to tobacco blends or to the cigarette paper. When sugars are burned, they form acetaldehydes, a group of carcinogens that are embryotoxic, teratogenic and induce respiratory tract tumours in hamsters when inhaled[276]. Acetaldehydes are weaker carcinogens than the polynuclear aromatic hydrocarbons, N-nitrosamines and aromatic amines that are also found in tobacco smoke but their concentration is thousands of times higher[277].
- Increasing the efficiency and rapidity of nicotine reaching the brain, by changing the pH of the smoke using ammonia chemistry (so-called "free-basing")[278].
- Reducing and masking unpleasant smells in sidestream smoke[161].
- Accelerating the rate at which cigarettes burn down. Burn accelerant chemicals (particularly citrates) are added to cigarette paper to cause it to continue to burn down when not being inhaled[279]. This has the simple commercial advantage of causing the cigarette to burn down faster than it otherwise might, thus causing the heavier smoker to consider lighting another one sooner.
- Reducing the yields of tar and nicotine as measured by the much criticised[280] International Standards Organization (ISO)/Federal Trade Commission (FTC) system while maintaining sufficient doses of nicotine to satisfy the smoker[281].

There is nothing new in the idea that tobacco products could be engineered to make them less harmful. Tobacco filters, incorporated into cigarette design from the early 1950s, were the first major embodiment of that idea, and as we will see, did not slow the growth of tobacco-caused disease and death. Spent cigarette filters show brown tar stains, so it is tempting to assume that filters trap material that would otherwise go into smokers' lungs. But as we will see later in this chapter, with the advent of filter ventilation, and the changes in puff topography that this caused, filters may well have caused smokers to pull more tar into their lungs than they might have when smoking unfiltered products. While filters visibly retain a proportion of the smoke particles that would otherwise enter the smoker's lungs, the industry was well aware that they did not, and indeed must not, trap everything. In a 1966 analysis of the market potential for a "health cigarette", Philip Morris noted that: "A large proportion of smokers are concerned about the relationship of cigarette smoking to health . . . The illusion of filtration is as important as the fact of filtration . . . Therefore any entry should be by a radically different method of filtration but need not be any more effective"[282].

Early pioneers

The late Ernst Wynder and his colleague Dietrich Hoffmann from the American Health Foundation, along with a tobacco industry that hoped it might be able to develop "safe" products, were the founders of today's harm reduction movement in tobacco control[283]. At a 1964 research meeting Wynder argued "The question has often been asked 'Can cigarette smoking ever be safe?' At present, an affirmative answer to this question would appear to be quite unrealistic . . . In view of the fact, however, that man may not always be willing or able to accomplish this objective [stop smoking], research efforts towards producing 'less hazardous smoking products' must be continued"[284]. Wynder and Hoffmann vigorously encouraged continued research efforts towards "reducing the experimentally established tumorigenicity of smoking products"[285]. The US National Cancer Institute accepted the challenge and between 1968 and 1980 spent over $50 million on contract research, of which 74% went into biological and chemical analysis of modified cigarettes[286]. Mark Parascandola's review[286] of the history of harm reduction catalogues numerous high-level statements of optimism from public health officials that were made about the programme until it was eventually phased out by 1980 after no significant breakthroughs had been made.

Michael Russell, a pioneer in nicotine addiction research, once observed that "were it not for nicotine people would be no more inclined [to smoke] than they are to blow bubbles"[287]. While the addictive properties of nicotine are cardinal to the industry's continuing profitability, the idea that the tobacco industry could have ever been happy that many of its best customers died years early is unsustainable. Plainly, it was always going to be in the tobacco industry's interests to try to manufacture highly addictive products that caused as little harm to their users as possible. Dead customers are very unprofitable. Products that allow strongly addicted users to live a normal lifespan in good health are a tobacco manufacturer's dream come true. If such products could be developed, only those who objected to addiction rather than to the collateral health harms caused by repeated nicotine delivery through "dirty" delivery systems like cigarettes, would continue to object.

However, the industry had painted itself into a corner because of its obdurate denial of health risks. For as long as it maintained the public position that tobacco's role in disease causation remained an unproven hypothesis, any implication about reducing risk invited the obvious question of "reduce *what* risk?" This caused at least one company to be highly cautious about any public statements about their private hopes for less dangerous products. As the then chairman of British American Tobacco (BAT) put it in 1986: "in attempting to develop a 'safe' cigarette you are, by implication, in danger of being interpreted as accepting that the current product is 'unsafe' and this is not a position that I think we should take"[288].

Enter lights and milds

In spite of the tactics of the tobacco industry, public concern about the harms caused by smoking continued to swell unabated. So the industry cleverly opted to have it both ways, throughout a disgraceful 30-year period of communicative duplicity.

While continuing to argue publicly that smokers should remain sceptical about smoking and disease claims[64], it developed and aggressively marketed light and mild cigarettes[289], knowing that many consumers unsuspectingly believed these to be risk-reducing products, as the following examples from internal industry documents show:

- Philip Morris "research shows Lights = Milds = Less harmful"[290].
- "The Australian company has found that smokers of the ultra low tar brands are very conscious of the S&H [smoking and health] controversy but that smokers of 6–9 mg tar brands split between those wanting mildness per se and *those wanting smoker reassurance*." [my emphasis][291]

The publication of "league tables" showing the tar readings of different brands was similarly seen by the companies as a way of promoting the idea that smoking could be "safer". In 1982 Brown & Williamson concluded: "The publication of a League Table heightens the awareness of the smoking and health controversy. It also gives the consumer a new frame of reference for judging his brand and this provides a new dimension in a brand's image. The perceived concept of "safer" is introduced."[291]

The industry negotiated this duplicity through the ruse of "taste". While privately knowing full well that many anxious smokers were switching to lights and milds out of concern for their health, its public policy was always to repudiate claims that it was effectively admitting its products were harmful by claiming that words like light and mild referred strictly to taste characteristics, and had nothing to do with toxic ingredient delivery. This was a clever move. Different brands of cigarettes can have differing taste characteristics, so to the ordinary person, it seemed reasonable that words like "mild" or "light" referred to taste.

An Australian billboard advertisement for *Kraft Light* peanut butter with 25% less fat, carried the caption "for health nuts" – people preoccupied about their health. Kraft is a subsidiary of Altria, Philip Morris's parent group. We are thus invited to believe that when Altria employees in the tobacco division use the word "light" they mean "taste", but when their colleagues in the Kraft food division use the word, they mean "reduced health risk".

With misleading terms like "light" and "mild" now becoming banned in an increasing number of countries, and attracting their own clause in the Framework Convention on Tobacco Control, the industry has simply selected a new generation of synonyms for the same concepts. Brand names incorporating words like "smooth" and "fine", packaged in the same pack colours in which their "light" and "mild" predecessors appeared, are now being sold[292]. The tobacco industry would be nothing less than delighted in being able to perpetuate the old, immensely profitable deception.

People do not smoke like machines

The cigarette yields that appear on packs are obtained from a testing protocol adopted by the US Federal Trade Commission (FTC) and the International Standards

Organization (ISO). The tar, nicotine and carbon monoxide yields of smoke emissions from test cigarettes are obtained by testing lighted cigarettes on a machine that uses the fixed parameters of a 35-mL puff volume and a 2-second puff duration at 1 puff per minute, and leaves a fixed butt length to which each cigarette is smoked[293].

However, people do not smoke like machines. The FTC/ISO ratings do not take into account large variations in tar and nicotine yields that smokers in fact obtain as they seek to maintain a particular intake of nicotine[294]. Smokers can increase the amount of nicotine (and tar) they obtain by taking more puffs per cigarette, unwittingly obstructing the ventilation holes (see below) around the filter with their fingers, smoking the cigarette further down, smoking more cigarettes per day and inhaling a larger puff volume more deeply into their lungs.

The tobacco industry knew from at least 1972 that people did not smoke like smoking machines. Following the publication in *Nature* of a paper[295] by a tobacco industry consultant[137], internal Philip Morris correspondence summarised that "The amount of nicotine abstracted from a cigarette by a smoker may be considerably different from the nicotine yield of the same brand as measured with a standard smoking machine. In the experiments with smokers, the puff size, 'puff profile' and butt length differed from those with the smoking machine"[296].

By 1977, the picture within the industry was very clear: "The standard puffs of 35cc repeated at one minute intervals are seldom seen among smokers. Of the 165 R&D smokers screened with profile recording units, there are fewer than 20% who take puffs of an average volume less than 35cc. Fifty percent take puffs that average 35–55cc and the remaining smokers take even large puff volumes on the regular brands. The vast majority of smokers show a comparatively large lighting puff and then a gradual stepwise decrease in puff volumes as they proceed down the rod . . . Average total volumes (puff count × average puff volume and tar deliveries for smoking panels at R&D are at least 45% larger than the standard CI values)"[297].

Ventilated filters

The factor largely responsible for all these differences in puffing behaviour between humans and smoking machines is the placement of barely visible ventilation holes around the filter to dilute the smoke with entrained air. Tobacco companies began test marketing cigarettes with filters perforated with pin-prick-sized ventilation holes in 1975[298] (see Fig. 4.2). Their use rapidly spread. For example, by the end of the 1970s, all three manufacturers in Australia were selling brands with ventilation holes[299], and by the early 1990s around 90% of Australian brands had filter ventilation[300,301]. The ventilation holes allow air to be drawn in each time the cigarette smoking machine draws on the cigarette, thus causing a dilution of the smoke that is drawn through to the smoke-collecting apparatus at the end of the cigarette. Under test conditions, these ventilation holes are not occluded by the test machine, allowing maximum dilution with air. However, when smokers use ventilated cigarettes, partial occlusion often occurs as smokers' fingers partially block the holes. A Philip Morris official observed in 1974 that "the consumer will not have his attention

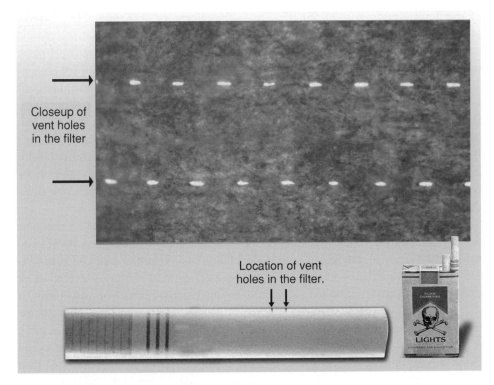

Fig. 4.2 Cigarette ventilation holes. Source: New York State Smokers' Quitline (http://www.nysmokefree.com/newweb/pageview.aspx?p=4040).

drawn to the fact that the tipping is indeed, perforated"[302], suggesting that the company would have appreciated their little secret as an advantage. Had smokers been aware of it, they may have been less confident that they were indeed smoking lower yielding brands.

Today, the ISO standard remains completely discredited as a means of assessing what exposures smokers actually obtain from cigarettes. An ISO working party report concluded "Smoke emission data from machine measurements may be used as inputs for product hazard assessment, but they are not intended to be nor are they valid measures of human exposure or risks. Communicating differences between products in machine measurements as differences in exposure or risk is a misuse of testing using ISO standards"[303].

Early harm reduced products

There have been several previous generations of so-called "safer" cigarettes, most of which have been abject failures in the marketplace. Perhaps the most infamous was *Kent's Micronite* filter, introduced in the 1950s in the USA and almost certainly exported outside the USA[304]. The Micronite filter contained crocidolite (blue asbestos) fibres[305], which caused cancer in users resulting in both death and successful litigation. On 31 December 1997, Lorillard Tobacco Company, manufacturer of the *Kent* brand, paid $1 556 851.75 to the survivors of *Kent* smoker Milton Horowitz.

The 1970s saw the promotion by the US-based Celanese company of its plans to develop an inorganic smoking "supplement" known as Cytrel, designed to generate less smoke[306]. Imperial Chemical Industries (ICI) also developed a supplement known as "new smoking material", which was a total market failure. The 1970s also saw the major tobacco companies energetically promoting brands like *Merit* (Philip Morris), *Kent Golden Lights* (Lorillard) and *Now* (R.J. Reynolds). Mark Parascandola reminds us that the then head of the National Cancer Institute, Frank Rauscher, told Congress: "If these cigarettes are acceptable to the public taste wise, we should see a diminution of the increasing curve of lung cancer incidence in the next years."[286]

However, the emerging epidemiology of tobacco-caused disease told a different story. Thun and Burns' 2001 review of the evidence as to whether 40 years of consumer drift towards machine-tested low-yielding cigarettes had changed tobacco-caused disease incidence concluded: "cohort studies in the USA and UK show that lung cancer risk continued to increase among older smokers from the 1950s to the 1980s, despite the widespread adoption of lower yield cigarettes. The change to filter tip products did not prevent a progressive increase in lung cancer risk among male smokers who began smoking during and after the Second World War compared to the First World War era smokers. National trends in vital statistics data show declining lung cancer death rates in young adults, especially males, in many countries, but the extent to which this is attributable to 'reduced yield' cigarettes remains unclear"[307].

Importantly, these same authors also considered whether the introduction of supposedly reduced risk products had slowed cessation and increased initiation, and concluded: "No studies have adequately assessed whether health claims used to market 'reduced yield' cigarettes delay cessation among smokers who might otherwise quit, or increase initiation among non-smokers", and finally that: "There is no convincing evidence that past changes in cigarette design have resulted in an important health benefit to either smokers or the whole population."[307]

PREPs: potential reduced exposure products

In the past 15 or so years there has been a renaissance of interest in nicotine delivery systems with potential to reduce the harm caused to users. This interest has never really waned in tobacco toxicological circles nor within the industry, where it remains the equivalent of the search for the Holy Grail, but has become more mainstream with the appearance in the US marketplace in particular of a multitude of alleged harm-reduced or "potential reduced exposure products" (PREPs), the publication in 2001 of the US Institute of Medicine report *Clearing the Smoke,* which examined the scientific base for harm reduction[258], and an accelerating rate of publications about Sweden's experience with the smokeless tobacco product, snus (see below). A growing research literature is illuminating key questions about the potential of these products to reduce particular diseases, the impact that manufacturers' claims are having on smokers and ex-smokers, and whether these products are making inroads into the cigarette market.

R.J. Reynolds introduced in the USA a cigarette-like nicotine delivery device called Premier in 1988, but withdrew it after it flopped with consumers[308]. A similar device, Eclipse, began to be test-marketed in parts of the USA in 1994, and Philip Morris test-marketed *Accord* in 1998. *Premier, Eclipse* and *Accord* differ radically from conventional cigarettes in that they heat rather than burn tobacco, via a central heat rod, which causes a nicotine-laden aerosol to be delivered to the user when they draw on the cigarette-like product[309]. I once tried a *Premier* and was reminded of an expression I once heard a smoker use about lights: "you've got to inhale so hard to get any flavour, you feel you'll wind up getting a hernia!" Apparently many smokers felt the same way.

Industry researchers from R.J. Reynolds claimed that *Eclipse* was less mutagenic and cytotoxic than conventional cigarettes of the sort also sold in the billions by their company[310]. However, *Eclipse* was shown to discharge glass fibres and particles from the filter into the smoker's mouth. These bioresistant fibres and microscopic glass dust could be then inhaled and/or ingested posing a potential and unnecessary health hazard to uninformed consumers. The authors of this study noted that "*Eclipse* is a paradigm of the health danger that may be imposed by technically complex tobacco articles and nicotine delivery devices promoted by an unregulated industry to smokers worldwide, many of whom are addicted to nicotine and who seek a less hazardous cigarette"[311].

Studies show that *Eclipse* could "dramatically decrease cigarette consumption without causing withdrawal symptoms or decreases in nicotine concentrations or motivation to quit altogether" but that it increased carbon monoxide intake[312–314], a factor relevant to heart disease (which kills more smokers than die from cancer). *Advance* is another PREP that has been externally assessed. One study observed a 51% reduction in urine NNAL (a nitrosamine biomarker) concentrations and no increase in carbon monoxide in *Advance* users[315].

Advertising claims

In nations like the USA, where cigarette advertising remains rampant, intensive advertising campaigns have accompanied the launch of PREPs. Brown and Williamson described *Advance Lights* as "a revolutionary breakthrough in cigarette technology" that provides "All of the taste . . . less of the toxins". Vector Tobacco promotes *Omni* as offering "Reduced carcinogens. Premium taste". *Eclipse* advertising states "the toxicity of [*Eclipse's*] smoke is dramatically reduced compared to other cigarettes".

For all their careful wording, these campaigns convey to smokers that the products are "safe". In one study, 1000 current cigarette smokers and 499 ex-smokers were read advertising descriptions for *Eclipse*. Nearly a quarter believed the product was completely safe, with 91% believing it to be safer than regular cigarettes. Exposure to *Eclipse's* claims was also followed by reduced interest in quitting, and interest in the product was higher among younger people who had recently stopped smoking. The findings from this important study provide evidence that the largely unregulated promotion of PREPs might reduce smokers' readiness to quit, and undermine adult cessation[316], an outcome that would be extremely pleasing to PREP manufacturers also marketing cigarettes. Another US study found 25% of smokers who were aware of reduced risk cigarettes believed them to be less risky than conventional cigarettes[317]. The most explicit embrace of this goal by the tobacco industry was seen in advertising for an early low-tar brand, True, featuring the slogan "Considering all I'd heard, I decided to either quit or smoke *True*. I smoke *True*".

Consumer failures

With the exception of the decades-long consumer fraud of lights and milds, which saw wholesale migration of consumers to these products, all other PREPs have been abject failures in the marketplace. In July 1977, Gallaher in the UK launched four brands containing the Cytrel substitute material. Gallaher told the British parliament that "None of these brands, nor those containing other substitute materials marketed by other cigarette manufacturers, were commercially successful. After one year of being on sale, the market share of all substitute brands was only 1 per cent of the total UK cigarette market. In 1978, *Silk Cut No 3* and *Benson & Hedges Sovereign Mild* and later, in 1982, *Silk Cut King Size* (all of which contained 25% Cytrel) and *Silk Cut Ultra Mild* (which contained 40% Cytrel) were withdrawn by Gallaher due to the reluctance of consumers to smoke them"[318].

A 2003 study of US adult smokers found "extremely low" use of PREPs, with only two people among 2028 adults having used *Quest*, and one each *Eclipse* or *Accord* in the previous 6 months[317]. Gary Giovino from the Roswell Park Cancer Center, Buffalo, recently asked two groups of US smokers about their use of PREPs. In a national sample of 1000 adult (aged 25+) smokers, he found 5.4% had *ever* tried PREP, but that only 0.5% had used them for over 30 days and none had used them in the previous 30 days. Similarly, a 2003 study of 2853 smokers aged 16–24 found that 0.6% had used a PREP in the previous 30 days (G. Giovino, personal communication). A recent focus group study of PREP users found that most had stopped using them, that those who were still using them did so infrequently and also kept smoking their regular brands of cigarettes[319].

Such data need to be kept in mind when assessing enthusiastic claims about the likely response of consumers to later generations of PREPs or indeed to smokeless tobacco if it were to be marketed as harm reducing. The current generation of products has seen sometimes intensive local advertising, resplendent with beguiling claims about reduced toxins. But this has failed to interest even tiny fractions of US smokers to use these products on anything other than an experimental, curiosity basis.

So why have PREPs so far been abject commercial flops? Some even go so far as to suggest that the major companies planned it that way and have little interest in their new products succeeding commercially. These cynics suggest their development and relatively low-key promotion confined mainly to US test markets are part of a broader legal defence strategy that runs "we offered consumers reduced risk products, but few were interested in taking them up. Yet again, consumers must therefore take full responsibility for the consequences of their choices".

However, this is a position that is becoming increasingly hard to reconcile against recent significant developments by the transnational majors. Facing ever-declining domestic markets for cigarettes in the USA, Philip Morris has begun to test market LNST (Taboka), BAT to test market *Lucky Strike* and *Peter Stuyvesant* snus, and R.J. Reynolds has introduced *Camel* snus and bought the US smokeless company Conwood for $3.5 billion – hardly a frivolous investment[320].

One important reason why the latter generation of PREPs have failed is that most in the public health community have bitter memories of being hoodwinked by the industry. We were kept in the dark about its internal knowledge of compensatory smoking that made a mockery of machine-measured yields, and as Nigel Gray put it, "measured the wrong thing" in tar[321]. This has engendered immense mistrust of any next generation harm reduction claims.

Swedish snus[ii]

Snus is a form of moist, ground oral tobacco that can be contained in a small thumbnail-sized portion pouch like a mini teabag, or used loose as a "pinch" and parked between the upper lip and the gum, allowing nicotine to be absorbed into the bloodstream via the buccal mucosa over about 30 minutes before being discarded (spent snus portion pouches and small balls of snus are a common sight on Swedish streets). The product has high pH, facilitating rapid absorption of its nicotine, which reaches levels about twice that found in nicotine replacement pharmaceutical products. There are critical differences between snus and oral tobacco products sold elsewhere in the world. Snus is made from tobacco blends that have been air- and sun-cured, while US moist snuff products tend to include blends high in fire-cured tobacco. Snus is also heat treated with steam for 24–36 hours (reaching temperatures of approximately 100°C), whereas US moist snuff is typically fermented, allowing continued formation of tobacco-specific nitrosamines (TSNA). In Sweden, snus is refrigerated immediately after production and is designed to be kept in refrigerators by retailers, a factor again thought to be responsible for maintaining very low levels of TSNA compared with smokeless tobacco sold in the USA and places like Sudan[265].

In 2001, Swedish Match, which manufactures snus in Sweden, announced a quality standard, the Gothiatek standard[322], for its snus products that includes maximum permissible limits for nine carcinogens and other toxic substances. Foulds and colleagues state that "It is unclear if all Swedish Match smokeless tobacco products produced in Sweden and abroad adhere to the Gothiatek standard".[265] The Gothiatek standard for TSNA stipulates a maximum of 5 mg/kg of snus. In 2001, American Health Foundation research found that two Swedish brands Ettan, and

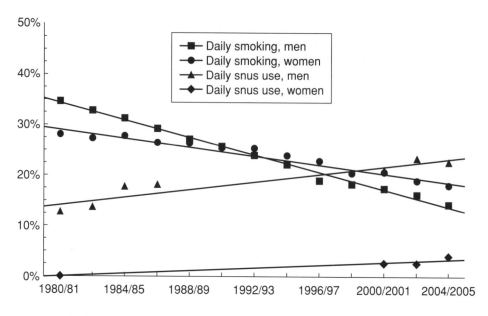

Fig. 4.3   Daily tobacco use in Sweden 1980–2005. Point observations and least squares regression lines. Sources: smoking data from STATISTICS SWEDEN surveys of Living Conditions; snus use data from NTS surveys (1980–1987) and ITS/FSI surveys (2000–2005).

Timber Wolf, a Swedish subsidiary, had far lower levels of TSNA than the standard US-manufactured brands available in Massachusetts. Ettan's TSNA levels were 2.8 μg/g and TimberWolf's TSNA levels were 7.5 μg/g, compared with domestic brand Silver Creek, which had a TSNA level of 127.9 μg/g[323].

Figure 4.3 shows Sweden's changing pattern of snus and cigarettes use from 1980 to 2005.

Evidence of reduced harm

Most of the intense interest in snus derives from evidence about the apparent association between Sweden's historic shift in male tobacco use away from cigarettes to snus, and the nation's relatively low rates of tobacco-caused disease (specifically lung and oral cancers and cardiovascular disease). The reductions in male smoking prevalence (attributable to both the nation's comprehensive tobacco control policies and the shift among men from cigarettes to snus) that have occurred in Sweden over the past 25 years have been among the largest of any nation: today 15% of Swedish men smoke daily, with an additional 20% using snus without smoking[266]. Since the mid-1970s there has been a pronounced reduction in the incidence of lung cancer in Swedish men compared with Norwegian men, comparatively few of whom use snus (5% of Norwegians aged 16–74 years use smokeless tobacco daily, and another 5% occasionally[324]. Snus use is less common among Swedish

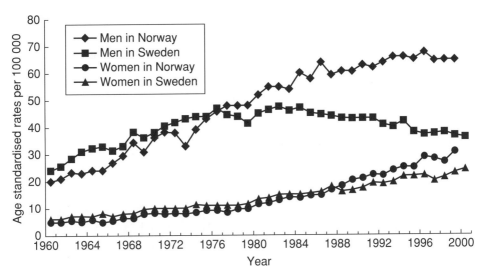

Fig. 4.4 Lung cancer incidence for men and women in Sweden and Norway from 1960 to 1999; age-standardised rates per 100 000 inhabitants based upon census population in each country. Source: Nordgren & Ramstrom[265].

women (about 2% are daily users) than among men (about 21%), and is uncommon in Norwegian women. The incidence of lung cancer in Swedish women is lower than that of their Norwegian counterparts (Fig. 4.4).

The incidence of cardiovascular disease is falling in most industrialised nations, including Sweden. However, in Sweden the rate of decline of myocardial infarction among men aged 30–64 (22%) has been about double that seen in women of the same age[325], inviting consideration of whether the historic move to snus in men but not in women explains that difference.

Many who are familiar with the epidemics of oral cancer caused by smokeless tobacco in nations from the Indian subcontinent and North Africa remain highly concerned about the potential for snus to generate such epidemics in other nations. This concern often reflects a lack of understanding of the significant differences between Swedish snus, with its low TSNA levels, and other forms of smokeless tobacco. A recent systematic review of the health effects of smokeless tobacco concluded: "Chewing betel quid and tobacco is associated with a substantial risk of oral cancers in India. Most recent studies from the US and Scandinavia are not statistically significant, but moderate positive associations cannot be ruled out due to lack of statistical power"[326]. Sweden's rate of oral cancer is little different from that of other developed nations and significantly lower than that in three nations (USA, India and Sudan) where oral tobacco use is prevalent (see Fig. 4.5).

"Far less" risky

In 2002 the Royal College of Physicians of London considered the harm reduction issue, calling for the establishment of a nicotine regulatory agency (discussed later). It concluded: "As a way of using nicotine, the consumption of non-combustible

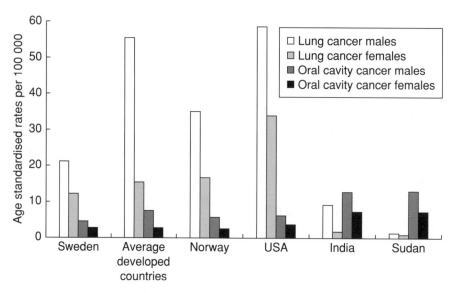

Fig. 4.5 Age-standardised rate of lung cancer and oral cavity cancer for males and females in selected countries and a global average for more developed countries based upon age-standardised rates for 100 000 based upon world population census. Source: Nordgren & Ramstrom[265].

tobacco is of the order of 10 to 1000 times less hazardous than smoking, depending on the product"[327]. The report provided no data or discussion to support this conclusion. More conservatively, a group of nine epidemiological experts in the cancer field estimated that compared with the risks from smoking, LNST promised "at least a 90% reduction in the relative risk" for all causes of mortality[259]. There is a world of difference between a risk being "90%" less and "1000 times" less. The 50-year follow-up of British doctors by Doll and colleagues found that about half of long-term smokers are killed by their smoking[47]. So among 100 000 long-term smokers, 50 000 would die of a smoking-caused disease. If the same group had used LNST instead of smoking, one expert panel[259] would suggest that "at least" fewer than 5000 would die, while the Royal College of Physicians' outer estimate of the risk being 1000 times less would see just 50 deaths. Given that both groups were referring to Swedish snus, this degree of imprecision points to wild divergence of risk estimation and provides a fragile basis for forecasting likely risk, given the critical but imponderable factors such as those I will discuss below.

Notwithstanding this imprecision, no review or expert group that has examined the comparative risks posed by LNST and smoking has concluded anything other than LNST is *far* less dangerous than smoking. Even on the "worst" case scenario, that snus is 90% less harmful than cigarettes, millions of lives could potentially be saved if a wholesale switch from cigarettes to snus across large populations could be affected. With whole populations like Europe denied access to snus-like products[328], such a scenario has no hope of even beginning until such total bans are modified.

Not "safe"

However, no one should argue that snus is "safe". For example, one recent study – heavily attacked but strongly defended[329] – demonstrated that the relative risk of pancreatic cancer among Norwegian male snus users was 1.67 (95% confidence interval = 1.12–2.50)[330]. Pancreatic cancer is a far less prevalent disease than heart disease or lung cancer, but it is an ugly and rapidly fatal cancer. Such reports need to be put in perspective against the potential for snus to reduce far more prevalent tobacco-caused disease.

David Sweanor, a strong advocate for tobacco harm reduction, has eloquently summarised how the harm reduction principle might operate here in a posting to the international tobacco control listserver, Globalink:

> The key concept behind a vast range of product regulatory initiatives is the recognition that there is a continuum of risk for various products and that there is the potential to reduce the risks for users. For example, auto safety standards do not mean that no one will be killed in an auto accident any more that FDA oversight of pharmaceuticals renders them benign. Similarly condoms do not completely eliminate the risk of contracting HIV and helmets do not make bicycling completely safe. The goal of policy in such areas is to reduce risk as much as possible . . . Were clean forms of nicotine to replace cigarettes there would still be harm caused to users, but the harm would be a very tiny fraction of the present carnage. So, just as we would be foolish to argue against auto safety due to the fact that all autos still have risks, we should not inadvertently help the cigarette companies continue their carnage by maintaining that no alternative to cigarettes should be considered unless the proposed alternative reaches the unattainable standard of being completely harmless.
>
> Post to Globalink, 15 May 2005

It is worth reflecting that there are medical procedures and therapeutics that elevate cancer risk (e.g. diagnostic radiation and the breast cancer preventive drug tamoxifen which, while reducing breast cancer risk, increases the risk of endometrial cancer[331]). Setting a demand for absolute zero risk for tobacco harm reduction reflects a way of thinking that has no parallel in product regulation.

How benign is nicotine?

Nicotine, in high doses, is extraordinarily toxic. However, at the dosage levels that are delivered to smokers, the accepted wisdom has been that nicotine is "not the problem" but rather the key pharmacological vehicle that delivers tobacco toxins to users[332]. Pharmaceutical companies have long been anxious to dispel widespread misconceptions[333] that nicotine is the component of tobacco smoke that causes cancer. But a growing body of recent research is beginning to cast serious doubt on the idea that nicotine is a relatively benign substance of little concern in itself. Two broad concerns have been identified. Nicotine has been demonstrated to stimulate various signal transduction pathways in cells, with various outcomes. First, nicotine has been demonstrated to inhibit apoptosis. Apoptosis is a form of cell death in which a programmed sequence of events leads to the elimination of cells without releasing harmful substances into the surrounding area. Apoptosis plays a crucial role in developing and maintaining health by eliminating old, unnecessary and unhealthy cells. Too little or too much apoptosis plays a role in a great many diseases. When programmed cell death does not work correctly, cells that should be eliminated may hang around and become immortal, as in cancer. When apoptosis works too well, it kills too many cells and inflicts grave tissue damage – the process by which damaged cells are killed[iii].

Second, nicotine also stimulates cellular proliferation[334]. This means that cells are replicating faster or more than they should be – and this can result in hyperplasia or excessive growth. Nicotine also stimulates signal transduction pathways causing an increase in vascular endothelial growth factor (VEGF), which has been shown to cause angiogenesis, arteriogenesis and promote tumour growth and atherosclerosis[335,336]. Significantly, one study concluded: "The steady-state serum concentrations of nicotine achieved with [nicotine replacement products] vary, but transdermal delivery of nicotine is virtually complete and can result in serum concentrations of nicotine that approximate those seen in active smokers. Although nicotine *per se* is not thought to be carcinogenic, *the risks of long-term supplementation are unknown.* [my emphasis] Our data and those of Heeschen et al. suggest that sustained exposure to nicotine might alter the phenotype of endothelial and/or epithelial cells in undetectable, pre-malignant lesions"[337]. Such emerging concerns need to be taken very seriously indeed.

We may never know if harm-reduced products reduce harm

The diseases caused by tobacco use, almost without exception, take decades to become symptomatic. The basic question therefore arises: when (and how) will we know that any putative risk-reduced product actually delivers the goods and *is* less harmful when used by large numbers of people throughout whole populations? While research using carcinogen and toxin biomarkers in blood, saliva or urine can show us whether tobacco users are taking in fewer toxins from harm-reduced products[338], this is not equivalent to saying that reduced concentrations of these toxins mean lowered disease rates. As the WHO Study Group on Tobacco Product Regulation put it in 2006: "assessing the relative harm of different tobacco products from biomarkers of individuals who use different products remains a future hope rather than a current reality"[339].

Importantly, we will probably never be able to answer the core question. Cigarette brand recipes are destined to keep changing and we will never be able to know what "dose" of any given soup of toxicants a cohort of, say, *Marlboro* smokers actually inhaled across time unless we were able to require the industry to fix brand recipes and refuse to allow changes, a totally fanciful scenario in an unregulated market. More sophisticated biomarkers may be developed to assist in the tracking of what toxicants research cohorts of smokers actually take in, but this remains speculative.

Gateway or "reverse gateway"?

Harm reduction critics also argue that the advertising and promotion of LNST like snus may attract young people into this form of tobacco use, and that a significant proportion of these will later "graduate" to smoking, people who, importantly, might never have taken up smoking were it not for their initial use of smokeless tobacco. These products, they argue, could be a so-called "gateway drug" that leads to smoking.

One piece of recent research, however, supports the opposite view: that snus use is more of a gateway *out* of smoking than into it[266]. In this study, over 90% of male daily smoking began before age 23, whereas 33% of people who started daily snus use were aged more than 22. Only 20% of male primary snus users who commenced their tobacco use with snus went on to become daily smokers compared with 47% of daily smokers who started their tobacco use by smoking. Moreover, 88% of smokers who later took up snus ceased daily smoking completely compared with 56% of smokers who had never used snus. Snus was the most common method used to try to quit smoking (24% of those reporting their latest quit attempt). Among men who used snus as their only method of quitting, 66% had succeeded in quitting completely, compared with 47% who used nicotine gum and 32% of those using the nicotine patch. Women using snus as an aid were also significantly more likely to quit smoking successfully than those using nicotine patches or gum[266].

US research[340–342] also suggests that a majority of tobacco users (as high as 66%) who commence tobacco use via smokeless tobacco do *not* go on to smoke. But harm reduction opponents point out that this means that 33% *do* progress: so the smoking gateway hypothesis is by no means a non-issue. Gateway theory is widely criticised as a too simplistic, reductionist account of the complexity of the factors that predispose to progression of drug use[343]. For example, 100% of infants who drink breast milk go on to drink fruit juice; and perhaps 80% of all Western children who drink fruit juice go on to try beer or wine, of whom a large proportion then go on to try alcoholic spirits. Positing that fruit juice "leads" to alcohol use like this would be plainly mindless. Gateway theory is usually blind to covariants like social context, social class, education, family variables and personality variables, which when taken into account are more predictive[341].

Consumer sovereignty vs paternalism

Those advocating the lifting of bans on the sale of LNST products like snus have marshalled some powerful arguments. Sitting on top of these are the results from the Swedish "natural experiment". Kozlowski and colleagues doubt "that any feasible clinical trial in another country can provide us with better evidence on the possible individual and societal effects of snus. Controlled experiments can be instructive, but the Swedish example is priceless"[344].

In my view, the strongest argument advanced by LNST advocates is the argument for consumer sovereignty in having the right to be informed about the potential of reduced risk from LNST, and being able to exercise choice on the basis of that information. As Kozlowski and colleagues sum it up:

> Individuals who do use or who are thinking of using cigarettes have a right
> to know that smokeless products are safer than cigarettes. [Lawmakers will have
> heard arguments] about increased use of a safer product being *potentially*
> able to lead to greater risk for society. For large reductions in risk, it is possible,
> or even likely, that use would not increase to a level that could cause net
> societal harm. Snus and medicinal nicotine are so much safer than cigarettes
> that net societal harm is very unlikely. Public health concerns should trump
> individual rights only when there is clear and convincing evidence of harm
> to society. Lacking that evidence, individual rights should prevail[344].

Kozlowski and O'Connor have been scathing about what they demonstrate to
be misleading information about the comparative harms of cigarettes and smokeless tobacco – claims that all tobacco products are equally harmful – that have been
placed on the websites of the US Centers for Disease Control and Prevention and
the Substance Abuse and Mental Health Services Administration[345].

Those who maintain that LNST products should remain totally banned need
to explain why they believe the potential harms outweigh the potential benefits.
However, for all these possible benefits, there are some extremely serious concerns
as well. I will now consider some that are relevant here.

How will consumers be informed about the new less dangerous products?

There could be two broad approaches to introducing reduced toxin tobacco
products into new markets. The first, to be discussed later, would be simply to
have governments set maximum levels for tobacco carcinogens and toxins for *all*
tobacco products, thereby levelling to mandatory values the harm playing field for
all companies. If this happened, there would be no point in informing consumers
that a given brand was lower in certain toxins, because all products on sale would
also have to conform to the same maximum levels.

For example, nations that mandate standards for pesticide residues on fruit do
not see advertising for bananas emphasising conformity to such a standard: all fruits
conform, or are banned from sale if discovered to be above the standard, and their
distributors heavily fined. As I will argue later, this would be a key element in the
preferred approach to harm reduction. However, it would seem unlikely to
happen without extraordinary resistance from powerful sections of the tobacco industry because many companies' brands (both smokeless and combustible tobacco)
would be banned under such regulation.

The second approach – one of competitive attempts to shift consumers to
reduced toxin products – is therefore likely to be the model preferred by most of
the industry (except those companies that would stand to benefit most from the
first approach). Under the model of influencing consumer demand, the core concern would be that there is little point in developing reduced-harm products if
consumers could not somehow be informed about their existence and the characteristics that justified their claims to harm reduction.

Much of the debate about harm reduction has been concentrated in the USA, where there are very few restrictions on tobacco advertising because of the prevailing legal view that banning tobacco advertising would violate the first amendment of the US Constitution on freedom of speech[346]. A wide variety of PREPs and smokeless products are being advertised in an environment that outside observers see as being virtually unregulated. However, there are many nations that already ban all forms of tobacco advertising. Plainly, global policy on harm reduction should not be set to accommodate a constitutional argument in a nation like the USA, which has extremely weak controls on tobacco advertising. The WHO's legally binding Framework Convention on Tobacco Control obliges each nation to "undertake a comprehensive ban of all tobacco advertising, promotion and sponsorship[347]. This will mean that no tobacco company in nations with bans will be able to use advertising or promotion of any form to attempt to inform or persuade smokers to consider switching to LNST or other harm-reduced products.

A wedge to unravel advertising bans?

Those who remain cautious about unleashing LNST and other PREPs into nations where tobacco advertising is banned know that this problem is already being used[348] as a wedge issue by tobacco companies and will be certainly used to try to pry open advertising bans, all in the name of the virtuous goal of providing consumers with important information about reducing harm. In nations like the USA, it will also be used as an argument to retain tobacco advertising.

In 2005 I listened to Philip Morris's David Davies talk about his company's interest in harm reduction, and use that special coded language that hinted at the importance of consumer information needing to be available ("And regulation should allow adults who choose not to quit *to receive information about the availability and attributes of such products* [my emphasis]"[349]. I have no doubt that if decoded this translates as a dialogue about rolling back advertising bans, although his company's test marketing of *Taboka* (see below) in my view illustrates an intriguing degree of responsible restraint in advertising.

Part of the caution shown by those who are leery of any effort legally to free up LNST in countries in which it is now banned, is that the issue could be a Trojan horse that will allow the industry onto a powerful "white hat" debating platform to argue for relaxing advertising bans, something that would be disastrous for wider tobacco control, potentially unravelling advocacy that has taken nearly 40 years from articulation to implementation.

PR spin

There are also other important ways in which the industry can talk to consumers. In all but the USA and New Zealand, prescription-only pharmaceuticals are not allowed to be advertised direct to consumers, but only to prescribing physicians and specialists through advertising media not accessible to the general public. In Australia, *Zyban* cannot be advertised to the general public, but its manufacturer was nonetheless able to mount huge media publicity about the drug through the generation of news. I was one in the public health community who made frequent radio and television comments about hopes that its clinical trial results would translate into "real life" cessation successes. Without direct-to-consumer advertising, Pfizer was able to get about one in ten Australian smokers prescribed *Zyban*[350]. *Viagra* similarly has been a massive global marketing success without most of its consumers ever having seen or heard a "legal" *Viagra* advertisement. *Viagra* spam in the in-boxes of millions of email users tells a different story. In many nations today, tobacco advertising is completely banned or heavily restricted. Even in such settings, only the most unimaginative person could foresee a situation where a tobacco company wishing to launch a PREP could not use the same sort of news generation and "stealth" marketing practices that they use today to promote allegedly "safe" tobacco products in settings where they cannot advertise directly to the public.

Some PREP advocates argue that public health officials will be able responsibly to control and moderate the flow of information to consumers, replete with all the appropriate caveats and qualifications that would be essential in any open and honest communication about the prospects of reduced risk. However, only the most gormless and innocent observers of the way the harm reduction debate is already unfolding in the media would predict that oceans of tempered and qualified evidence-based talk from health officials will dominate the news on these products. Tobacco companies will use every trick in their public affairs arsenals to get the message stretched from the ultra-cautious talk that most in tobacco control would see as appropriate, to a message designed to go way beyond the evidence. A new generation of high-profile "independent" scientific consultants will emerge to talk up the potential virtues of harm reduction products while avoiding the important caveats being discussed here.

A perfect illustration of this occurred in 2005 when the *New York Times* magazine published a large, balanced and appropriately qualified feature article on a new PREP, Fact, manufactured by a Hong Kong-based company, Filligent[351]. Two days later, the *Pakistan Times* reported on the article under the headline "Finally there's a safe cigarette". Not, "a cigarette that reduces some of the many toxins in tobacco smoke". Not, "a cigarette that needs to be monitored for the next 40 years to see if its reduced delivery of toxins makes any difference to disease rates". Instead, simply, with no complications, "a *safe* cigarette". As Stan Shatenstein, an astute analyst of global tobacco control, succinctly put it: "this is where the rubber meets the road" in the debate about how the complexity of the harm reduction debate will be communicated to smokers. For every detailed, qualified, cautious, caveat-laden public discussion of PREPs, we can expect many more swashbuckling, irresponsible news items like the Pakistani one, driven by journalistic ignorance or the need to simplify because of the constraints of space. This is how most of the community will encounter news about harm reduction.

Philip Morris's *Taboka*

In 2006 Philip Morris began test marketing its LNST portion-packed product *Taboka* in Indianapolis. The product is as low, or lower, in tobacco-specific nitrosamines than Swedish snus. *Taboka* is being promoted as an alternative to cigarettes, which "lasts twice as long as a cigarette" and unlike most US smokeless tobacco, is "spit free". Its advertising slogan is "Instead of a smoke, tuck a *Taboka*".

Advertising and pack information on the product makes no mention of any reduced levels of toxins, and indeed the pack states "This product is not a safe alternative to cigarettes" – a claim that demands a consistent response from aggressive harm reduction advocates who were scathing of a recent US Surgeon General making the same comment. In not making any harm reduction claims, Philip Morris would appear to be seeking to demonstrate its willingness to exercise restraint and differentiate itself from other companies that are making strong imputations that their PREPs *are* less dangerous than cigarettes.

The intriguing aspect of the *Taboka* campaign is that it is devoid of any argument as to why smokers might want to start sucking tobacco instead of smoking it. Philip Morris must be entirely confident that public relations efforts will fill in the dots and get word about fast that the reason why smokers should consider using *Taboka* is that it has greatly reduced toxins. Philip Morris has launched the product as part of an approach it calls its "adjacency growth strategy . . . This strategy looks at potential moves into complementary tobacco or tobacco-related products that would allow PM-USA to use its existing core infrastructure". "Adjacency" means "the state of being adjacent; contiguity", suggesting that the company sees itself as being in both the combustible and smokeless tobacco business.

Who will use the new reduced-harm products?

Most who advocate that the tobacco control community should support the availability of LNST seem to be primarily attracted to the idea that a significant proportion of smokers might switch from their very harmful cigarettes to the new reduced-harm products. We know that a large proportion of smokers smoked "light" cigarettes believing that these products reduce risk: of 12 285 ever-smokers questioned in the 2000 US National Health Interview, 37% "reported having used light cigarettes to reduce health risks". Importantly, current abstinence was less often reported by ever-smokers who had previously used light cigarettes than by ever-smokers who had never used lights (37% vs 53%, $P < 0.01$)[352], demonstrating the massive potential for products promoted as risk reducing to effectively retard cessation.

The appeal of the new products has mostly been considered in terms of existing smokers, and there is persuasive evidence that snus in Sweden has indeed caused a reduction in smoking[266], mainly from smokers switching. But no manufacturer of any product would ever consider developing a new product that would only be used by people already using that category of product. Industry executives have always claimed that cigarette advertising is only directed at current smokers, and that it never crosses their minds that it might also be made to appeal to those who have not yet started. We are meant to believe that when *Marlboro* sponsors a Formula 1 racing team, they have no interest whatsoever in whether teenage non-smoking motor racing fans notice the *Marlboro* sponsorship. They are only interested in whether smokers notice it and either stick with *Marlboro* or switch to it.

If you are tempted to think this sounds reasonable, imagine if the product was not *Marlboro*, but *Hyundai* cars. Imagine the marketing director of *Hyundai* making a presentation to the board about the marketing plans for a new model *Hyundai* and saying "We only hope that existing owners of *Hyundai* will decide to upgrade to this new model, and that owners of other brands of car might switch to *Hyundai*. We are not at all interested in first-time buyers choosing a *Hyundai*, or in seeding the idea in people as yet too young or unable to afford a *Hyundai* that one day they might like to own one. We leave all thoughts about those markets to all other manufacturers". Anyone thinking this way would last a nanosecond in their job, yet this is the nonsense that the tobacco industry would have us believe about their marketing ambitions.

This sort of argument is sometimes dangerously close to nonsense in the harm reduction debate too. While the net impact of snus in Sweden has seen more smokers switch to snus than non-tobacco users take it up, anyone who thinks tobacco companies would not be delighted if they were able to see LNST become as popular as mobile phones with youth is very much missing the point. Recall that in Sweden, 67% of people whose tobacco use started with snus were aged under 22 years[266].

The manufacturers of LNST and other PREPs include "Big Tobacco" companies such as BAT (*Lucky Strike* and *Peter Stuyvesant* branded snus being test marketed in South Africa and Sweden), Philip Morris (*Taboka*) and R.J. Reynolds (*Camel* snus). We are already seeing the exact same claims about the target markets for PREPs: that they are only intended to appeal to current cigarette smokers: "It will be marketed fully in line with our International Marketing Standards, which focus strongly on making sure that all our marketing is only directed to adults who have chosen to be tobacco consumers."[353] This, of course, is nothing but blather coached by lawyers and public affairs people. The companies will certainly hope that some smokers will switch to PREPs and LNST − particularly those contemplating quitting because of health concerns about smoking. But many of these smokers will be smokers of the same companies' cigarette brands, so the commercial benefit of having customers stop buying one company brand in favour of another will bring little if any gain to each company. The main commercial goal will be in diverting people away from cessation, and to induce dual use to plug times when people can't smoke.

Starters and relapsers

In addition to switchers from cigarettes, the companies also have intense interest in the potential of two groups of consumers: those who have not yet started using tobacco (i.e. mainly young people) and those who have stopped smoking and might be tempted back into it. BAT and Reynolds, by naming their snus brands with cigarette names, will not be disappointed if some young people who take up snus will drift into its cigarettes with the same names as well: after all, the branding and imagery are identical. Many former users of tobacco look back on their smoking with mixed emotions. They will be glad to have quit, but often miss smoking and identify situations and cues when they become particularly nostalgic for a cigarette.

Relapse among ex-smokers is extremely common. PREP manufacturers know this well and will seek to exploit this potential market by directly appealing to the same health concerns that they used when marketing light and milds. Is there anyone who seriously thinks that the industry's filing cabinets are not already bulging with projections about enticing new and former tobacco users to use PREPs as well? And should we all be comfortable that new tobacco users and former smokers relapsing into snus would only stay with snus/PREPs and not drift over to cigarettes?

Dual use

Several brands of PREP and smokeless tobacco are advertised for use by smokers to tide them over with nicotine during times when they can't smoke, such as during office hours:

- *Lucky Strike* snus: "can't light up/can snus" (Fig. 4.6).
- *Revel*: "Anytime. Anywhere. A fresh new way to enjoy tobacco when you can't smoke."
- *Ariva*: "When you can't smoke."

There is no suggestion anywhere here about switching from smoking. *Dual use* is being promoted. We know that policies that restrict smoking opportunities cause falls in smoking frequency, but importantly for the argument here, cause smoking cessation as well[148]. The investment advisors Morgan Stanley suggested that one of the factors responsible for the recent rapid growth of the smokeless sector in the USA was perhaps "the increased prevalence of more highly-restrictive state and/or local indoor smoking bans (e.g., particularly those including bars, restaurants, etc.".[354] If harm reduction advertising succeeded in convincing continuing smokers who otherwise might have quit (because of smoking bans) to keep smoking with the support of smokeless tobacco use during times when smoking was banned, the net effect of this on overall tobacco-caused death throughout populations would be unquestionably negative. Harm reduction supporters who embrace policies that encourage such products, promoted by advertising saying "don't quit. Use this when you can't smoke, so you can keep smoking", are in effect working to retard smoking cessation, which is an unintended effect of their primary concern to allow harm-reduced products to be made available to smokers. Such products are in effect harm *increasing*, not reducing, products.

There is likely always to be a group of smokers who will keep on smoking. Chapter 8 considers what proportion of the population such a group is likely to be. Some of these will be smokers who claim to know the risks they are running, but who nonetheless openly choose to take those risks. Others will be profoundly addicted smokers who have made repeated unsuccessful attempts to quit, but who have continued to fail. Should we deny such smokers who want to keep on dosing themselves with nicotine, products that greatly reduce some of the carcinogenic load they would otherwise obtain? To answer "yes" here is effectively to behave like the moral puritans who say to injecting drug users "we will deny you access to clean needles so that your already risky behaviour will be even more risky".

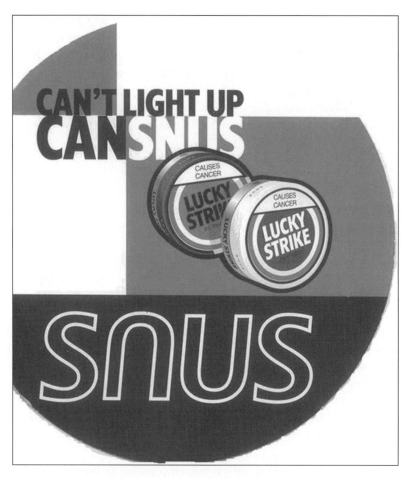

Fig. 4.6 *Lucky Strike* advertising from South Africa.

The important consumer sovereignty argument discussed earlier would say here that consumers who want to keep using nicotine during times when they can't smoke, should be able to exercise that right and choose smokeless products that fully satisfy their nicotine cravings. But the consequence of that argument for public health is likely to be a diminution of cessation stimulated by situations where people can't smoke. Responsible health policy will need to balance the consumer sovereignty argument that allows smokers wanting to reduce their risk with wider population concerns about stamping on the brakes of cessation and possibly opening up a total new gateway to smoking.

Will smokeless tobacco transpose to cultures with no traditions of use?

Every culture has its own peculiarities in food and drink that are widely enjoyed, sports that are popular locally but have never appealed to other nations, and musical styles that never develop significant global appeal. In Australia nearly every kitchen has a jar of a black, salty, yeast-based spread called *Vegemite* (made by Altria's Kraft division). Australians cannot get enough of it, but overseas visitors typically find it a form of culinary torture inflicted on them in "see if you are ready to be a real Australian" kitchen initiation ceremonies. Similarly, Swedes and Norwegians are fond of eating fermented herring (*Surströmming*), a dish that smells like rotting fish. Asians love the fabled durian fruit, which charitably could be described as smelling like an open sewer and is banned from being taken into many Asian hotels. Chinese laud the liqueur *mao-tai*, which most Westerners find as appealing as castor oil. I have eclectic tastes in world music, and while I remain incredulous at the popularity of rap music, I am confident that Tuva throat singing from southern Siberia will never catch on globally, much as it is loved by many Tuvans. Such examples abound, and while globalisation provides many examples of products and tastes once indigenous to particular nations but now universally appreciated, there remain many that don't "travel". In speculating about the potential for snus to make a serious contribution to reducing tobacco-caused harm globally, it is important therefore to consider how likely it is that snus could ever migrate beyond its Scandinavian base.

Snus is sold in two forms: as loose, moist tobacco, and in small tea-bag-like sachets. The tea bags are relatively unobtrusive and can be quickly placed between the upper gum and lip, barely showing as a mild bulge to others. Loose snus is a different proposition, involving the rolling of a pinch of tobacco into a small ball, and then placing it under the lip. Over the course of the typical 30 minutes in which the user absorbs nicotine from the ball, adjusting it occasionally with the tongue, loose fragments of tobacco can come away from the ball and become lodged between the teeth. It can be a sight some way from notions of oral hygiene, teeth whitening and freshness promoted in toothpaste and breath freshener product advertising. At the 13th World Conference on Tobacco or Health in Washington, Dr Gunilla Bollinder from the Karolinska Institute reported that typical snus users carry the product in their mouths for 13–15 hours a day. Taking snus in this form presents considerable challenges as to whether such a product is ever likely to migrate successfully out of its Swedish cultural origins. My gut instinct is that it won't. One only has to look at how the product has performed outside Sweden to date to gain this impression.

Probably the least examined but among the most elementary questions in the snus debate is why the practice of using smokeless tobacco has not spread more widely than it has. Much is being made of the inability of tobacco companies like Swedish Match to gain access to the European market and to markets in a handful of other nations like Australia, New Zealand, Hong Kong, Japan, Switzerland and Israel, which have banned the sale of smokeless tobacco products. The European Union ban plainly remains a massive blow to companies like Swedish Match, but nonetheless there are many vast marketing opportunities where tobacco companies wishing aggressively to promote snus-like products could do so if they chose.

There are vast regions of the world where replications of the natural experiment of Swedish snus could happen today, unhindered. For example, in the USA there is aggressive competition, assisted by advertising, for the smokeless tobacco market. In 2001, the five main smokeless companies spent $236.68 million on advertising for smokeless products[355]. But again, it is salutary to keep some perspective on the size of this market in a nation that has had largely uninhibited advertising opportunities to grow that market. One report shows that the market for smokeless declined in the USA during 1993–2002 faster than that for cigarettes, and from a much smaller base. Among males, smokeless use dropped by 37% from 2.3% in 1992/93 to 1.5% in 2001/02 while that among females declined 63% from 0.43% to 0.16%. During the same period, male smoking fell 13% from 26.8% in 1992/93 to 23.3% in 2001/02. Female smoking declined nearly 17%, from 22.6% to 18.8%[356]. However, more recently, financial advisors Goldman Sachs reported that for the half year ended June 2006, the smokeless market grew 7.8%, on the back of a 4.5% growth for the last half of 2005. In September 2006, Morgan Stanley confirmed this ("US moist smokeless tobacco category total unit volume growth was approximately 8.5%, more than double the category's average 3.6% growth rate from 1995 through 2005")[354]. Most of the US smokeless market is a loose tobacco "chaw", which generates fetid brown juice, regularly spat on the ground by users. This is not the same product as contemporary snus, which is sold in compact "tea bags" and does not cause users to spit. If the US market responds to the greater availability of spitless tea-bag-style smokeless, this growth may well continue.

While some cavalier forecasters infer that *all* smokers could switch from cigarettes to harm reduced products like snus and thereby eliminate all tobacco-caused deaths ("How shameful that the United States is willing to allow almost a half-million Americans to die each year, and that the World Health Organization is prepared to allow up to 5 million annual deaths worldwide – all because of a delivery device, cigarette smoke, whose hazards are well known and largely avoidable")[357], it would seem obvious that despite the best efforts of smokeless tobacco companies to promote their products in markets where there are few restraints, smokeless tobacco is an extremely challenging product to sell to the majority of tobacco users.

Advocates for LNST imply that skilled marketers will convince significant numbers of smokers from cultures with no history of oral tobacco use to start sucking tobacco. But to date, there are no major examples of where this has occurred, despite the absence of legal constraints on either selling or promoting such products in most nations. Even in India, where there is a long tradition of smokeless tobacco use, Swedish Match's efforts to interest Indians in switching proved very challenging. Bo Aulin, Senior Vice President, Secretary and General Counsel at Swedish Match, was reported as saying that less than 1% of his company's sales were in India: "Gradually, I guess we've got the insight that it takes time in India, and one shouldn't expect some type of 'explosion'. India is not a place where we make money from the snus today . . . Of course, for this project as for all other projects, you reach some point when you have to decide whether to continue."[358] My strong sense is that were snus-like products to be made legal in those nations where they remain banned today, that uptake would be marginal.

So if snus is unlikely to catch on with many consumers, then removing all access barriers to those consumers who may want to choose to use it will not unleash a major outbreak of use and possible harm, however remote that might be. Making it freely available will allow choice, and given what is known from Sweden about its association with reduced harm, almost certainly no net harm will be caused by such a move, with benefits (reduced harm) being much more likely. The logic of this seems unassailable, provided the deregulation of availability was accompanied by appropriate regulation that controlled advertising and other publicity. And this of course, is where a whole different set of major problems arise because such a major consumer shift is almost inconceivable without also unleashing advertising.

Regions and nations with catastrophic epidemics of cancers caused by moist snuff oral tobacco, such as the Indian subcontinent[359] and Sudan[360], have no meaningful means of regulation or market conditions to replace the present inexpensive products, produced by small-scale vendors, with anything like the Gothiatek standard, and are likely to be understandably derisory of this discussion. The notion that the "Swedish experience" could be exported to such regions or that the views of some in Sweden, the UK and the USA should apply in these nations would be the height of Western arrogance.

Good vs bad companies?

There are some who argue that talk of "the tobacco industry" obscures key differences among companies. Scott Ballin argued at the 13th World Conference on Tobacco Control in July 2006 that "While much of what we have called the 'tobacco industry' remains the same, there are major changes and shifts that have taken place over the last decade that warrant the consideration of the development of new strategies and the redefining or clarification of who the tobacco industry is and isn't. Gone are the days when it was easy to see who wore the white hats and who wore the black hats and when the industry was a monolithic economic power that stuck together every step of the way. Cracks have developed. New players have entered the market place. Big Tobacco spends an increasingly large amount of time fighting amongst themselves. These are opportunities that need to be assessed and explored. Instead of talking in terms of the 'tobacco industry' as being all the same, we need to start asking the 'what, why, when, and how' we might engage segments of a more broadly defined 'industry' . . . segments that just might be advocates for forcing change in Big Tobacco."

The idea being promoted here is that there are some tobacco companies that should be trusted to work towards genuine harm reduction and others – Big Tobacco companies that continue actively to undermine effective tobacco control – that should not be trusted. The implication is that we can assist in levelling the playing field so that the "good" tobacco companies selling genuinely harm reducing products will be encouraged to compete with the big, evil companies that sell products estimated to cause a billion deaths this century. PREPs will become so successful that competition will see the "bad" companies take harm reduction products seriously, thereby reducing their own contributions to tobacco-caused disease.

For all the virtues of Philip Morris's Taboka, we can be assured that the company will keep on manufacturing and marketing its "bad" cigarettes, stimulating demand for them and resisting any tobacco control policies that would see people abandon or reduce tobacco use. This means that in any negotiation about PREPs, Big Tobacco's interests in safeguarding its interests in continuing to sell these products will never be far from the foreground.

Swedish Match is said by some to be the model of a "good" tobacco company. However, in South Africa the company ignored the country's Tobacco Products Control Act, 1993. When it first introduced snus into the South African market its product, Tobaccorette, did not carry the mandated health warning "Causes Cancer". Today Tobaccorette places the label on a paper seal that is destroyed when the tin is opened. Catch dry from Swedish Match places the label on the side, but the lid does not have the sign as required, allowing the user easily to miss the sign when in use.

Ayo-Yusuf and others report that the percentage of free base nicotine in South African commercial snuff "is higher than that from most of the leading US or Swedish brands. The pH and percentage of free base nicotine reported for the *Taxi* and *Singleton* menthol brands [both Swedish Match products] . . . study is indeed the highest ever reported for any industrialised snuff brand."[361]

High-delivery nicotine replacement therapy

For all the effort that has gone into advocating for restrictions on snus to be lifted, surprisingly little has gone into urging the pharmaceutical industry to raise the levels of nicotine in its nicotine replacement delivery products. A group of some of the most experienced nicotine addiction experts working in tobacco control recently stated: "There exists a broad spectrum of nicotine replacement products with respect to dosing characteristics and form. However, a broader spectrum is possible and warranted to accommodate the broad diversity of needs and preferences of tobacco users. For example, there is no true inhaler which delivers nicotine to the lung in the same way as the cigarette does. There is no oral nicotine delivering product which can compete with the 10 mg nicotine containing, highly buffered oral tobacco products that are popular among smokeless tobacco users. Whether a clean nicotine product such as gum, lozenge, patch, or inhaler (by "clean" we mean free enough of tobacco toxicants to pass regulatory approval) can or should be made to deliver nicotine as efficiently and palatably as tobacco products is an unresolved question."[362]

The latest update of the Cochrane smoking cessation database identified 123 clinical trials involving different forms of nicotine replacement therapy (NRT), with 103 of these contributing to the primary comparison between NRT and a placebo or non-NRT control group. The review concluded that these trials demonstrated that NRT "increases the odds of quitting approximately 1.5- to 2-fold regardless of setting."[363]

A review of studies of unaided cessation showed that if 1000 smokers try to quit unaided, in 10 months time approximately 73 will not be smoking[364]. If the clinical trial data reviewed by the Cochrane group applied to smokers in "real life" settings (showing a 1.5–2-fold increase), then between 110 and 146 smokers in

1000 using NRT will have quit 10 months later (i.e. 10.1–14.6%). However, the real figure is likely to be somewhat less than this because clinical trial results almost always produce better results than the performance of a drug outside the highly supervised conditions of a drug trial where participants are subject to lots of attention from researchers in a way that would never happen in "real life" settings. This extra attention can cause participants to do better because they are aware that they are being studied[365].

Putting this another way, at best 85–90% of smokers using NRT to stop smoking will still be smoking 10 months later. Such an outcome immediately invites awkward questions about just *how* successful NRT is in assisting smokers to stop. Another reasonable question is to ask whether the current generation of NRT has sufficient nicotine "grunt" to satisfy the nicotine hunger in those long addicted to nicotine.

Figure 4.7 shows the very different patterns of blood nicotine levels in cigarette smokers compared with those taking nicotine via various nicotine replacement therapies and as oral snuff. Smokers obtain far higher levels of nicotine (Fig. 4.7a shows the case of an individual who obtained very high levels) than NRT users.

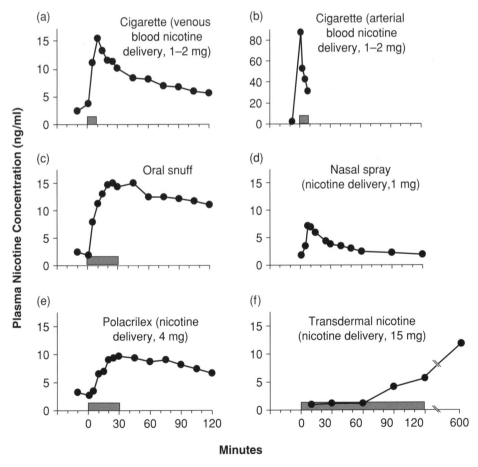

Fig. 4.7 Plasma nicotine concentrations for different forms of nicotine delivery systems. Source: Jack Henningfield, Pinney and Associates.

They also get a rapid bolus of nicotine – a "spike" – that users of NRT gum, patch or nasal spray do not get. Part of what cigarettes do is to enable very high but precisely titrated doses – puff by puff. So the obvious question arises as to whether the word "replacement" in "nicotine replacement therapy" is very misleading. Smokers do not obtain the same levels or profiles of nicotine from NRT that they get from cigarettes, which may explain a great deal about the suboptimal effects of NRT in cessation and why so many smokers stop using it. Cryptically, Shiffman and others concluded a recent paper of theirs examining the impact of a high-dose 35-mg nicotine patch on withdrawal symptoms by writing "we found that treatment with high-dose NRT significantly reduced, and in several cases completely eliminated, withdrawal symptoms and craving during smoking cessation. This raises the question of why NRT is not even more successful than it is."[366].

An obvious retort to this is to note that the highest dose NRT available to smokers today is 4 mg, nothing remotely like 35 mg. It further invites the question of why the pharmaceutical industry does not develop nicotine delivery products that would provide sufficient nicotine "grunt" to satisfy smokers' appetites. One company – Niconovum – founded by a pioneer in addiction studies, Karl Fagerström, is apparently developing NRT formulated for faster release, featuring alkaline pH for more rapid absorption. Such a product has been used in one trial[367], which reported significantly reduced craving in subjects using the fast–release version compared with those using regular NRT. Big Pharma has also provided trials with high–nicotine NRT (as high as 44 mg), showing improved withdrawal symptom relief and no apparent toxicity other than in light smokers[366,368]. However, such trials have not shown high levels of cessation. Colleagues I consulted believe Big Pharma is nervous about the possible safety issues I raised earlier in this chapter arising from marketing high-dose NRT, and believe that government drug regulators would be unwilling to approve such products in any schedule other than prescription only, which would not predict a large sales volume and hence mean that such products would be commercially unattractive to the industry.

Jack Henningfield suggested to me that:

> Although a new chemical entity or a truly big time advance in efficacy in an NRT (much more than tweaking up the nicotine yield) might generate a substantial market, there is not a lot of reassurance [for the industry to develop such products] based on past experience. Gum and lozenge could be made to deliver much higher and faster but would almost certainly be given prescription status in the US. Probably many other countries would follow. That's not much of an incentive for the pharmaceutical industry nor promise for public health. If any system comes too close to being considered a cigarette it risks control in the US by the Drug Enforcement Administration. Nasal NRT came within a hair's breadth of this fate.
>
> There is even a risk of international control because it might trigger application of the 1971 International Psychotropic Convention – UN Drug Control Treaty. The WHO Expert Committee on Drug Dependence considered regulating NRT in the 1990s when assessing the NRT systems we have today, without lozenge . . . So you might see why the pharmaceutical

industry would be less than enthusiastic about going a route that offers uncertain benefits to health or market, and the risks of tainting the whole market with an official "controlled substance" addiction label.

Henningfield added that the pharmaceutical industry "often makes decisions by weighing the US heavily. Because for better or worse our high drug prices mean the US market floats other countries where the profits are much lower. We are sort of the business class of pharmaceutical pricing".

Yet again, the above assessment confronts the core regulatory paradox in tobacco control, where high nicotine delivery devices (cigarettes), which kill millions, remain unregulated and can be sold in most countries by anyone, while "clean" nicotine delivery devices that might stand a chance of competing with cigarettes in their ability to quell nicotine craving, are nowhere in sight through fear of being rejected as too dangerous or so heavily regulated as to make them uninteresting to the drug industry.

I have often heard colleagues speculating that it is not in pharmaceutical industry interests to have smokers quit. The argument runs that it would be far more in their financial interests to have smokers recycling through repeated episodes of pharmacologically assisted cessation attempts where they purchased cessation aids, used them for as long as possible, relapsed and then tried again later – perhaps cycling through this pattern on several occasions. A customer who uses NRT and quits quickly, is not a valued customer.

Some argue that the pharmaceutical industry should make a major policy turn and embrace NRT use for nicotine maintenance as an additional objective to promoting it in smoking cessation. Might not this inadvertently have potential to promote the same "dual use" with cigarettes that I have argued tobacco companies would welcome and that could thereby dramatically slow cessation? My view is that provided any company does not in any way promote "clean" nicotine maintenance as way of continuing to smoke, that it fully informs users about the possible adverse consequences of nicotine use described earlier, and that access to the high-delivery product is regulated through under-the-counter pharmacy distribution, this could have potential to wean smokers off cigarettes.

Internal tobacco industry documents show that in the past tobacco companies have been able successfully to put pressure on some pharmaceutical companies to limit their targeting of NRT only to smokers wanting to quit, and not to engage in any "anti-smoking" activity designed to increase the size of the smoking cessation-ready population[369]. The apparent reluctance of the pharmaceutical industry to enter the harm reduction debate as a main player casts something of a shadow over whether such influence still persists today.

Combustible tobacco: enter the dragon

So far, I have spent most of this chapter considering smokeless tobacco, and the potential for significantly harm reduced forms to make serious inroads into the cigarette market. I have argued that such inroads are likely to be marginal at best.

Other than a bold call by the minnow Smokeless New Zealand group[370], in all this no one is imagining either that governments will order the phasing out of combustible forms of tobacco (principally cigarettes) or that tobacco companies will voluntarily go the same way.

A realistic scenario sees tobacco companies taking a long-term view of the global demand for tobacco as one where health concerns and tobacco control policies steadily erode uptake, accelerate quit attempts, and continue to limit smoking opportunities, causing significant falls in consumption by continuing smokers. This scenario is already a reality in many Western nations, and with the impetus that the FCTC will provide, it should spread quickly into developing nations in the next decade.

A major goal of the companies will therefore be again to seek to arrest the decline in smoking primarily via a dual smokeless/smoking policy and a "switch, rather than quit" strategy. For the reasons outlined above, I do not see smokeless tobacco use as likely ever to capture a major proportion of current and future smokers. This leaves combustible products as the most likely "main game" in the harm reduction debate. Can smoked products ever be made significantly less dangerous?

The precautionary principle

One of the most basic principles underscoring the protection of public health is the precautionary principle, which states: "When an activity raises threats of harm to human health or the environment, precautionary measures should be taken even if some cause and effect relationships are not fully established scientifically. In this context the proponent of an activity, rather than the public, should bear the burden of proof . . . [The process] must also involve an examination of the full range of alternatives, including no action."[371] The principle is often invoked in areas of environmental health for issues such as water quality contamination[372] to justify the removal of pollutants before definitive evidence of harm is established. The WHO's TobReg Committee has said of the principle:

> Wherever possible, this approach moves towards a general reduction of known harmful constituents of any product to the extent technically feasible, as part of good manufacturing processes. It does not require, for the substance under consideration, proof of the specific linkage between a lower level (dose) of any individual constituents and a lower level of human disease (response). It merely requires that the substance be known to be harmful and that processes exist for its diminution or removal. Evidence of actual reduced harm is not required for this approach; and correspondingly, compliance with these regulations does not support a claim that a given brand is safe or safer than other brands."[339]

To date in tobacco control, the principle has never been applied by governments in even a rudimentary way. Early in my career, I criticised government inaction on a report[373] that showed high levels of organochlorine pesticide residue on Australian-grown tobacco. Years later, tobacco industry documents from around this time confirmed this concern[82]. One 1978 Philip Morris document stated that "extremely high pesticide residue levels have been found on all samples submitted by PM-Australia: eg: DDT group >330 ppm; HCH group – up to 100 ppm; Dieldrin – up to 22 ppm".[374] Government officials' response at the time was simply to say that policy was to discourage everyone from using tobacco. One said that the extra potential harm from pesticide residue was "like being in hell, and turning the temperature up one degree". The prevailing attitude about regulating the content of tobacco has always reflected this attitude, with the result that tobacco has escaped all the regulatory requirements on health and safety that food, drinks and pharmaceuticals are obliged to meet. We know from internal tobacco industry research[375] and emission monitoring from several identically named brands sold in different countries[376–380] that the tobacco industry is capable of manufacturing cigarettes with radically different levels of several carcinogens.

The attitude that all tobacco use is unhealthy, and that people should simply not smoke, is a total abnegation of all responsibility for setting consumer standards for dangerous goods. Motor cycling is a very risky activity and easily avoided if zero risk is the objective. But many people find motorcycling economical and enjoyable. The equivalent policy stance on motorcycling would see government officials doing nothing about crash helmets, speed limits, graduated licensing schemes, or drink-driving, all premised on the *caveat emptor* proposition that consumers should be aware that there are inherent dangers lurking in the activity.

The seduction of reductionism?

Public health has a long and successful history of requiring the modification of consumer goods to make them less harmful to consumers and the environment. Removing lead from petrol and modifying car, toy and furniture design to reduce injury are obvious examples. Examples also abound with food where countless product formulation standards have been changed over the years to reflect emerging knowledge about the harms of ingesting various ingredients and the benefits of consuming others (e.g. iodising salt and changing the formulation of foods to reduce or increase ingredients like fats, sodium, fibre and various minerals). It is important to note that these standards are continually evolving, and it rarely occurs that an initial standard remains unchanged. New knowledge about risk and new manufacturing capabilities allow for changes to occur.

This product modification paradigm comes to tobacco control as a result of the notion that tobacco can be manufactured for consumption in a host of different ways to increase, reduce or eliminate many of its components. Tobacco smoke is rich in carcinogens, most being generated when tobacco is burned. The International Agency for Research in Cancer (IARC) produced a mammoth 1452-page report in 2004 in which it reviewed the evidence on tobacco smoke and involuntary smoking. Table 1.14 of that report lists 64 chemical compounds evaluated as present in mainstream cigarette smoke and known from animal studies to be carcinogenic. These include:

- ten polynuclear aromatic hydrocarbons;
- five heterocyclic hydrocarbons;
- eight *N*-nitrosamines;
- four aromatic amines;
- eight *N*-heterocyclic amines;
- two aldehydes;
- two phenolic compounds;
- seven volatile hydrocarbons;
- nine miscellaneous organic compounds;
- eight metals and metal compounds.

Hoffmann and Hoffmann[381] consider that there are 38 major carcinogens or cardiovascular/respiratory toxins in cigarette smoke. The Canadian province of British Columbia requires mandatory disclosure of emissions for these 38 carcinogens and toxins, as well as tar, nicotine and carbon monoxide for any brand variety that has a market share of 1.25% or more[382].

Among all these, considerable focus has been placed on tobacco-specific nitrosamines, particularly NNN (*N*-nitrosonornicotine) and NNK [4-(*N*-nitrosomethylamino)-1-(3-pyridyl)-1-butanone], which are found only in tobacco products. NNK is known to be the only carcinogen in tobacco smoke that induces lung tumours in each of rats, mice and hamsters – the three commonly used rodent models[383]. As discussed above, snus has very low TSNA levels, and its rising use in Swedish men has been associated with declining lung cancer deaths. Many of the 64 listed carcinogens mentioned above are present in smoke because they are by-products of combustion. Because snus is not burned and is low in TSNA (because of the way it is manufactured), it delivers fewer carcinogens than cigarettes.

Because the tobacco industry *can* reduce TSNA, polycyclic aromatic hydro-carbons (PAH), benzopyrene and various other toxicants, an emerging expert voice within tobacco control is now saying that – because of the precautionary principle – they should be *required* to reduce all toxicants as soon as practicable to the lowest possible levels, in much the same way that lead reduction levels were set for petrol. The core recommendations of the 2006 WHO TobReg report were that:

- Maximal limits be set for specific toxic constituents per milligram nicotine with a prohibition on the sale of any brands where the levels in the smoke exceed these limits.
- NNK and NNN should be the first constituents for which maximum levels should be set, because there "is marked variation across brands in the level of these nitrosamines within countries as demonstrated in the Massachusetts Benchmark data, internationally as demonstrated by the comparison of inter-national brands published by Counts and colleagues[375], and between countries as demonstrated by data from Canada and Australia as compared to the U.S. and the International data."
- Maximal limits of 72 ng NNK per mg nicotine and 114 ng NNN per mg nicotine be set for these constituents. These values reflect the mean values

currently produced by a range of international brands, as reported by Philip Morris scientists[375].

- Maximal limits for a more complete set of constituents should be developed as a next step, with those constituents thought to contribute to cardiovascular disease, chronic lung disease and cancer being the prime candidates.

- "Any regulatory approach specifically prohibits the use of the results of the testing in marketing or other communications with the consuming public, including product labelling. It is also recommended that communicating the relative ranking of brands by testing levels and/or the statement that the brand has met governmental regulatory standards be prohibited."

Importantly, the TobReg report also noted that a recently developed PREP, *Marlboro UltraSmooth*, is apparently being test marketed in at least three US locations in different formulations. The version being sold in Salt Lake City, Utah, "is an example of sufficient charcoal present in the filter to maintain reductions in yields of volatile compounds . . . however the *Marlboro UltraSmooth* cigarette marketed in Atlanta, Georgia . . . [and the version] marketed in North Dakota have less charcoal, and there is a breakthrough of the volatiles at more intense puffing regimens resulting in higher yields".

So what should we make of these recommendations? I believe that the precautionary principle, together with knowledge that the tobacco industry can reduce the various toxicants in its products, makes it indefensible to allow the industry to continue to market products that have unnecessarily high emission levels. The tobacco control community should unite to demand that the industry be required to reduce all reducible toxins to the lowest levels possible. That said, major concerns remain about the way in which such recommendations will actually play out for consumers.

The recommendation to set NNN and NNK maximum limits at the median level reported for all brands would see the 50% of brands above this mark forced to leave the marketplace. It will be vital here to implement international monitoring to ensure that companies do not meet these standards in some countries and then export their high TSNA leaf to unsuspecting developing nations. Those companies whose major brands are below these median levels will naturally see this as a major coup, and lobby hard to see such a regulatory policy implemented. Philip Morris is predicted to benefit most from such a policy, which is why it is lobbying hard to support such regulation for what some are facetiously referring to as "the Marlboro Monopoly Act" in the USA.

The TobReg Committee Report[384] set thresholds at the mean of NNN and NNK values for brands known to be already on sale in different parts of the world. This decision reflects a pragmatic marriage of policy with science. Regulatory practice generally compromises between the theoretically ideal and the commercially unacceptable. To have recommended that the maximum limit be set at the *minimum* levels already being manufactured would have driven almost all brands out of the market – an outcome that would have attracted little support from government and massive protests from the industry. TobReg's plan is to review the maximum permissible levels every few years, progressively reducing the levels each time. This process will play out for years, if not decades, over which time smoking prevalence is almost certain to fall further and further.

Importantly, the TobReg report also recommends that manufacturers be prohibited from communicating any statements to consumers that the products they are buying contain reduced levels of toxins. The idea is that if all brands on sale conform to the maximum emission standards described, then there is no point in any manufacturer being able to make statements that might imply that their brands were somehow different, or less dangerous, than other brands – and all would conform equally. By analogy, we don't see water authorities advertising that their water contains "reduced arsenic" levels.

At first blush, this would seem an eminently sensible recommendation. But it is one that I fear would present few difficulties to the well-oiled publicity and public relations machines of the tobacco industry. If we assume for the moment that the TobReg principles go forward, we will first witness several years of intense debate between companies concerned about the potential removal of their products from the marketplace. Much of this debate will be orchestrated in public by the potentially losing tobacco companies, and so consumers will unavoidably be exposed to a large amount of deliberately misleading information implying that "safe" cigarettes are just around the corner. As the TobReg report makes emphatically clear, reduced emission products of the sort they are describing present completely unknown risk reduction potential. This fine distinction will be lost on the great majority of consumers, to the obvious delight of the tobacco industry.

Risk swapping?

On the basis of comparing published emission data for Canadian and Australian cigarettes, Bill King and colleagues[385] have recently posited two possible models of emission reduction. The preferred "spring mattress" model would see all or any carcinogens able to be reduced without seeing any compensatory increase in others. Alternatively, the more problematic "water bed" model would see the lowering of some carcinogens generating a corresponding rise in others. They suggest that the goal of establishing emission limits for particular carcinogens could be undermined by two important problems. The first is "risk swapping", where the emission load of some carcinogens is reduced, while that for others rises because of the manufacturing process involved in reducing the first group. Neil Collishaw has said of this: "there is no public health benefit to getting cancer caused by PAH (polynuclear aromatic hydrocarbons) over cancer caused by nitrosamines"[386]. The second is "risk shifting", where exposure to specific carcinogens or toxins is reduced for smokers in one market area, but increased for smokers in other areas; this arises when the tobacco industry exports cigarettes that will not pass maximum emission levels in one country to another county where such levels do not apply. King and his colleagues believe that Canadian and Australian data show that there is a "waterbed" model in operation: "Our findings concerning the inverse relationships in adjusted emissions also suggest that some apparent achievements could actually constitute large-scale risk swapping, where specific populations gain lower exposures to one agent at the cost of higher exposures to another. This possibility is clearly illustrated in the negative relations between benzo(a)pyrene (BaP) and NNK emissions. Selecting out brands with high emissions of one agent from a pool of conventional cigarettes would generally mean selecting out brands with low emissions of the other, and selecting out brands with high emissions of both agents would leave only those with middling emissions of both. That would be a dubious accomplishment."[385]

Several PREPS are promoted in the USA as having reduced emissions of both PAH and TSNA, such as the commercial failure *Omni*. Hatsukami and colleagues (2004) found significantly reduced TSNA biomarkers but non-significantly reduced PAH biomarkers in 22 subjects who switched to *Omni Light* for 4 weeks. Hughes and others (2004) found non-significantly reduced TSNA and PAH biomarkers in 34 subjects who switched from their regular brands to *Omni Regular* or *Light* for 6 weeks. Importantly, in both these studies, the exposure reductions to both carcinogens from smoking *Omni* were modest compared with those implied in promotional material, based on emission figures. Furthermore, both studies found CO intakes increased when subjects moved to *Omni*. King and colleagues comment here that: "Unless *Omni* is a poor example of what PREPs can achieve, even putatively radical innovations will not substantially reduce combined PAH/TSNA exposures and there may be significant risk swapping with other agents, such as CO."[385]

As to the key question of whether variation in brand emissions as determined and promoted by PREP manufacturers means that some brands are more or less harmful than others, King and colleagues state "we believe we would be moving way ahead of the available evidence if we offered such answers without greater knowledge of how emission patterns vary over time and how emission measures relate to actual intakes, along with greater knowledge of emissions of agents not included in the disclosures. In other words, we do not believe there is currently any advice to offer to smokers interested in brand switching rather than quitting".[385]

As we have seen, studies on both *Eclipse* and *Omni* have shown that while users have decreased levels of TSNA biomarkers, they also show elevated levels of carbon monoxide compared with regular cigarette smokers. Cancers account for 36.9% of tobacco-caused deaths in developed nations, and vascular diseases for 33.3%[42]. Carbon monoxide is a key component in the development of cardiovascular disease caused by smoking. Important questions therefore arise about the net impact on health of harm reduced products that might reduce cancer, while elevating the risks of cardiovascular disease. A very recent paper examining smokeless tobacco use in 52 countries found an odds ratio for acute myocardial infarction of 2.23 in smokeless users, although the authors noted that the numbers involved were "too few to allow conclusive results"[387]. The US Cancer Prevention Study (CPS-II) found that use of smokeless tobacco products "was significantly associated with death from CHD, stroke, all cancers combined, lung cancer, and cirrhosis. The associations with cardiovascular and other non-malignant endpoints were attenuated, but not eliminated, by controlling for measured covariates"[388]. A large 10-year Swedish cohort study found that the development of metabolic syndrome was "independently associated with high consumption of snus, even when controlling for smoking status".[389]

This "swings and roundabouts" disease risk-benefit concern is seldom addressed by today's PREP-focused public health community, whose preoccupation is overwhelmingly on the potential for reducing carcinogenic risk.

The beta-carotene lung cancer prevention story

The perils of reductionist thinking (where the whole is simply the sum of its parts) are perhaps no better illustrated than in the case of one of the most salutary predictions-gone-wrong in cancer epidemiology: the saga of beta-carotene and hopes that it might, through dietary supplementation, be able to prevent cancer.

Epidemiologists have long observed that populations and individuals with diets rich in fruit and vegetables have lower rates of some cancers than populations and individuals who eat fruit and vegetables infrequently[390]. Because of their anti-oxidant properties, carotenoids were suspected of having anti-carcinogenic potential, and in studies of dietary differences between populations, dietary intake of beta-carotene has been shown to be inversely associated with the development of lung cancer[391]. A 16-year prospective cohort study (the Nurses' Health Study), which involved 1 793 327 person-years of follow-up, found that eating carrots showed a strong inverse relation to the risk of lung cancer: women who reported consuming five or more carrots per week had a relative risk of 0.4 (95% CI 0.2–0.8) compared with the risk for women who never ate carrots[392].

Such findings fired the imaginations of cancer epidemiologists, who speculated that if beta-carotene were increased in diets, reductions in cancer incidence might follow. This led to trials of dietary supplementation, to see whether taking beta-carotene pills could produce the same protective effects for cancers, including lung cancer. One randomized, double-blind, placebo-controlled trial of beta-carotene (50 mg on alternate days) commenced in 1982 and involved 22 071 male physicians; by 1995 it was found that "there were virtually no early or late differences in the overall incidence of malignant neoplasms or cardiovascular disease, or in overall mortality"[393].

However, in two other similar large trials[394,395], beta-carotene supplementation actually led to *increases* in lung cancer. As the authors of one of the studies summarised: "The Beta-Carotene and Retinol Efficacy Trial (CARET) tested the effect of daily beta-carotene (30 mg) and retinyl palmitate (25 000 IU) on the incidence of lung cancer, other cancers, and death in 18 314 participants who were at high risk for lung cancer because of a history of smoking or asbestos exposure. CARET was stopped ahead of schedule in January 1996 because participants who were randomly assigned to receive the active intervention were found to have a 28% increase in incidence of lung cancer, a 17% increase in incidence of death and a higher rate of cardiovascular disease mortality compared with participants in the placebo group."[396]

In discussing these unexpected outcomes, it has been argued that beta-carotene may "require the presence of other factors also found in fruits and vegetables"[392] and that "Beta-carotene may also be a biomarker for critical carotenoids and phyto-chemicals in fruits and vegetables . . . We do not know what it is in fruits and veget-ables that protects. There may be a number of factors. Initially, attention was given to the nutrients beta-carotene and vitamin C. Then people started to think about fiber, vitamin E, and folate. Recently, people have turned their attention to the other carotenoids, such as lycopene and lutein. However, a wide variety of other compounds have the potential to be protective".[397]

The above story should be salutary to those who believe that by reducing or even eliminating *particular* carcinogens from the menu of 64 known to be in tobacco smoke, let alone the many other toxins in tobacco smoke, that risk reduction will follow. The beta-carotene story is a classic case study in the risks of reductionist thinking.

Scepticism inside the industry

At least one senior scientist within BAT shared these views. In May 1999 Derek Irwin wrote to his industry colleagues about meetings BAT was having to discuss the Star Tobacco company's recent development of a PREP: "the Star process inter-feres with the curing process. Details are not clear but it seems to involve micro-wave treatment of green tobacco. There must be some concern that other chemical differences between green and cured tobacco could lead to other or enhanced hazards. This is quite different to use of a novel filter that would selectively remove TSNA. That would be a safer route but unfortunately TSNA cannot be filtered selectively relative to tar . . . My own opinion . . . is that . . . *we need to think of smoke holistically. Its biological effects are not due to some simple sum of the parts. This would ignore the probability of substantial interactive effects between those many parts. For that reason, the regulatory initiatives to control or reduce levels of specific substances are missing the point* [my emphasis]. The "across the board" [tar reduction] approach used by the industry is right in principle but subject to criticism on compensation arguments."[398]

In January 2000, Irwin reiterated his concerns in another memo:

> 1. There are other carcinogens in tobacco smoke. We cannot claim "99% car-cinogen free", to draw an analogy with another regrettable case and I remind you of the consequences of that case. 2. A non-specific mechanism, such as long-term irritation from many different components of tobacco smoke, acting additively or synergistically, may be more likely in such a complex system. 3. Epidemiology shows that lung cancer is strongly associated in all markets where this has been studied . . . 4. TSNA are one of the few substance classes that show substantial variation by blend style and therefore in some cases by market, yet differences in lung cancer between USB [United States style blend] and Virginia have not been glaringly obvious."[399]

By this time though, Irwin had been assigned to other responsibilities within BAT, and he signed off his memo with an apparent sense of himself as a lone voice in the harm reduction wilderness: "If I am 'off message' on this, either of the points themselves or because I am persisting too far, then it would be better to take me off the SRG. I believe the same issue was the reason I was removed from the Smoke Science Team in 1998, so there is a precedent."[399]

In May 2000, Irwin became even more forthright. After viewing a BBC documentary on tobacco where harm reduction was discussed, he wrote to three senior scientists inside BAT: "I disagree with just about every point made by every speaker, including our own. Our main problem appears to be that 'the technology exists to make cigarettes which are appreciably less lethal and that many tobacco companies appear to be looking for any excuse not to use it.' The technology does not exist, despite the impression given by the patent record or Star Scientific. It will not exist. All four BAT R&D Centres have overstated to the Company what they can do in terms of product innovation. This has gone on over a number of years. This is now being picked up by outside pressure groups, through patents etc. It is being exacerbated by statements by BAT personnel such as those in this programme. Internal overstatement is one thing, externally it is even less in the Company's interests. We should tone down future expectations. Firstly, it is not ethical and secondly we shall be asked to explain our failures at some point in the future."[400]

Other scientists within BAT were (and are today) presumably happy to go along with the company line, intent on reducing a limited number of carcinogens within the total carcinogenic load with a view to publicising this to smokers as implying that reduced emissions of selected carcinogens mean reduced total health risk.

Ingredients

There is an old joke about *Camel* cigarettes being the only brand of cigarettes with a picture of the factory on the packet. *Camel* cigarettes almost certainly do not contain camel dung, but there is no law or regulation of which I am aware in any nation that would actually prevent manufacturers from adding such an ingredient if they wished to do so.

Cigarettes and other tobacco products contain chemical additives. Under the Tobacco Control Act (1990) the New Zealand Government requires tobacco companies operating there to supply the Health Department with an annual list of all additives that they might be using in their tobacco products. The list is not released to the public and does not specify which additives are selected for use from this list. Two identical lists of 2168 additives and chemicals, for the year 1991, were submitted by the two main companies operating in New Zealand, W.D. & H.O. Wills (New Zealand) Ltd (then a BAT subsidiary) and Rothmans of Pall Mall (New Zealand) Ltd. The list shows additives approved for use by the industry in Europe. The New Zealand government had apparently sanctioned the list for local use.

The list includes a veritable gastronomic checklist of herbs, spices and flavours but also includes chemicals found in rat poison, fungicides, urine and sheep dip, creosote (the poison painted onto fence posts to deter borers) and even ambergris, a grease obtained from whales[401].

Table 4.1 The weights of additives in tobacco products, based on submissions to the New Zealand government for 1991 by W.D. & H.O. Wills (New Zealand) Ltd and Rothmans of Pall Mall (New Zealand) Ltd.

	Tobacco weight by product class (tonnes)	Weight of additives in total by product class (tonnes)	Percentage of additives by weight of product class
Wills cigarettes	879.219	1.803	0.2
Wills cigarette tobacco	366.036	82.456	22.5
Wills pipe tobacco	6.695	2.227	33.4
Rothmans cigarettes	2271.04	10.184	0.4
Rothmans cigarette tobacco	280.495	30.108	10.7
Rothmans pipe tobacco	21.862	3.565	16.3

The document submitted by Wills included a letter making it plain that the company did not want smokers or the wider public to know about the additives (". . . the information is provided in confidence and may not be communicated to others"). Attachments to the submissions showed the weights of additives added (see Table 4.1). The data showed that pipe and roll-your-own tobacco were heavily adulterated, putting an end to the myth espoused by many roll-your-own smokers that the tobacco they use is "more natural" and additive-free.

In a few nations today, consumers are given access to information that companies are prepared to disclose. A voluntary disclosure agreement between the companies and the Australian government was signed on 20 December 2000[402,403] providing for brand-by-brand disclosure of ingredients by descending order of weight. However, significant exclusions were "flavourings that give each brand its unique characteristics" and "processing aids and preservatives that are not significantly present and do not functionally affect the finished product". Nowhere were such terms as "significantly present" or "functionally affect" defined.

Today, every brand of cigarette sold in Australia marketed by BAT and Philip Morris is described as including these unspecified "processing aids"[81]. Effectively then, the voluntary agreement revealed nothing that the industry wanted to remain secret, and so Australian consumers continue to be unable to make informed choices about the brands they select. An internal BAT document in 1994 noted that "BAT is happy to disclose information on ingredients so long as brand recipes [sic] are protected"[404].

Among industry documents are occasional glimpses of the sort of additives the industry does not wish to reveal to the public. In 1981 Philip Morris noted that "Marlboro concentrate, Alpine exotic, P.M. flavour, BD-1 additive" were being imported into Australia[405]. If these are still being used, none appears in the lists released in 2000. Similarly, a 1993 letter from R.J. Reynolds USA to Rothmans Australia requested ". . . further information regarding the mixing formulas and the actual application rates for the top flavors being used on Blends 9 and 13 . . . the amounts of these materials which are added to the Quest DC05162, IFF

GA502544 and the ITC-14 concentrates to produce the final top flavor (which is applied to the tobacco) . . ."[406]. None of the Australian industry websites list any of these ingredients.

Indeed, Australian companies were themselves kept ignorant of what it was they were adding to the local blends. For example, in 1984 W.D. & H.O. Wills Australia wrote to Brown and Williamson about "ingredient MGE-7"[407]. Wills was introducing a "total Quality Assurance . . . involv[ing] routine inspections of incoming materials. Because of the confidentiality we appreciate you would not be able to provide us with full specifications for Ingredient MGE-7 but whatever specifications you are able to pass on to us, preferably with corresponding tolerance, would be appreciated. One detail of particular use in facilitating our test procedures would be the molecular weight of the product"[407].

Despite the companies continually insisting that the additives are safe, some documents suggest otherwise. In 1993, Rothmans Australia wrote to R.J. Reynolds International requesting a product information sheet for "ITC 14 flavour used to manufacture *Now* cigarettes", an ultra "light" brand that Rothmans was distributing in Australia[408]. The Material Safety Data Sheets provided stated: "The composition of this product is considered to be a trade secret by R.J. Reynolds Tobacco Company" and that "No Federal OSHA exposure standard or ACGIH TLV [American Conference of Government Industrial Hygienists threshold limit value] has been established for this material." Nonetheless, Reynolds was aware that "Ingestion during pregnancy resulted in birth defects and reproductive effects in laboratory animals"[408].

Perhaps no document yet discovered is so disturbing as a report written in 1977 by Dr Sydney Green, then BAT's Senior Scientist for Research and Development[409]. In a memo on scientific developments Green wrote: "A way-out development is that of compounds (such as etorphine) which are 10 000 times as effective as analgesics as morphine and which are very addictive. It is theoretically possible (if politically unthinkable) to add analytically undetectable quantities of such materials to cigarettes to create brand allegiance. But this thought may suggest the possibility of such compounds occuring [sic] naturally"[410]. Etorphine, known among veterinarians as elephant juice because a small drop will kill an elephant, was used in race horse doping because a very small dose can produce hyperexcitability in horses.

The above brief glimpse into the current anarchic situation of tobacco ingredient regulation should appal anyone with even rudimentary concern for the consumerist principles of the rights to safety and to information. Tobacco companies, excuse the cliché, remain a law unto themselves. Any attempt at comprehensive tobacco control policy that avoids engagement with this on-going scandal will continue to shirk a major challenge that astonishes anyone hearing it plainly for the first time: why should manufacturers of products that kill some 4.9 million people each year remain totally unaccountable to any product safety standard when such accountability is taken for granted in every other area of product regulation?

A spoonful of sugar helps the tobacco go down

The path ahead will require tough political decision-making to meet the ultimate challenge of placing public health above industry profitability. The issue of adding flavourings to make cigarettes more palatable to children starting to smoke[411,412] epitomises the irreconcilable differences between the tobacco industry's commercial ambitions and public health. As Greg Connolly has said: "Using candy flavours in cigarettes is like adding a sachet of sugar to a side of rancid meat. The FDA can forbid sweeteners for masking the taste of rotten meat but not the 'Berry Bayou Blast' or 'Crema Mint' in Camels"[413].

The industry would not sit idly by while public health regulators sought to ban any ingredient designed to make smoking more palatable to starters. Companies will continue to display the same ruthless determination to dominate the market by making their products more appealing to smokers, and particularly to starters without established brand preferences. We will see the same cynical, self-interested posturing about responsibility that we have seen for years. In 2006, for example, BAT Australia stated in a submission to the New South Wales parliament that it would support the banning of "fruit flavoured" cigarettes: "we support the policy of removing products designed to specifically appeal to minors – such as those manufactured by Trojan Tobacco with overt fruit flavours"[414]. BAT's own brands draw from flavours that include apple concentrate, apricot, caramel, chocolate, honey, liquorice, orange, peppermint, plum and vanilla[415]. Naturally, BAT is not prepared to support banning its own brands.

Moreover, BAT scientists have recently reported results suggesting that the net effect of additives might even be to *reduce* the toxicity of certain tobacco emissions. Additives might be good for us! Examining emission data after adding flavourants and other ingredients "at or above the maximum levels used commercially by British American Tobacco" they found that:

> the effect of the ingredient mixtures on total particulate matter and carbon monoxide levels in smoke was not significantly different to the control [cigarette with no additives] in most cases, and was never more than 10% with any ingredient mixture . . . For the test cigarettes with ingredient mixtures containing casing ingredients, there were again no significant changes in smoke analyte levels in most cases. Those changes that were observed are as follows. Decreases in smoke levels were observed with some ingredient mixtures for most of the tobacco specific nitrosamines (up to 24%), NO(x), most of the phenols (up to 34%), benzo[a]pyrene, and some of the aromatic amines and miscellaneous organic compounds . . . Increases were observed for some test cigarettes in smoke ammonia, HCN, formaldehyde and lead levels (up to 24%). The significance of the ammonia and lead increases was not present when the long-term variability of the analytical methodology was taken into account. The yields of some carbonyl compounds in smoke were increased in one comparison with an additives mixture containing cellulosic components; in particular, formaldehyde was increased by 68%.[416]

The scientists did not recommend that carbonyl compounds be *not* used as additives.

Summary and conclusions

So, how do we reconcile the above cautions that should be flashing bold amber lights to harm reduction enthusiasts keen to tinker with setting limits to a limited number of carcinogens, with the inviolable precautionary principle that would demand that we reduce all harmful constituents known to be reducible? Combusted tobacco produces such a plethora of harmful emissions that to embark on a programme, perhaps decades long, of requiring the reduction of just a handful of them may be of little consequence to the health of the general population. Rather like a programme of ensuring that the decking of the *Titanic* was non-slip and its handrails splinter-free.

Nigel Gray has laid down some plainly spoken, unavoidable challenges: "To those who are hesitant to require tobacco products to be regulated, I ask: are we really to believe that . . . levels of nitrosamines such as NNK (that vary between 35 ngm per cigarette and 325 ngm per cigarette within a single brand, in this case *Marlboro* in 1996) should be uncontrolled? That polyaromatic hydrocarbon yields, plus lead and arsenic do not matter? That ventilated filters . . . should not be outlawed? That nicotine dose delivered to the smoker should be misleadingly labelled on the packet and facilitated by ammonia technology? That the real nicotine dose should be uncontrolled? That sugars that produce acetaldehyde when burnt are acceptable? That sophisticated flavourings that appeal to children are OK?"[417]

My own position is to agree with Gray and other colleagues that tobacco products should be regulated to reduce all harmful constituents known to be reducible as soon as possible to the lowest levels found in products now being sold in different global markets. I support this for three reasons. First, it is simply incongruous and absurd that tobacco companies should continue to be accountable to no one for product standards. Second, while remaining profoundly sceptical that reducing a handful of the many carcinogens and toxicants in tobacco smoke will do much to reduce harm, a strong regulatory régime where all tobacco companies were bound to the precautionary principle would be an effective Trojan horse to, in the process, disallow a large range of additives designed to make smoking more pleasant and palatable.

As stressed earlier, the tobacco industry will not countenance any form of product regulation that threatens the consumer acceptability of its products. But tobacco control has a long and often victorious history of being told repeatedly of other policies that the industry will not countenance either. If that was all that mattered, we would have lamely walked away from tobacco advertising and smoke-free indoor air battles too.

The third reason for supporting product regulation is that it would need to be a central focus of an overall regulatory approach to tobacco. This would see packaging, health warnings, nicotine content[418], retailing regulations, public information campaigning and perhaps one day smoker licensing[116] organised through a government tobacco regulatory agency, linked to a global network of similar agencies committed to harmonising regulation of what is increasingly a transnational product. Advocacy for the establishment and cooperation of these should become a major platform of contemporary tobacco control.

Borland[419] and Callard et al.[420] have both proposed radical approaches to the regulation of the tobacco industry, based on the establishment of central tobacco regulatory agencies. When it comes to product regulation, each national agency would license manufacturers to supply to retailers tobacco products that met specified standards of emissions. Liberman[421] is highly critical of the need to establish any new "green fields" regulatory agency, arguing that the same regulatory objectives could be better pursued through the use of existing laws or amendments to them.

Such proposals today remain in the radical realm of futuristic tobacco control. But if the momentum to regulation continues as it must, the merits of these and alternative models will need to come under close scrutiny. The worst possible outcome would be to see systems of product self-regulation perpetuated whereby manufacturers remained free to declare only those aspects of brand recipes that they chose and accountable to no one.

Conclusions about smokeless tobacco

Low-nitrosamine smokeless tobacco products like snus and nicotine lozenges, which deliver cigarette-level nicotine equivalents to smokers, are means for cigarette smokers to obtain satisfying levels of nicotine while greatly reducing their exposure to carcinogens and other toxins that combusted forms of tobacco like cigarettes deliver. Changes in Swedish tobacco-caused disease rates would appear to be associated with the historic shift by a large proportion of Swedish male smokers to snus. There remain important concerns about whether snus might cause pancreatic cancer and more general concerns about the role of nicotine in apoptosis. This latter concern is highly relevant to projections about encouraging nicotine maintenance through higher yielding NRT or LNST.

However, the Swedish snus experience has to date not shown that it is transferable to any other nation, despite many nations presenting few if any regulatory barriers to the opportunity for companies to market and promote it as a less dangerous alternative to smoking. In the tobacco industry advertising paradise of the USA, where domestically the recent end to billboard advertising was considered radical, the use of smokeless tobacco has recently been declining faster than that of smoking, although the most recent signs suggest some growth. New-generation PREPs are proving to be a minor side-show in the tobacco market, not gaining consumer acceptance, even in environments where they can be promoted quite freely.

Smokeless tobacco has been more of a gateway drug out of smoking than into it in Sweden and the USA, but still a third of primary smokeless tobacco users become regular smokers. The Swedish experience does not guarantee that this would be repeated in any other nation. Companies like Philip Morris, R.J. Reynolds and

BAT – which also market old-generation highly toxic products – would pop the champagne if ex-smokers flocked back to tobacco use via smokeless, if the product became as fashionable as mobile phones with youth, or if large cohorts of smokers intending to quit switched instead to smokeless. Anyone who imagines that these companies have not modelled the impact of all these scenarios on their bottom lines is certainly naïve.

Interestingly, no one in tobacco control has yet produced any mathematical models showing projected disease reduction gains under different realistic best- and worst-case assumptions of uptake by both smokers and new tobacco users, dual smokeless/cigarette use and ex-smoker relapse into smokeless. The results of such modelling would need to be compared with those obtained from projections of the reduced health burden from smoking being generated now in some nations as a result of falling smoking prevalence.

Unbridled optimism about snus and other non-combustible PREPs being a major route out of smoking is not supported by the situation of any nation other than Sweden. For this to happen, there would need to be a major programme of government information, designed to persuade smokers not contemplating smoking cessation to switch to smokeless. This would immediately raise concerns about a confusing or diluted message being sent to smokers by governments: at 7 pm on television we would see an anti-smoking advertisement designed to persuade smokers to quit. At 8 pm we would see another message from the government saying "well, perhaps you don't need to quit . . . consider smokeless instead".

To rely on the industry to develop and run such campaigns would be to risk unravelling tobacco advertising bans where they have occurred and provide a further excuse to delay their introduction where advertising still occurs. It would also place trust in the industry to behave ethically when that industry has written the textbook on unethical business conduct.

So do I support the lifting of the bans on snus? Unequivocally but not unconditionally, yes. The subtitle of this book is "making *smoking* history". The consumer sovereignty argument (that smokers wanting to continue to smoke should be able to be informed about the emission differences between combusted tobacco and LNST, and able to buy those products) is compelling, even sacrosanct. But as we have seen, the arguments about the need to inform consumers that will accompany lifting of bans, risk letting the evil genie out of its bottle.

A compromise in the form of tightly controlled distribution of LNST products, unaccompanied by any form of advertising, would seem sensible. Countries that have methadone and needle exchange programmes typically allow distribution through accredited pharmacists. The entire system of controlling public access to potentially dangerous pharmaceuticals through the mediation of a doctor's prescription and/or under-the-counter pharmacy-only access is well established in nearly every nation. Pharmacies are conveniently located in every town and suburb, providing ready accessibility for consumers in an environment where smoking cessation products are also sold. Pharmacists in many nations do not sell tobacco products, but the challenges of persuading their professional associations to review this policy to allow LNST are likely to be minor.

A giant distraction from the main game?

Smoking "culture" is in free fall in many nations, thanks to a comprehensive approach that today translates into smokefree environments, high prices, total advertising bans, in-your-face awareness campaigns, and generally an environment where the tobacco industry gets clobbered every time it raises its head with its dissembling contributions. Most people whom I respect in tobacco control would see 10% smoking prevalence as very possible by 2010 in such nations. After that, it's anyone's guess. Smoking could remain entrenched in an ever smaller section of the community, or it could go the way that public spitting went early last century, via anti-tuberculosis campaigning[2].

So, against this background, proponents of harm reduced products are urging that we should somehow support the lifting of bans on (some forms) of smokeless tobacco. A serious consideration is "why, with smoking being in freefall thanks to the traditional approach of promoting abstinence through prevention and cessation, would one risk distracting perhaps significant numbers of people who might otherwise quit, by allowing the tobacco industry to use advertising (especially in the USA where tobacco advertising remains rampant) and public relations strategies elsewhere, to promote switching, or worse, dual use, rather than quitting?"

Given the scenario of this decline, that there is little evidence of the smoking population "hardening" in countries where prevalence is falling[422] (considered in Chapter 5), and that the Swedish evidence points to major harm reduction effects, how much of the tobacco control effort should be diverted to trying to lift the ban on smokeless in, say, Australia and the European Union? Should we invest more effort into whipping governments into a proven pathway to reducing tobacco-caused disease premised on a prevention and quitting model? Or should we take our foot off that throttle and focus on a model that would seem likely to slow the rate of cessation by diverting some smokers who might quit onto harm reduced products, which in some cases would become dual use or a holding pattern before reverting to smoking? The speech by David Davies of Philip Morris on harm reduction to the Australian National Press Club in 2005[349] was totally premised on a steady-state model of smoking prevalence. He repeatedly referred to "the one in five Australians who choose to smoke", as if this was the way it would always be. In fact a few weeks after his talk, newly released government data showed a further slide.

If we conceptualise all our tobacco control efforts as 100%, should we decide to put 10% of all this effort, resources and money into harm reduction? A quarter? A half? How much? More specifically, how much of a national tobacco control budget should be allocated to communicate the advantages of reduced harm products in nations where there are total tobacco advertising bans and so where the manufacturers would not be able to communicate this themselves?

Harm reduction has become a huge absorber of energy among sections of the global tobacco control movement. My feeling is that the smokeless issue is worth possibly 10% of effort in countries with rapidly reducing smoking prevalence, and given the small budgets that almost all nations have allocated for tobacco control,

10% would buy very little public awareness campaigning. Inevitable pressures would arise to have the issue absorb a disproportionate amount of resources to help it climb out of such marginality.

A decision to make LNST available under the counter through pharmacies would seem a sensible way of addressing both the consumer sovereignty argument and placing a major brake on tobacco industry marketing excesses. Consumers would be informed about its availability through news generated by both health agencies and (inevitably) the manufacturers. Public health agency communications (websites, brochures, etc.) would describe the potential advantages of smokers switching to these products in ways that would both keep harm reduction in perspective and avoid the ludicrous and misleading demonisation of the products that is too frequent today[345].

Notes

i   Tobacco product manufacturers could not add proscribed substances like illicit drugs, but beyond that, almost anything would be possible.

ii I have drawn here from a review of snus: Foulds J, Ramstrom L, Burke M, Fagerstrom K. Effect of smokeless tobacco (snus) on smoking and public health in Sweden. *Tob Control* 2003;**12**:349–59.

iii Description of apoptosis from MedicineNet.com (www.MedicineNet.com).

Chapter 5

Accelerating Smoking Cessation and Prevention in Whole Communities

In the first lecture I give to medical students each year, I ask them to raise their hand if they believe that "prevention is better than cure". Nearly all hands in the room go up. Preventing smoking has to have more priority than "curing" its use, surely? But the correct answer here depends on your goal. If the concern is to prevent new cohorts from ever developing smoking-caused disease, prevention is the correct answer. But if the concern is more focused on the short to medium term – up to the next 50 years – and the primary goal is to reduce the number of tobacco-caused deaths, then the importance of cessation leaps out, as Richard Peto's famous projections so dramatically illustrate[423]. If we halved the number of people who took up smoking by 2050, Peto calculates that 20 million deaths would be avoided globally between now and 2050. However, if we halved adult tobacco consumption between now and 2050 (principally by promoting cessation), 180 million deaths – nine times more – would be avoided.

Efforts to motivate and assist people to stop smoking are therefore at centre stage in comprehensive tobacco control policy. Cessation is also the area of tobacco control that attracts most investment – including massive amounts from the pharmaceutical industry – and has most people working in it. Globally, hundreds of millions who used to smoke no longer do so. In nations now into their third or fourth decade of concerted tobacco control effort, it is typical that there are more ex-smokers in such populations than there are smokers. For example, in the USA in 2004, 24.5% of the adult population consisted of ex-smokers, while 20.9% were smokers. Just over half (52.4%) of all people who have ever smoked in the USA have quit (in Connecticut and California this rate is as high as 62%)[424]. In Australia in 2004, 26.4% of all people aged 14 and over were former smokers, compared with 19% who still smoked at least once per week[5]. In Canada in 2005, 20% of all people aged over 15 smoked and 26% were former smokers[425]. Britain lags somewhat, having 20% former smokers but 25% still smoking[426]. However, the phenomenon of widespread quitting throughout populations is by no means universal: in most nations, smokers outnumber ex-smokers, so many nations today face immense challenges as to how they can best influence many millions of people to stop smoking.

In those nations where smoking cessation is widespread and accelerating, the data illustrate the classic "is the glass half full or half empty?" dilemma. They show that cessation on a mass scale *can* occur. But when coupled with data on failed attempts, massive expenditure on therapeutic aids to assist with cessation and perennially high reported levels of intention to quit, they also show an unparalleled level of substance addiction that thwarts millions of cessation attempts each year. In Australia, around 60% of smokers quit smoking for at least one day per year, with nearly three-quarters of these relapsing within one month[427].

Why and how do smokers stop smoking?

The most fundamental questions to ask about such vast numbers of ex-smokers are why and how did they stop smoking, as well as questions about how we can keep adding large numbers to their ranks, as cost-effectively as possible. Understanding *why* most people quit will provide useful information about which motivational levers might be pressed more cleverly to stimulate more people to quit throughout whole populations. Similarly, a better understanding of *how* most of these people have stopped may provide important guidance to smokers wanting to quit about how to approach the task, and about the wisdom and cost-effectiveness of policies that might best facilitate this to happen.

If our concern is to maximise cessation throughout whole populations, it is vital to understand the natural history of smoking and its decline in populations, giving most attention to those factors that can maximise the *numbers* of people who quit. One of the most elementary perspectives that a population-wide lens provides is that policies and interventions that have low success *rates* can be much more important than those with higher success rates when the different *reach* of those interventions is considered. An intensive quit smoking programme that sees 20% of participants quit may seem far more promising than an intervention that results in only 2% of people quitting. But if the intensive intervention is only ever run with small numbers of people willing to commit to attending groups or counselling, whereas the intervention with 2% success influences an entire population, the latter will be immeasurably more important than the apparently more "successful" intervention. A 40% success among 2000 participants yields 800 ex-smokers, but 2% of 2.9 million smokers translates to 58 000 ex-smokers.

For this reason, the most important question that always should be asked of interventions (including policies) designed to reduce smoking is "what is the potential *reach* of this intervention?" The impact of any cessation aid or intervention is measured by multiplying its efficacy rate by its participation rate, or its ability to penetrate into the population of smokers in the community. As we will see, interventions that fail to reach large numbers of smokers, no matter how high their success rates, have an insignificant impact on smoking throughout a population.

Biener and her colleagues in Massachusetts studied recent quitters' differential use of different smoking cessation interventions, calculating both the penetration, or reach, of each method (how many were exposed to each aid), and its "impact" (defined as the proportion of recent quitters who reported being helped by the aid (Table 5.1)[428]. While some methods had much higher success rates, Table 5.1 shows which methods had greatest impact in the Massachusetts population.

However, there is a kind of "inverse impact law" that operates in smoking cessation research. Attend any major conference on tobacco control and you will find

Table 5.1 Massachusetts recent quitters who accessed various cessation aids and proportion who reported being helped by each aid ("impact").

Cessation aid	Penetration (%)	Impact (%)
TV ad	90.6	30.5
NRT	22.9	20.8
Professional help[a]	14.3	11.1
Self-help	8.7	7.6
Prescription	8.3	6.8
Programme	6.4	5.9
Website	3.9	3.6
Quitline	0.8	0.5

[a]Doctor, counsellor or other professional.

legions of people employed to run and evaluate interventions at the lower end of population impact which, even when aggregated, barely produce a surface ripple in reducing smoking prevalence in whole populations, as we will see later in this chapter.

In 1985 I wrote an article in the *Lancet* provocatively entitled "Stop smoking clinics: a case for their abandonment"[429]. I argued that:

- the contribution of dedicated, labour-intensive smoking cessation services could only ever make a negligible contribution to reducing smoking in communities;
- such services siphoned off scarce resources that could be used more efficiently to achieve the same ends throughout communities via mass reach campaigns;
- such services, as Ivan Illich[430] might have said, risked reinforcing a *disabling* message that said to smokers "if you want to quit smoking, you will need help".

Moreover, I wrote that paper before the advent and mass promotion of nicotine replacement therapy (NRT), bupropion, or the latest pharmacological hopes in cessation, rimonabant[431] and varenicline[432]. The evidence from clinical trials of these products has always provided cause for optimism, but the acid test is whether widespread access to them in the community has translated into large numbers of extra cessation successes. I also wrote the article before bans on smoking in workplaces became widespread and began causing both widespread cessation[148] and reduced daily consumption[95], as I have described earlier in the book. In this chapter, I will reprise the arguments I ran in the *Lancet* article, considering their merits in today's very different climate. I will consider the hypothesis that in communities where smoking prevalence has fallen to 20% or less, smoking is confined to a "hard core" who are impervious to the sorts of influences that caused millions of smokers to quit when smoking prevalence was much higher, and so who need additional help to quit today.

I will also consider the track records of several other policies and interventions that hold potential to stimulate large numbers to quit: tobacco tax rises, mass-reach quit (advertising) campaigns, quit and win contests, internet-delivered cessation programmes, quitlines, NRT giveaways, physician/primary health care-mediated cessation efforts and dedicated smoking cessation centres, of the sort that have recently proliferated in Britain. Finally, I will consider several interventions and policies that have been advocated within tobacco control circles, designed to prevent the uptake of smoking, including those programmes currently being promoted by tobacco companies.

Avoiding the elephant in the living room

Anyone new to tobacco control research who expects to find major research into the two fundamental "why" and "how" questions posed above will be disappointed. There is relatively little information about the experiences of the millions who have successfully quit unassisted, easily the most common route out of smoking. Instead, the international research literature on smoking cessation is dominated by studies into the characteristics and experiences of people undergoing smoking cessation interventions such as individual therapy, various motivational and support groups, workplace programmes, physicians' cessation counselling, telephone quitlines, and medications such as NRT and bupropion. In short, the research literature is preoccupied by ways of fine-tuning the professionally mediated smoking cessation experience: examining how smokers can be encouraged to do anything but go it alone when they want to quit.

Most research effort is focused on smokers who have tried to quit but who still smoke. There is comparatively little attention focused on what can be learned from the other side of the coin: people who *have* quit. Here there are important questions that are less commonly asked in the smoking cessation literature:

- What is the "natural history" of all this widespread unaided smoking cessation?
- What lessons are there here for stimulating others to emulate such patterns?
- What are smokers' demonstrated preferences for help with smoking cessation?

On the occasions that researchers explore the experiences of people who have made quit attempts without assistance, they almost inevitably draw two conclusions: those who try to quit without assistance have lower success rates than those who are assisted (by almost any means); and that greater efforts should therefore be made to encourage people to seek assistance in quitting. Strangely in all this, sight is lost of the elephant in the living room here: that most ex-smokers quit alone and unaided.

The attitude seems to be one of "smokers who can quit alone will just do it and are not a fruitful focus of study, whereas those who try to stop but later relapse, almost by definition, need assistance". There is no doubt from clinical trials that assistance improves the prospects of successful cessation. But against this, overwhelmingly, people who are quitting elect repeatedly to try to do it alone, with hundreds of millions around the world having succeeded. The virtual silence about this undeniably positive news probably reflects the domination of the field by those whose careers depend on continuing to offer and evaluate labour-intensive regimens, and the influence of the pharmaceutical industry. I have heard drug industry employees casually referring to unassisted, cold turkey cessation as "the enemy", seeing a smoker contemplating quitting without help as a lost marketing opportunity and doing all they can to promote the idea that serious quit attempts should be pharmaceutically assisted.

However, it is critical that in trying to promote cessation, we do not allow the tail to wag the dog; that is, to allow the experience of the minority who undergo labour-intensive mediated smoking cessation to influence how the majority will stop smoking. As described below, only a small proportion of smokers ever become engaged with any form of dedicated smoking cessation service. There is no country where the aggregated successes of such services count for anything significant in population-wide terms.

Quitting smoking is traditionally framed as agonisingly difficult, characterised by sequences of attempts and relapse, and tortured accounts of nicotine craving and "nicotine nostalgia" that can last years. For many, this is definitely how it happens. But again, much of this information derives from study populations who are often drawn from self-selecting populations of cessation intervention attendees. People who seek help to quit may differ in important ways from smokers who want to quit but do not seek help. Conclusions drawn from study populations of people who have sought help are not conclusions that necessarily apply to the experience of most people who have tried to quit or who will later attempt to stop.

Why do people stop smoking?

If tobacco use had not been found to be harmful, tobacco control would have remained where it was for its first few hundred years as essentially a moral crusade against a vice, decried largely by people with religious objections to defiling the "temple" of the body with intoxicants. Today's Niagara of bad news about smoking and health started as a trickle in the 1950s and then began pouring out of research journals throughout subsequent decades; this has always been the principal motive for people to want to stop smoking.

In spite of ever-changing fashions in tobacco control circles for emphasising the many reasons for quitting, health reasons continue to dominate ex-smokers' accounts of why they quit[151,427]. Table 5.2 emphasises that smokers' accounts of *why* they quit typically reflect a synergy between a numbers of factors, as I emphasised in the "day-in-the-life" narrative of a hypothetical smoker in Chapter 2. Over the years, there have been many highly creative ways of proposing to smokers that they smell, pollute the air and endanger others' health, and over the years set light to a small fortune. But "concern for your own current or future health" is mentioned by more than nine in every ten smokers and is so far out ahead of the next most nominated reasons for quitting (expense and concerns about the effect of your smoking on others), that it merits special attention.

So, where do smokers encounter information or influences about the many and varied health risks of tobacco use that turn so many of them to thoughts of quitting? In Chapter 3, I examined the importance of news in conveying

Table 5.2 Reasons given by ex-smokers for quitting. (Source: US COMMIT study of 20 communities, 2001[151].)

Reason	Percent nominating
A. Health related	
Concern for your own current or future health	91.6
Advice from doctor or dentist	49.9
Illness or death of a friend or relative	24.3
B. Social unacceptability	
Concern for the effect of smoke on others	55.7
Setting a good example for children	51.8
Pressure from family, friends or co-workers	46.5
Bad breath, smell or taste	35.7
Smoking restrictions at work	19.5
C. Expense	58.7

information and debate about tobacco to the community, arguing that this was so pervasive and important that it deserved to be taken far more seriously by tobacco control advocates and policy analysts. The other major vehicle for communicating motivating information to large numbers of smokers is through "health scare" campaigns.

Can you scare people out of smoking?[i]

Ever since Janis and Feshbach's influential research on the unproductive use of fear in dental hygiene education in the early 1950s[433], several generations of health educators have uncritically accepted as near holy writ that you should not try to scare people into adopting healthy practices, including smoking prevention and cessation. Evidence from ex-smokers has repeatedly affirmed that personal concern about "scary" health consequences is the primary motivation for smoking cessation and predicts cessation[434], so interesting questions arise about whether this dogma is empirically grounded or whether it reflects a profession–wide neurosis intent on avoiding opprobrium from those who believe it is somehow not "nice" to deal in gory imagery in the name of persuasion[435].

A mass media-led campaign – "Every Cigarette is Doing you Damage" – launched in Australia in June 1997 and since used in over 25 nations, has been seen by many as "the mother of all scare campaigns", described repeatedly as "hard-hitting", "gory" and something smokers will "see once and never forget". To some, the campaign has been seen as something of a health promotion profanity in the wake of previous so-called "positive" practice – campaigns using every manner of wholesome non-smoking role models, and general proselytising about "healthy lifestyles", freshness and so on. The campaign represents the culmination of a painstaking formative research process undertaken in the context of a 1990s stalled decline in smoking prevalence and a historical return to the more hard-hitting Australian campaigns of the early 1980s[436].

The brief to the advertising agency proposed a communication model based on "personal agenda" about smoking. The model was based on the following assumptions:

1   Day-to-day actions of individuals are largely explained by the existence of an unwritten personal agenda with items on it implicitly ranked for importance/urgency and grouped along the following lines: today, tomorrow, sometime soon, if I ever get the chance, when I eventually get around to it.
2   For intentions to become actions they must at least make it to today's agenda.
3   Behaviours (like quitting smoking) that require action over many days and are difficult, require resources and reinforcements external to the individual.

Most smokers "intend" to quit, but clearly for most smokers, for most of the time, quitting is not on today's agenda. Hence, the major communication objective in the brief to the agency was that the campaign should put quitting higher on smokers' personal agendas. The brief listed seven key facilitators of behaviour change. It stated that to potentiate an existing intention, an individual should be stimulated toward some or all of the following. Smokers should:

- gain *fresh insights* on the recommended behaviour;
- reassess the *importance* of the behaviour;
- reassess the *urgency* of carrying out the behaviour;
- reassess the *personal relevance* of the behaviour;
- have confidence in their own *ability* to carry out the behaviour (self-efficacy);
- *remember* or be reminded to do it;
- for long-term change, *gain* more than is lost by carrying out the behaviour (response efficacy).

Further, the campaign should: (a) show the damage of smoking in new insightful ways that are both enlightening ("Now I see what the doctors are on about") and chilling ("I can't bear to think of that happening to me"); and (b) develop a conditioned association between the images of bodily harm and the act of smoking such that those images are evoked when smoking is contemplated or seen. Unlike traffic accidents where people "know" the mechanisms of cause and effect, knowledge of the serious consequences of smoking are known to most smokers only in the abstract. Most know the long-term effects of smoking only because they have been told third-hand what scientists have discovered. People have poor ability to perceive, understand, evaluate and respond to statements about risk[75]. The evidence about smoking is often stated in probabilistic terms, but we know this lets people distort and objectify the hazard, and "exempt" themselves with various rationalisations[48]. Past campaigns may, paradoxically, have been weakened by emphasising how "risky" smoking is. Given that people are more likely to act on the basis of what they experience than what they are told, the communication challenge for this campaign was to translate the scientific knowledge about smoking into "felt" experience, rather than cognitive appreciation of risk.

Because people do not think probabilistically or behave "rationally" in relation to probabilities[437], it was considered that it may be more effective to describe the *certain* consequences of smoking, even if they are less dire than the uncertain ones, such as lung cancer and heart attacks. This was a core rationale behind the content of the campaign as executed.

To convey a doctor's-eye view of the damage caused by smoking, it was felt important to bring the advertising agency's creative team into contact with medical specialists in workshops where the agency pressed relentlessly for images and words that describe disease processes due to smoking, particularly little or unknown aspects. Persistence from the creative team yielded dividends, best exemplified by the cardiologist who said of atherosclerotic damage: "I suppose you could liken a severe case of atherosclerosis to squeezing brie cheese from a toothpaste tube, except it's an artery." And so was born the advertisement known as "aorta", which features fatty deposits (atheroma) being squeezed by a surgeon's gloved hand from a human aorta. Other ads have covered emphysematous damage, the recent discovery of a mechanism by which smoking damages the P53 tumour suppressor gene in lung tissue[438], macular degeneration (blindness)[73], peripheral vascular disease leading to amputation, and oral cancer. Each advertisement brought smokers some compelling "new news" about smoking, but more than this the message was framed in a way to maximise the effect on behaviour.

First, the emphasis was on relatively certain rather than less probable effects. The campaign slogan was: "Every cigarette is doing you damage", with the advertisements focusing upon continuing damage (the things that happen as you smoke now, rather than clinical outcomes). Second, because beliefs about consequences of actions can only determine behaviour if they are salient (top of mind) at the time the behavioural decisions are made, a device was needed to bring these consequences to mind at the time smoking was contemplated. To achieve this, the advertising agency created a journey into the lungs. The viewer travels with the smoke as it is inhaled down the trachea and into the lungs where it begins its deadly work. This scene in each of the advertisements immediately follows a brief typical moment in which the smoker lights up and inhales, ignorant, it seems, of the damage being done.

Fear or threat appeals have great potential for stimulating behavioural change, if used correctly[439–441]. Fear can be dealt with adaptively by a behavioural response that removes the reason to be fearful, such as quitting smoking, or maladaptively by a psychological response meant to dispose of the fear, for example, denying the truth or personal relevance of the message. To maximise the chance of the intended behavioural response, each advertisement carried a Quit Helpline number. Smokers who were stimulated to quit, but wanted assistance, could (and did in large numbers[442,443]) contact a telephone counselling service.

How to fund campaigns

As we will see below, mass-reach public awareness campaigns are an important component of comprehensive tobacco control. But their cost precludes them being run by most low-income nations, where governments still devote most of their relatively meagre public health budgets to communicable and vector-borne disease control priorities. As a result, public awareness of the harms of smoking is typically rudimentary, smoking by doctors often is very prevalent (see Chapter 8), and immediate prospects for improving widespread public awareness of reasons for not smoking remain low.

In such circumstances, the solution that screams out for adoption is the hypothecation of an increment on tobacco tax, whereby the resulting funds are guaranteed by the accompanying legislation to be devoted to funding wide-reaching public awareness anti-smoking campaigns. This model was first developed in Victoria, Australia[444], used to fund the massively financed California[445] and Massachusetts[446] campaigns as well as those in Arizona and Oregon, and has since been adopted by several other governments, including Thailand, Switzerland, Malaysia and Tonga.

How do most people stop smoking?

As mentioned, the research literature on the great majority who quit without any formal help (medication or professional advice) is rather scant, but it is very instructive. In the late 1980s, when the availability of NRT was in its infancy, about 90% of ex-smokers in the USA had used no form of organised cessation programme or assistance: most of these had succeeded by going "cold turkey". Moreover, among smokers who had attempted to quit within the previous 10 years, 47.5% of those who tried to quit alone succeeded while only 23.6% of those who used cessation programmes succeeded[447]. This probably reflects self-selection bias in that people with greater nicotine dependency are likely to perceive themselves as needing help, whereas those with higher self-efficacy (belief in their own ability to quit unaided) just "get on with it". But how much has the widespread promotion and availability of cessation pharmacotherapies changed things? Various studies have reported different levels of increased use.

The US COMMIT study reported on a cohort of 12 435 smokers followed for 13 years between 1988 and 2001. During this time NRT was to emerge as the most heavily promoted approach to smoking cessation ever advocated. In 1993, 35.2% of smokers attempting to quit reported having used some form of medication to stop smoking (but not necessarily that they succeeded). This proportion increased to 52.3% by 2001. The report did not give success rates by method used[151].

In 1996 in California, a study of 4480 smokers who had attempted to quit, found that 19.9% had used some form of assistance, up from 7.9% in 1986, and that 12-month abstinence rates were 15.2% in those who had sought assistance and 7% among those who had tried to quit unaided[448]. Shu-Hong Zhu, the study's lead author, provided me with unpublished data for those respondents who reported a minimum of 12 months abstinence using each approach (data column 3, Table 5.3). Extrapolated to a population of one million smokers attempting to quit, this would mean that 26 330 people would still be not smoking when

Table 5.3 Estimated cessation rates and numbers at 12 months in a population of 1 million smokers attempting to quit (extrapolated from Zhu et al.[448]).

Method	Percent using	Number using in 1 million smokers trying to quit	Percent quit at 12 months	Number quit at 12 months
Unassisted	77.9	779 000	7	54 530
Using self-help materials	3.0	30 000	16	4 800
Total without professional help	80.9	809 000		59 330
Counselling	3.1	31 000	15	4 650
NRT without counselling	13.6	136 000	14	19 040
Counselling plus NRT	2.4	24 000	11	2 640
Total with professional help	5.5	55 000		26 330
Total		1 000 000		85 660

followed-up a year later after being assisted by a professional, compared with 59 330 who had sought to quit unaided – more than double the number. Moreover, if we consider those who quit for more than 12 months using NRT without the addition of special counselling to have also largely self-managed their own cessation, then those who quit for at least 12 months after receiving counselling (*n* = 7290) constitute only 9.3% of long-term quitters.

Such "yield" data need to be factored into cost-effectiveness planning on how to maximise the number making quit attempts and balanced against the temptation to simply pour more resources into those methods with higher success *rates*.

In 2000 in the USA, only 1.3% of smokers who had quit for at least a day in the previous year had used any form of behavioural intervention, group or booklet, compared with 21.7% who had used pharmacotherapy.[449]

Efficacy of unassisted cessation

Self-managed, help-free cessation remains the most common way that smokers use to quit. But how efficacious is trying to quit alone? A meta-analysis of the abstinence rates observed in 14 different studies of smokers researched in primary health settings who had received either no cessation intervention or usual care (typically, brief advice to quit) found the estimated rate of stopping smoking without intervention, over an average 10-month period, was 7.3%[364]. A later Swedish study reported an identical figure[450]. This estimate provides a baseline to judge the effects of other smoking-cessation interventions; hence, for every 100 smokers, just over seven will not be smoking 10 months later without having received any cessation intervention.

A significant number of these will later relapse, even after 6 months' abstinence[451], while some will never again start smoking. Of course, the same applies for any method of cessation. The net effect of all aggregated efforts at cessation, taking relapse into consideration, is that a country like the UK sees a "background" quit rate of about 1% a year[452] (although this seems to have increased in the UK – see

Tocque et al.[453]). Hughes and colleagues reviewed the available prospective studies literature (where cohorts of smokers were followed to examine outcome) on how likely it would be that an unassisted smoker would quit at a given attempt, lamenting the paucity of studies in the research literature on this fundamental question. They concluded that 3–5% achieve prolonged abstinence[150] and that because about 50% of people who have ever smoked quit permanently at some point, on average it takes a smoker 10–14 attempts finally to stop (although they recognise that many will succeed after fewer attempts).

So anything better than 3–7% continuous abstinence after 10 months might be thought of as progress. But, recalling the yield data in Table 5.3, we need to consider questions of efficiency: which policies on cessation will generate *most* successful quitters, and at what marginal cost utility?

The UK smoking cessation experience

Since a major report, *Smoking Kills*, was published in 1998 outlining the case for government support of cessation, the UK has seen the world's biggest ever per capita injection of funding into the cessation area. Table 5.4 shows recent expenditure by the UK government on this venture.

The UK's expenditure is heavily focused on dedicated smoking cessation centres, requiring attendance at individual or group counselling sessions. A 2005 report examining the contribution of this massive programme to meeting a target national smoking prevalence of 21% by the year 2010, stated:

> contribution to the [21% target] is not being achieved effectively in areas where the number of smokers is highest. These areas . . . will require additional funding to meet the national target . . . Nationally, stop smoking achieved a reduction in prevalence of 0.51% in 2003/04. If persisting up to 2010, this success rate would lead to a reduction in prevalence of 3.6% – i.e. from the current level of 26% to 22.4%. For stop smoking service alone to meet the

Table 5.4 Expenditure (£ million) on the UK government's treatment and quit campaign, England, 1999–2006. Sources: ASH UK[454]; G. Tunbridge, UK Department of Health.

Year	Stop smoking services	NRT	Bupropion	All treatment	Mass campaigns	Total	Ratio campaigns to treatment
1999–2000	5	0.142	–	5.142	6.18	11.322	1:0.83
2000–01	21.5	0.931	14.7	37.131	8.97	46.101	1:4.14
2001–02	24.7	21.7	7.3	53.7	7.79	61.49	1:7.89
2002–03	24.7	25.6	4.7	55	7.88	62.88	1:7.98
2003–04	36.2	32.5	4.5	73.2	17.76	90.96	1:5.12
2004–05	46.8	40.9	5.2	93.2	25	118.2	1:4.73
2005–06	52.0	43.5	4.6	100.1	23	123.1	1:5.35
Total	210.9	165.273	41	317.37	96.58	514.05	1:532

target of 21%, in England the number of successful quitters each year would need to be 50% greater.

However, in a remarkably understated next paragraph, the report continues:

> since successful quitting [in these calculations] is measured by a self-report at 4 weeks and only 25% of smokers remain quit at 12 months . . . all the estimates of reduction in prevalence calculated in this report *could legitimately be divided by four* [my emphasis] – producing an overall reduction of 0.13% per year or around 1% (from 26% to 25%) by 2010 for England.[453]

The above statement that "only 25% of smokers remain quit at 12 months" also contrasts with a published evaluation of the programme's cessation rate where, after one year, one in seven (14.6%) of smokers who had attended the English tobacco treatment services were still not smoking[455]. In 2005, Milne[456] examined the use of government-supported smoking cessation services in two English regions with the highest numbers of smokers using such services. Comparable with the above caveat, he calculated an annual reduction in smoking prevalence in the region attributable to the cessation services of 0.12%, (a figure corrected later by others as 0.15%[457], whereas the background quit rate was 1.5–2%, 10 to 13 times higher.

Thus, the expenditure data in Table 5.4 show that the UK government is currently spending 2.26 times more on treatment services than on efforts to motivate cessation, while the impact of these services contributes between 10 and 16.7 times less to reducing smoking in the UK than the background quit rate in the community.

These figures show that unprecedented funding of smoking cessation services across a whole country will help a considerable number of people to quit permanently, but will do virtually nothing to reduce smoking prevalence, yet again illustrating the difference between a clinical and population health perspective.

Cost-effectiveness

Advocates for dedicated smoking cessation services emphatically promote their importance as a component of a comprehensive approach to tobacco control, never as a substitute for it. They argue that these cessation interventions are among the most cost-effective clinical interventions known to medicine, and therefore should be fully supported by government by the same logic that is advanced to support any cost-effective intervention in medicine. They point to favourable cost-benefit comparisons between other routine therapeutic interventions in medicine, arguing that "this is a bargain". For example, Parrott et al. calculated that the most intensive smoking cessation services would cost £873 per life gained[458], compared with a median cost of £17 000 for 310 different medical interventions[459]. Advocates invoke pejorative imperatives about the injustice of denying smokers effective treatment, and analogies with humanistic treatment budgets for narcotic users. They often concede that while the contribution of such interventions to reducing smoking in whole communities might be negligible, wealthy nations can afford both[422]. It is hard to argue against this and my call 22 years ago for such clinics to be "abandoned" seems churlish and dispassionate today, in the case of affluent nations like the UK.

But nonetheless there remain huge dangers in all this. First, health officials in poor nations with relatively homeopathic levels of tobacco control funding risk being mesmerised by the "bricks and mortar" attractions of tangible cessation service facilities, so favoured by politicians and so affordable in wealthy nations like the UK and USA. It would be tragic if models like this became enshrined as serious best-practice strategy for tackling smoking in nations where smoking prevalence remains stratospheric and mass-reach smoking cessation campaigns almost non-existent. The embrace of individual-oriented smoking cessation programmes, like QuitAssist[460] by Philip Morris, underscores the irrelevance of such approaches in seriously promoting cessation.

Second, while affluent nations might well be able to "afford both", the UK ratio of expenditure on mass campaigns versus smoking cessation services and pharmaco-therapies shows how distorting the imperatives of the rule of rescue[15] can become. Five times more has been spent on assisting cessation than on trying to encourage more smokers to make quit attempts, and instil in them the confidence to do so. In Australia and Canada two decades of quit campaigns see smoking prevalence today about 10 years ahead of where the UK is today. Economic evaluations of the cost-effectiveness of various smoking cessation strategies often fail to consider self-directed cessation[17] and the effectiveness of mass media efforts that stimulate this. Clinical practice guidelines on cessation tend to define the role of the primary health care worker (PHCW; e.g. doctors, nurses, dentists) in cessation entirely as what they do when coming face to face with a smoker, and in doing so limit the PHCW's sense of personal relevancy in advocacy processes that would see more resources put into efforts capable of significantly reducing use. In most nations, there is a desperate need for advocacy for mass-reach campaigns far more than for assisted cessation centres.

Zhu has demonstrated that "For the annual cessation rate in a given population an increase in quit attempts matters more than the same level of increase in the use of help"[461]. He argues that "any promotion that makes smokers feel that they cannot quit smoking without treatment can be potentially harmful" at the population level and that campaigns should put more energy into promoting quit attempts.

Role of the pharmaceutical industry

No analysis of contemporary smoking cessation can avoid considering the huge role of the pharmaceutical industry. The industry-supported Pinney & Associates in Washington DC estimates that the current global sales of NRT plus other prescribed medications are worth between $1.5 and $2 billion, with the prescription sector comprising about 10–15%. "Big Pharma" is the juggernaut of contemporary tobacco control, responsible for placing more messages about quitting in front of smokers than those from any other source. Recently in the USA, the average person saw 10.37 pharmaceutical cessation advertisements per month compared with 3.25 government and NGO ads[462]. While industry policy has never shifted from one of providing products to assist people trying to quit (as opposed to overtly proposing that smokers should consider quitting) their advertising messages directed to quitting contemplators are also seen by many smokers who are not currently considering quitting. Bit by bit, this "normalises" cessation and it becomes harder for smokers to avoid seeing that there is a lot of it happening out there, and that maybe they should consider quitting too.

Before NRT went over the counter (OTC) without prescription, Big Pharma had armies of drug salespeople visiting physicians, plying them with information and samples. Now that it has gone OTC in many nations, every second pharmacy has prominent in-store advertising material for NRT products, and the products are advertised direct to consumers in peak viewing times, soaking up advertising budgets that most public and NGO sector agencies could only dream of. Prescription-only smoking cessation drugs like bupropion are not allowed to be advertised to the public except in the USA and New Zealand, but even when the advertising is restricted to physicians, the industry's public affairs strategies ensure than that there is abundant news and commentary out there about these products. Collectively, all this adds up to an unparalleled number of smoking cessation messages circulating in communities.

Recent research suggests that many[463] – even a majority[464] – of smokers make quit attempts without any conscious planning attempts, and that these attempts have a greater chance of succeeding than those that are planned, creating some rather fundamental problems for the "stages of change" orthodoxy that has dominated theorising on cessation. Constant exposure to discourse about quitting via news, advertising and everyday conversations about cessation fuels this momentum.

But there is an important downside to the dominance of quit-through-medication messages. It has been a long time since any smoker heard a message suggesting that they might quit unassisted, like the great majority of ex-smokers have done. This produces an entirely distorted and potentially *disabling* message about smoking cessation, which is under constant pressure to be defined as a process that is entirely commodified and serviced by professionals.

Has NRT accelerated cessation in whole populations?

So what impact has nearly 20 years of NRT had on smoking prevalence? Cummings and Hyland recently reviewed the evidence on the impact of NRT in the USA[465]. Clinical trials of the various forms of NRT show that the products increase quit rates by about 1.5- to 2-fold that of placebo, regardless of setting or use of adjunct treatments. When NRT moves from prescription-only access to over-the-counter availability, sales jump by up to 250% in the first year[466], with eight studies showing that the efficacy of OTC use compares well with NRT obtained via prescription[467].

Given this, we might expect that proliferating use of NRT would be associated with increasing rates of cessation in whole communities, but according to

Cumming and Hyland, this has not happened. They summarise that: "Time series analyses of national cigarette consumption and NRT sales from 1976 to 1998 suggest that sales of NRT were associated with a modest decrease in cigarette consumption immediately following the introduction of the prescription nicotine patch in 1992[468]. However, no statistically significant effect was observed after 1996, when the patch and gum became available OTC . . . annual quit rates as well as age-specific quit ratios remained stable."[469] Similar conclusions were reached for the state of Massachusetts[470] and California[471], although the Zhu et al. study cited above[448] (see Table 5.3) shows that more than one in four smokers in California who quit for more than 12 months used NRT.

So why have clinical trials so consistently shown benefit while community studies have not? Clinical trials see participants subjected to often extraordinarily "unreal" conditions. Trialists, unlike those quitting in real-world settings, do not have to pay for their medication, reflect on several questionnaires, have their urine, blood or saliva, or expired carbon monoxide regularly checked, undergo physical check-ups or receive reminder phone calls. All of this creates higher levels of compliance, which exaggerate the effectiveness of drugs in trial conditions. Other suggestions are that many community NRT users do not use the product long enough, and simply not enough people are using it to demonstrate a population-wide effect. Many smokers regard NRT as too expensive and potentially unsafe[472]. Another hypothesis is that widespread awareness about the availability of stop-smoking medication may have caused a "boomerang" effect whereby many smokers might delay quit attempts, believing that medication will be available to "do the trick" at a later date when they are ready[473].

Should cessation be subsidised?

In most industrialised nations, a 3-month supply of NRT costs about half as much as a year's expenditure on smoking, whereas in developing countries, where cigarettes are much cheaper, 3 months' NRT can cost as much as 1 year's (and to up to 7 years', in the case of Indonesia) supply of cigarettes, placing them totally out of the reach of all but the wealthy[474]. NRT would thus seem to be largely irrelevant to population-wide cessation in most poor nations.

In addition to the UK experience described above, there have been several major trials of providing free NRT to large numbers of smokers. In New Zealand, all smokers consuming more than ten cigarettes a day are entitled to receive a course of NRT, for which they are charged only a small dispensing fee. About 41 000 smokers from a national smoker population of 740 000 take up the offer each year, with 70% reporting that they complete the 4-week course[475]. An evaluation of the programme, which assumed that a conservative 9% of participants quit for 6–12 months, estimated that there was a net 1.5% increase on the background quit rate, at an estimated cost per quitter of $NZ7120, "a highly cost effective program".[476]

In 2003, the New York State Department of Health provided up to 6 weeks supply of NRT gum or patches to 40 090 smokers, at a cost of $2.7 million[477]. Twelve months later, the 7-day non-smoking prevalence rate for those who received the NRT was 1.78 times higher than the quit rate among a comparable group of callers to the New York Quitline who did not receive NRT[478].

The strong demand for subsidized NRT products demonstrated in such campaigns and the highly cost-effective outcomes, strongly suggest that for many smokers, despite cigarettes costing far more than NRT in many wealthier nations, price may well be a psychological barrier to cessation. NRT giveaways deserve far more research attention than they have to date received.

Are today's smokers "hardened"?

It is often said that in nations with several decades of tobacco control policy and programmes behind them, today's smokers are more "hard core", having remained impervious to everything that has been thrown at them through public policy measures, scare campaigns and anything else. These smokers are said to be either intractably resistant to wanting to quit or so dependent that they have been repeatedly unable to stop. If this were shown to be true, important implications might arise for changing emphasis more towards intensively targeted programmes of assistance for these hard core smokers, and easing off broader population-wide efforts at promoting cessation. The seminal review of the evidence for hardening in the US smoker population by Warner and Burns[422] found "little evidence that the population of smokers as a whole" was hardening; that population-wide cessation rates have not decreased and smoking prevalence again continues to fall after stalling in the early 1990s; that the average number of cigarettes smoked per day has fallen in recent years by about 20%; and that "truly hard-core smokers necessarily constitute a very small fraction of the population". Importantly, they noted that in California and Massachusetts, which for a time ran well-funded mass-reach programmes, prevalence fell more rapidly than in other states (see below). In Chapter 8, I will summarise evidence from several nations on the question of how low smoking prevalence might fall, but it will suffice to say here that in all nations, there remains huge scope for lowering smoking prevalence and frequency before population-wide approaches become unacceptably inefficient.

Warner and Burns' analysis should be read thoroughly by anyone tempted to believe that quit campaigns have somehow exhausted their potential and that countries that have run them for several decades are now down to a hard core of smokers who will only change with intensive help. This is not the case and is a myth that needs squashing whenever it is raised.

Price, tax and cessation

There is a large research literature examining the influence of price on tobacco consumption. Overall, this shows a figure of around −0.4 for price elasticity[479], meaning that an increase in retail price of 10% causes reduced demand of 4% in high-income countries and up to 9% in low-income nations[480], effected through both reduced consumption and quitting. Young people, having low disposable income, are particularly responsive to price[481]. Tax increases are the most cost-effective intervention known, with a recent study concluding that raising the real price of cigarettes by 10% worldwide through tax hikes would prevent between 5 and 16 million tobacco-related deaths, and could cost a remarkably low $US3–70 per disability-adjusted life year (DALY) saved in low-income and middle-income regions[482]. The World Bank's report on the economic case for tobacco control, including tax policy, is an ideal summary of this research[3].

Tobacco industry documents[483] repeatedly reach the same conclusion:

- **1983:** "The most certain way to reduce consumption is through price"[484]
- **1985:** "Of all the concerns, there is one – taxation – that alarms us the most. While marketing restrictions and [restrictions on] public and passive smoking do depress volume, in our experience taxation depresses it much more severely . . . It has historically been the area to which we have devoted most resources and for the foreseeable future, I think things will stay that way almost everywhere."[485]
- **1993:** "A high cigarette price, more than any other cigarette attribute, has the most dramatic impact on the share of the quitting population."[486]

For all the plain lessons for tobacco control in this, concerns are sometimes expressed that advocacy to raise the price of cigarettes ought to be tempered because of its regressive impact on addicted low-income earners whose continuing expenditure on tobacco will erode their ability to buy other things, including essentials like food. While the poor are more responsive to price rises than those who are more well off[487], many poor smokers obviously continue smoking in the face of price rises[488]. But *as a group*, poor smokers will reduce their consumption when price rises.

Those counselling that we should keep cigarettes more affordable to the poor by not advocating tax rises are in effect arguing for a policy that will increase use. Tobacco control should be wary of efforts to make it a sacrificial lamb to wider government policy on inequitable income distribution – something that deserves the attention of all in public health. All commodities are less affordable to low-income earners, so steps artificially to restrain price rises of just one commodity, which will cause increased use and consequent harm, is a perverse way of trying to be compassionate to the poor. Concerns about the poor being "harmed" by high tobacco prices, when lower prices will harm them just as certainly, are best addressed by advocacy to make the quitting choice more compelling and easier for low-income groups by having quit aids more affordable (as described above).

Raising prices can introduce other changes in consumer behaviour. In the UK, where tobacco prices are the highest in the world, there has been an unprecedented drift towards cheaper hand-rolled tobacco. In 1990–91, 18% of men and 2% of women smoked hand-rolled cigarettes. By 2004–05 this had increased to 34% and 14%[489], with half of men in the lowest socioeconomic group hand-rolling their cigarettes. Such developments need to be monitored so that taxation schedules are periodically revised to prevent hand-rolling tobacco becoming so obviously more attractive.

Similarly, in developing nations where black market, smuggled and counterfeit cigarettes are common, high prices can see consumers turn more to illicit products. More efforts are needed to expose tobacco industry participation in smuggling[490], its dealings with the criminals involved, and the damage to national tax receipts. Collaborative efforts with packaging companies to design counterfeit-proof packaging (including marks on cigarettes themselves) will also be critical. This is a relatively neglected issue in tobacco control, but is of vital importance in preventing the erosion of the impact of price policy. In 2000, an estimated 6% of all global cigarette sales (318 billion sticks) were smuggled[491].

Cessation in response to mass-reach media campaigns

Between 1967 and 1970 the USA saw a large number of anti-smoking television advertisements broadcast as a result of a court ruling on the fairness doctrine, which required that balance be demonstrated on what was broadcast about controversial issues. This was at a time when tobacco control as we know it today was far less developed, with basic pack warnings and routine news coverage being the main ways that Americans would have encountered anti-smoking messages. The impact of the broadcast ads was therefore less confounded than occurs in many studies today, where it is difficult to tease out the specific effects of campaigns from all other tobacco control inputs that often occur simultaneously. The founder of ASH USA, John Banzhaff, had argued successfully that because cigarette smoking was a controversial issue, advertising for cigarettes should be balanced with anti-smoking advertising. This intense period of anti-smoking advertising was followed by a substantial increase in cessation rates of both men and women, across all age and racial groups[156]. The industry secretly volunteered to remove its advertising if Congress would exempt it from antitrust action for collusion. Congress refused, instead passing the Public Health Cigarette Smoking Act of 1969, which banned broadcast advertising of cigarettes[492]. This resulted in the withdrawal of the requirement that the anti-smoking advertisements needed to be run, and cessation rates levelled off or actually declined[493].

Since that time there have been many large-scale, mass-reach anti-smoking campaigns run in many different nations. Hard–hitting, sustained media campaigns rank with tax rises, smokefree laws and advertising bans as causes of tobacco industry apoplexy. The industry has a long history of attacking any campaign or policy that its sales intelligence shows is biting its bottom line. Attacks on campaigns in the form of legal challenges, massively increased expenditure on advertising and political donations, and funding third-party attacks have occurred in Australia[64] and the USA, where the Californian[494], Massachusetts[495] and the American Legacy Truth campaigns[496] have been targeted.

Several generations of Australian campaigns[436,497] have driven down smoking prevalence. Perhaps the most-researched campaigns have been those in California and Massachusetts in the 1990s, reviewed by Siegel[498]. Smoking prevalence in the USA was falling at a rate of about 0.8% per year prior to the commencement of the Californian campaign in 1999. In California this decline accelerated to 1.1% between

1989 and 1993, with the rest of the USA falling at about 0.6% during that period. However, in the later phase of the Californian campaign, when the tobacco industry increased its advertising, these declines ceased[499]. Econometric analysis of the relative impact of the media campaign and price showed that 21% of the overall reduction in consumption in California during 1990–92 was based on the media campaign. Sales of cigarettes were reduced by 819 million packs (or 27.3 pack per capita) from the third quarter of 1990 through the fourth quarter of 1992 because of an additional 25-cent state tax increase, while the anti-smoking media campaign reduced cigarette sales by 232 million packs during the same period[500].

In Massachusetts, a similar experience occurred. Prior to the campaign, which commenced in the early 1990s, adult smoking prevalence had been declining in the state at the same rate as 41 comparison states, but while the campaign ran (1992–99) prevalence declined by 0.43% per year, while increasing in the comparison states by 0.03% each year[446].

Cessation effected through interventions of primary health-care workers

In 1979, Michael Russell published a landmark paper[501] in which he concluded that if every British general practitioner (GP) were to offer brief cessation advice to every smoking patient, about 25 of each GP's patients would quit permanently. He concluded that if every British GP were to do this, it would generate 500 000 quitters a year, equivalent to the yield that would be generated by opening 10 000 smoking cessation clinics. The paper inspired global interest in the potential to have primary health-care workers (PHCWs) routinely raise smoking cessation with all smoking patients. Asking about smoking status and then following up with advice on quitting should be as routine as gathering information on age, weight and blood pressure in any medical consultation.

Since that time, a massive amount of work has gone into researching how to increase PHCWs' engagement with smokers, particularly through the development and promotion of clinical practice guidelines and the activities of the pharmaceutical industry in developing prescribable smoking cessation therapies. Nearly 30 years on, the picture that has emerged is decidedly depressing.

A decade after the Russell paper, a study of the detection of smokers by 50 randomly selected GPs in Australia found that they identified only 56.2% of their smoking patients – a just better than chance result. Smokers with a smoking-related disease fared better (65% were identified) but only 41% of smokers aged under 30 were detected[502]. By the late 1990s, only 34% of Australian GPs provided advice to quit in every consultation with smokers – probably an optimistic figure, given the 27% non-response rate to the study[503].

Even among GPs who have been motivated enough to attend a training programme on smoking cessation, smoker recruitment rates can be appallingly low. Of 38 Australian GPs who had attended workshops on the use of a programme and were contacted 12 months later to find out what use they had made of the programme, only 18 had recruited smokers to the programme. These 18 doctors had recruited 121 smokers in 12 months: just 7% of all their patients who smoked.

The authors concluded that "Limited health-promotional funds may be deployed better in general community awareness and mass-media programs"[504].

Similarly depressing findings were reported in a British study from the early 1990s of patients' recall of advice: only 47% of smokers with a history of cardiovascular disease had received advice on smoking – a less than chance result. In true British understatement, the authors concluded that the "low rate of lifestyle advice reported by patients implies that more preventive advice could be provided in primary care"[505].

Most recently in Great Britain, despite huge government commitment to support smoking cessation implemented from 1998, a national study showed that the proportion of smokers who recalled receiving any advice on smoking from any health professional between 1996 and 2002 fell from 46% to 42%. In 2002, 36% of British smokers had sought some form of advice or help for their smoking[506].

In the USA, in 1992–93, 54.7% of smokers (n = 19.63 million) who saw a doctor in the previous year were advised to quit. By 1995–96, this number had increased to 59.2% (n = 20.5 million). Physician advice was calculated to produce about 189 000 additional quit successes, if the odds ratio (1:3) from clinical trials of minimal physician advice was assumed[156] – something for which there is poor evidence in "real life".

However, the 2000 US National Institutes of Health Monograph that reviewed population impacts of various smoking cessation approaches concluded of physician interventions: "it is not clear that additional resources would add to the number of individuals encountering these interventions . . . the promise of these interventions as established in clinical trials is not fulfilled in their real-world applications."[156] As mentioned, the pharmaceutical industry has a large sales force who visit doctors and are highly trained in ways of "getting to" doctors about their products, including smoking cessation drugs like bupropion. Public sector initiatives aimed at getting doctors to focus on cessation need to demonstrate why their far more modestly funded efforts have any real hope of significantly improving on what the pharmaceutical industry has been trying to do for many years.

Telephone quitlines

Telephone quitlines are an increasingly popular way of delivering support and advice to people wanting to quit. There is a large body of research on quitlines and whether different ways of providing support can better lead to higher rates of cessation and relapse prevention[507]. In Australia, all cigarette packs show the national smoking cessation quitline number; every tobacco retailer is obliged by law to display prominently a sign showing the quitline number; and every quit smoking advertisement run by the federal and state governments ends with the quitline number. I know of no other country where such widespread publicity is given to quitlines. Yet in spite of this, in a one-year period when an intensive national quit campaign was run, only 3.6% of adult Australian smokers made the small effort to call the quitline[443]. This lengthy experience in an environment strongly supported by publicity (often demystifying the process of calling the quitline by showing how unthreatening and supportive the experience of phoning will be), is a telling reminder that the great majority of smokers do not appear to be interested in receiving *any* form of assistance.

This small proportion (3.6%) nonetheless translates into large numbers of smokers. Quitlines remain highly cost effective[508] ways of attracting large numbers of intending quitters, particularly when they are integrated into hard-hitting motivational TV campaigns, and allow access to free NRT[509].

Internet-based interventions

Increasing interest has been attracted to internet-based interventions because of burgeoning internet access and the convenience this brings. One review described them as "the industrial revolution in smoking cessation programmes", with 7% of US internet users having searched the internet for advice on smoking cessation[510], and there being over 200 sites now operating, most completely unevaluated[511]. A review reported that over half of studies showed no improvement in outcome, with 47% of 19 published studies on internet interventions showing statistically improved outcomes relative to comparison groups[512]. There is no certification of standards for internet cessation programmes and many dubious sites that are little more than product-pushing sites or tobacco industry PR exercises in cyberspace. While their mass-reach potential is plain, little is known about how many smokers would be interested in seriously engaging with such sites, as opposed to surfing them out of curiosity.

Quit and win (Q&W) interventions

These are interventions in which smokers trying to quit enter a draw for a valuable prize. They are great vehicles to publicise cessation and can attract a large number of entrants. Many nations now run these events. While winners whose names are drawn typically have to undergo some sort of verification process to ensure that they were in fact a smoker before they entered (typically, just signing a statement affirming that they are a smoker), the same verification seldom (if ever) occurs with entrants at large. I examined this issue after running a Q&W event in Australia: at least 34% of a sample we interviewed long after the contest had ended admitted to being non-smokers at the time of entry[513], and so, disregarding the clear requirement to sign a verification slip on entry that they were smokers, more than one in three tried to enter deceptively.

Another significant problem in Q&W evaluations is that few research designs examine the question of whether smokers who enter and quit are simply "borrowing from the future" (i.e. are people who are likely to have quit anyway within (say) the next 6 months, and have brought forward the date of the quit attempt[514]. Quitting earlier is a good thing of course, but in considering whether Q&W contests have the ability to increase the quitting population over a year, bringing the date forwards may simply reduce the number who quit later, and over a year there may not be any net gain. Such questions are elementary in considering whether it is worth the effort to set up and run such interventions, yet are rarely considered.

Preventing the uptake of smoking in children

Most smoking starts in childhood or adolescence. It is uncommon for adults who have never smoked as children to start smoking. Efforts to prevent uptake are therefore seen as vital to tobacco control. The traditional vehicles for getting preventive messages to children about smoking are through school and mass media campaigns. School health education curricula have seen an enormous variety of approaches evaluated against outcomes like changes in knowledge, attitudes, intentions not to smoke and smoking itself. Two recent systematic reviews of the research literature on the effectiveness of school-based educational interventions in reducing smoking initiation and prevalence in the long term produced sobering findings.

In one review[515], 94 randomised controlled trials were identified, of which only 23 were in the highest category of rigour. For interventions that focused on "social influences on smoking", half of the most rigorous studies showed that "the intervention group smokes less than those in the control, but many studies failed to detect an effect of the intervention . . . The largest and most rigorous study, the Hutchinson Smoking Prevention Project[516], found no long-term effect of an intensive eight-year program on smoking behaviour". A second review concentrating on sustained effects[517] located 177 studies, of which only eight followed up to age 18 or 12th grade. Only one of these showed decreased smoking prevalence in the intervention group.

This track record provides little confidence that investing heavily in school programmes is a sensible way to reduce smoking in young people. However, more "oblique" approaches do show encouraging results. In Australia, despite the "myth that will not die" that smoking is rising in children, smoking prevalence among the young has been *falling* in all age groups since the mid-1990s, after rising briefly in the early 1990s[518]. This change has not been associated with any significant youth-oriented campaign activity.

The likely reason for the positive change is that youth smoking is being indirectly influenced by falling adult smoking. Because parental and sibling smoking is highly predictive of youth smoking, efforts to increase cessation are likely to impact on youth uptake[519–521]. Similarly, there is evidence from Australia[522] and the USA[523] that children see and respond well to ostensibly adult-targeted mass-reach campaigns. David Hill has eloquently summarised the case for downplaying the emphasis on youth smoking prevention in comprehensive tobacco control campaigns, noting that "elected representatives may get most praise for campaigns their adult electors see as transparently directed at teenagers, yet . . . such campaigns are likely to be the least effective, and they may even be counter-productive. Non-transparent strategies to reduce teenage smoking will need to be sold skilfully to legislators and to the public"[524].

Perhaps the most telling indictment of the ineffectiveness of overtly teen-oriented prevention campaigns is their embrace by tobacco companies[525], which would never support any intervention that undermined their economic future. As R.J. Reynolds' Claude Teague said in 1973: "Realistically, if our Company is to survive and prosper we must get our share of the youth market . . . We need new brands designed to be particularly attractive to the young smoker, while ideally at the same time being appealing to all smokers."[526]

Anodyne "decision-making" school programmes, virtually devoid of any information on why anyone would decide to not smoke, such as the Philip Morris-sponsored "I've got the power" programme, are typical[527]. A BAT advertisement run in Germany a few years ago showed an open pencil case used for storing cigarettes. The copy read "That shouldn't be normal. Dear young people: you can hide the cigarettes as best as possible and refresh your breath with a peppermint, but your parents and your teachers will find out that you smoke. Above all: smoking in the early ages can be quite harmful. Because growth has not been yet completed and because school requirements and education mean a heavy burden for young people. On top of that, smoking with a guilty conscience can never be delightful. And every cigarette that you do not smoke consciously, is one too many."

These sort of lame gestures have been developed by the industry as a cynical public relations strategy designed to show governments and the public their great concern for youth smoking, knowing full well that such initiatives have no impact on their bottom line. As one company representative put it: "This is one of the proposals that we shall initiate to show that we as an industry are doing something about discouraging young people to smoke. This of course is a phony way of showing sincerity as we all well know"[528].

Moreover, the industry's wolf-in-sheep's-clothing strategy on youth smoking allows it, in the name of prevention, to access young people for the ostensive purpose of researching youth smoking prevention while gathering potentially invaluable information about barriers to greater uptake.

Reducing sales to minors

Over the last 15 years, several nations have embraced efforts to reduce the selling of cigarettes to minors by education and law enforcement campaigns involving compliance monitoring of illegal sales to children. The tobacco industry also supports the educational components of such campaigns. The objectives of industry's "It's the law" campaign against selling to children were described internally as "1) to provide an alternative to legislated/mandated policy actions; 2) to improve PM's image regarding the youth issue".[529] No mention was made of the initiative actually reducing youth tobacco *use*.

A 2002 Canadian review of the evidence on whether compliance checking reduces tobacco *use*, as distinct from *sales* to youth, concluded there was "limited evidence" that these efforts reduced youth smoking[530], and Glantz and colleagues have argued powerfully for these programmes to be abandoned[531,532]. The main problem with prevention programs targeting sales to minors is that young people easily obtain their supplies by other means, particularly by using older friends to purchase for them. Many of the studies on youth access prevention have been undertaken in relatively small rural communities where children cannot easily move to the next town to obtain cigarettes when high retailer compliance is achieved in the town where they live. Small communities are much more easily subject to blanket surveillance, and shopkeepers known to be selling to children are more conspicuous and vulnerable to prosecution than are shops in large cities. I know of no large city anywhere in the world where tobacco control workers claim to be able, even remotely, to cause shopkeepers to think that they are highly likely to be "stung" in a compliance monitoring exercise. In nations where the majority of the population live in cities, young people are able to move easily from suburb to suburb.

The main thing in favour of these programmes is that they can generate a lot of news coverage, which is typically very negative about tobacco, and cynical of the tobacco industry's token efforts to reduce sales to kids. These not insubstantial benefits contribute to the climate of negativity about tobacco companies, which lends support to other more effective controls on tobacco.

If we want to draw attention to this issue in a way that has more "upstream" potential, research efforts should be made to calculate the under-age tobacco spend in each country, portioned out by retailer, manufacturer and government share[533]. The results can then be used as a wedge issue to taunt all three sectors to "put their money where their mouth is" and annually hand back all these "unwanted profits" to an independent foundation (completely detached from any tobacco industry membership or influence) that could use the money to run hard-hitting media campaigns that we know can drive smoking down.

Note

i   This section is an edited version of Hill D, Chapman S, Donovan R. The return of scare tactics. *Tob Control* 1998;**7**:5–6.

Chapter 6

The Denormalisation of Smoking

When I started work in tobacco control in the late 1970s in Australia, it was totally normal to see tobacco advertising in every medium imaginable (although direct tobacco advertising on radio and TV had been banned from September 1976). The main international cricket and national football competitions, production car racing and many horse races were sponsored by tobacco companies. Cultural citadels like art galleries, the opera and ballet were awash with money from tobacco-sponsored exhibitions and events. Grateful recipients lined up everywhere to do the tobacco industry's bidding against proposals for advertising bans. Tobacco sponsorship was normal. Today, in Australia and in an increasing number of nations, it is nowhere to be seen.

Before 1987, people smoked uninterrupted in their offices. They lit up cigarettes in restaurants without blinking. When smokers came to your house, some would ask if you minded if they smoked (which in effect meant would you mind if *you* smoked), but many would light up a cigarette with the same nonchalance with which they would pour a drink or pass the olives. Every party you went to was thick with cigarette smoke. If your hotel room had been last occupied by a smoker, you knew it immediately you unlocked the door. Your taxi driver was likely to be smoking when he picked you up and throughout the trip. It was not unusual to see someone in a television studio being interviewed while smoking. Tobacco company chief executives received civic honours from governments as model businessmen. In the early 1960s, 20%–30% of Australian doctors still smoked[534]. Today, only 2% do[535]. Smoking then was entirely normal.

A modern Rip van Winkle waking today from a 35-year sleep would be amazed at the changes that have occurred to differing degrees in dozens of nations. All offices, shops, shopping malls, sports stadia, public transport and, in an ever-growing number of nations, all restaurants and bars are likely to be smokefree. A smoker would no sooner light a cigarette inside your house as brazenly pocket your best cutlery. Instead, they surreptitiously slip outside on the pretext of fetching something from the car or getting some fresh air. Many smokers are embarrassed and most deeply regretful[536] that they smoke.

While everyone else is enjoying food, wine and conversation in a restaurant, smokers are thinking about how they might quietly get outside to stand in the street, sometimes in the cold, wind and rain, to relieve their discomfort from lack of nicotine. At airports smokers are forced to go outside the terminal and stand among the taxi and bus fumes, so that everyone entering sees their desultory, exiled status. They know they are being asked to move away from others because most people think they smell and because normal people do not want to be exposed to their toxic smoke. Some might reflect too, that before the law required them to go outside, many smokers were too self-absorbed to voluntarily decide not to smoke inside places like air terminals, despite over a decade of public debate: others just had to put up with it. Smokers were long presumed to be indifferent to their own health, but smoking had also become a symbol of indifference to others.

At the start of every flight, millions of smokers annually are warned on the aircraft public address system that smoking is banned and not to smoke in the toilet lest they set the plane on fire. Each smoker who contemplates the coming long hours without relief from their nicotine withdrawal must often reflect on just how much they still want to be a smoker. When each flight ends, it is then seen as necessary to remind the smokers that they can't light up until they get to a dedicated smoking room inside the terminal. The message is plain: here are desperate addicts.

The tobacco industry knows what a bad image this smokers' exile gives the public face of smoking, and so lobbied for the construction of smokers' rooms inside airports. The worst of these I've seen are in the Bangkok terminal. Smokers huddle in small glassed-in rooms, thick with acrid smoke and overflowing ashtrays, while other passengers move past freely outside looking in on this pathos. Inside, the smokers have time to reflect yet again on their "otherness", and why they feel compelled to subject themselves to such indignity. Fishbowl smoking rooms are living anti-smoking billboards. Even the more discrete ones I've visited out of curiosity are sullen, out-of-sight places where smokers are directed, away from other travellers. Everyone sitting in them must occasionally pause to reflect: "I'm sitting here in this awful room because I smoke." There can be few smokers who've sat inside such places wondering if they really enjoy smoking. Smokers sometimes say they feel like social lepers. Their analysis has become an accurate one.

A prescient BAT memorandum from 1976 summed up accurately where things were heading: "It seems likely that smoking will become increasingly a socially unacceptable and working-class habit, as it was in the 1860s. 'Men had to indulge in the practice out of doors or else . . . sneak away into the kitchen after the servants had gone to bed and puff up the chimney.' In the 1840s the working classes accounted for 90% of tobacco consumption. A similar trend is setting in at the present time."[537] By 1984, a Philip Morris executive had seen the writing on the wall: "It is our opinion that the single most important issue facing our industry is the erosion of the social acceptability of smoking . . . Today it is probably true to state that even a majority of smokers feel that theirs is an undesirable habit."[538]

Many car manufacturers now make cars without ashtrays or cigarette lighters. Those advertising on dating websites overwhelmingly specify that they are looking for non-smokers[147]. Shared rental accommodation ads request non-smokers more than any other characteristic[146]. Hotels declare whole floors smokefree, and in 2006 the entire Westin hotel chain and the Marriot group in Canada and the USA went smokefree. Holiday guest houses and cabins advertise that guests must not smoke indoors. The list goes on. In many nations today, smoking has become a *remark-able* activity, and the remarks about it are nearly all negative. Smoking in countries with comprehensive tobacco control programmes is rapidly becoming abnormal. If you want to smoke in a public place, you mostly have to do it by yourself or with other smokers, away from others. Smoking is no longer a convivial and integral part of everyday life. In large part, it has become an activity removed from routine human interaction.

The final insult is that in a growing number of nations, smokers today must take their cigarettes out of a pack that might show a colour photo of a gangrenous leg, a frightening looking mouth cancer, a reminder to not harm others around them with their smoke, or a suggestion that the man with the pack may have erectile dysfunction problems (Fig. 6.1). Cigarette packs were once elegant accoutrements of style, but today have their designer boxes desecrated with images that have tested strongly in focus groups to repulse and unsettle smokers. People are used to seeing strong health warnings on household goods like drain cleaning chemicals, rat poison and garden pesticides. But even these don't carry pictures showing damaged alimentary tract organs after ingesting such products. For all the whistling in the dark in which smokers engage ("the warnings have no effect on me whatsoever"), only the most self-deluded smokers must escape questioning what they are doing.

But in the great majority of nations, the picture of smoking painted above is far from true. In France, where I have been living for 5 months writing this book, I've found people to be unfailingly polite and friendly, but many French smokers think nothing about lighting a cigarette next to you in restaurants (although some

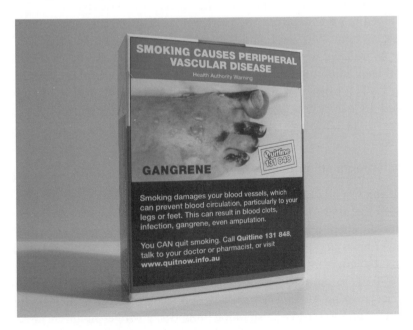

Fig. 6.1   Gangrene caused by peripheral vascular disease, on an Australian pack of cigarettes.

restaurateurs offer a choice of *fumeur* or *non-fumeur* sections). However, the same subversive beginnings that inexorably led to comprehensive smokefree public spaces are already well established in France and in many other nations. You can't smoke on public transport. French restaurants and other indoor spaces will go smokefree at the end of 2007.

Smoking restrictions have caused massive damage to the tobacco industry, not just because of the way they have changed the public face of smoking. When you can't smoke at work, on public transport, in shopping malls, in restaurants, in bars and in an increasing number of private homes[539], times and opportunities for smoking are radically reduced. When workers can't smoke indoors, they step outside to feed their brain's hungry nicotine receptors in a cheerless ritual that is the daily visible antithesis of every promise ever made in a cigarette ad. All-weather smokers outside buildings never make up the number of cigarettes they would otherwise have consumed despite smoking "harder"[45]. The global tobacco industry was quick to see a train wreck of implications in all this. Smoking rapidly moved from being a personal health issue to a very public one where others' actions – for all the protests about their rights – could harm you. As far back as 1979, the US Tobacco Institute predicted that if smoking restrictions caused every smoker to light just one less cigarette a day, 18 billion fewer cigarettes a year would be consumed at a cost to the US industry of $US500 million[540]. That forecast of one less cigarette a day turned out to be hugely conservative. In 1992, an industry insider noted: "Total prohibition of smoking in the workplace strongly affects industry volume. Smokers facing these restrictions consume 11%–15% less than average and quit at a rate that is 84% higher than average . . . Milder workplace restrictions . . . have much less impact on quitting rates and very little effect on consumption . . . If smoking were banned in all workplaces, the industry's average consumption would decline 8.7%–10.1% from 1991 levels and the quitting rate would increase 74%".[155]

Over 25 studies have shown that across 24 hours, smokefree workplaces reduce smokers' daily consumption by about 21%[95], and that workplace bans stimulate quitting[148]. The impact of social unacceptability on smoking has recently been calculated to have about the same impact as raising the price of a pack of cigarettes in the USA by $1.17[541].

The "half-pregnant" principle

Those living in countries where smokefree workplaces are in their infancy should not despair that their own nations are "different" and that such a change can never be achieved. There remain few nations today where there are *no* restrictions on smoking. This is important because once any restrictions have been legislated or regulated by governments, precedents are thereby set for the argument that smoking needs to be restricted. Ordinary people understand that if it is important to ban smoking for office workers to protect their health, then by the same argument, is important to ban smoking around *any* worker in an enclosed environment, including those working in restaurants and bars. This understanding can be usefully termed the "half-pregnant" principle: one cannot be half-pregnant, and attempts to portray such policies as rational and defensible will always be highly vulnerable to ridicule.

The rot set in for public smoking in the early 1970s when evidence emerged that babies whose parents smoked indoors had a greatly increased incidence of respiratory problems[159]. Some died. As if killing babies wasn't enough, over the next 30 years the "bad hair day" for passive smoking turned into decades. In 1981, the first study appeared showing that if you did not smoke and lived with a smoker, you stood a significantly increased chance of getting lung cancer, an uncommon disease in non-smokers[160]. Dozens of similar studies followed, with the evidence spreading to include stroke, heart disease, cot death and asthma.

As the media carried news of more and more studies, governments and employers soon started responding to the resulting public annoyance at being forced to smoke and to a string of workers' compensation cases. Smoking restrictions for enclosed public spaces have been progressively introduced in a growing number of nations as the evidence of the harms of passive smoking accumulates and public preference for smokefree air grows. Even tobacco companies[542] and their legal firms don't allow smoking indoors.

Yet throughout the world, hospitality venues – particularly pubs and bars – have staunchly resisted this momentum, as we saw in Chapter 2. Somehow, pubs and club bars were said to be different. Romanticised as the last bastions of smoking, their representatives stood their ground. Studies of the greatly elevated blood nicotine levels of bar staff came and went[543], as did stratospheric measures of toxic tobacco smoke particles in pub air. This was received as all namby-pamby nonsense by pub industry officials. Reports of the improved respiratory health of Californian bar staff[174] after that state banned smoking in bars in 1998 continue to produce shrugs in nations that still allow smoking in bars.

The immortal "magic line" system of controlling smoke, once favoured on planes, was resurrected for pubs. For a time in Australia, you could not smoke within two metres of a bar, this being deemed sensible to protect bar staff from harm. But at 2.01 metres, the idea was that they can breathe easy. There was the small problem that everyone forgot to tell the smoke it had to keep back. Anyone with an IQ a point higher than it takes to grunt understood that something was very wrong here (Fig. 6.2).

While all other workers breathed smokefree air, the group most exposed and at risk of disease were the last to be protected and told that it was their duty to risk their health as a sort of patriotic duty to the economy. The club and hotel industries fed governments, and an often unblinking media, a diet of empty bars and cataclysmic job losses if smoking were to be banned. That non-smokers outnumber smokers by as much as four to one and that many might go to pubs more if they could come away without a dry-cleaning bill and stinging eyes meant nothing to the leading lights in the pub trade, whose myopic outlook saw only their present smoking customers as their future. Bar workers are a highly casual, largely non-unionised, powerless workforce. Being predominantly young, many smoke themselves. They didn't have to work there, ran the unvoiced neo-Dickensian subtext.

The situation today in many nations is an object lesson in how public health law should not be made. Those *least* exposed – the relatively transient patrons of

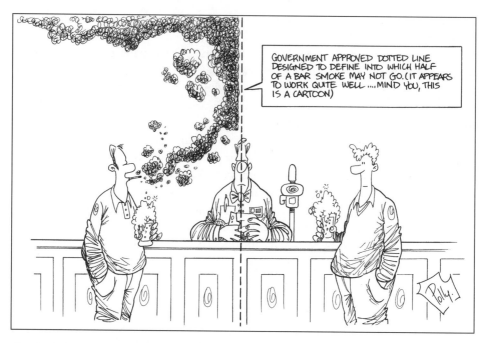

Fig. 6.2 Physics, as understood by some bar owners. Cartoon by John Farmer, Hobart Mercury. Reproduced with permission.

restaurants, public transport, cinemas and shopping malls – have often full legal protection from passive smoking. Yet those *most* exposed – bar and casino staff – are the least protected. In effect, government inaction says to them "we'll protect citizens from passive smoking even when their exposure is brief. But notwithstanding your unparalleled high exposure, we'll offer you no protection". It is unimaginable that workplace health protection could proceed in such a fashion in relation to toxic fumes, loud noise or asbestos.

The values inherent in this occupational health practice are being championed by two interest groups whose contempt for bar staff's occupational health rights is being driven entirely by misguided economics. The tobacco industry has a direct financial interest in discrediting the scientific basis for smoking restrictions, and since the 1980s has spent "vast sums of money to keep the controversy alive"[544], funded dozens of scientists who trivialized the risks, highlighted alleged confounders and promoted ventilation as the solution[177]. Massively funded consultancy programmes designed to attack the science of secondhand smoke (SHS) have been bankrolled by the tobacco industry in the USA[202], Europe[545], Latin America[546] and Asia[136]. In 1995, Philip Morris's global budget for regulatory affairs – mainly to attack restrictions on smoking – was $US91 476 000[547].

Nicotine classrooms

Bars represent much more than a last-ditch stand for the tobacco industry. They are where many graduate from occasional to regular smoking, and are an increasingly exploited venue for sales promotions. A Melbourne study showed that 70% of regular nightclub and bar patrons report smoking more than normally in these settings, and one in four said they would probably quit if smoking was banned in bars[548]. To the tobacco industry, bars are nicotine classrooms where a combination of alcohol and teams of glamorous tobacco company sales staff work to induct and consolidate smoking as an integral part of a good night out. If they lose bars, they lose a key venue for sales promotion.

As we saw in detail in Chapter 2, sections of the hospitality industry have also been prominent in opposing an end to smoking in bars. Their public line is that bans will see customers walk out the door, preferring to drink at home, where they argue many will subject their families to secondhand smoke. This argument of course seeks to have it both ways, in acknowledging that secondhand smoke can harm families, but implying that it doesn't really, which is why it is acceptable to expose bar staff. Perhaps the most bizarre argument is one recently advanced by BAT in Australia, which in 2006 argued that smokers risked having their drinks spiked with drugs when they went outside on the footpath to smoke[414].

Industry funding of "fuming bar owner" groups in the USA[181] has generated a reliable stream of PR-driven anecdotes about the commercial ruination of bars caused by anti-smoking zealotry, but these are not borne out by dozens of studies using before-and-after ban sales tax data[175], which show either no downturn in bar custom or small increases. Most telling of all, an internal Philip Morris document states "the economic arguments often used by the industry to scare off smoking ban activity were no longer working, if indeed they ever did. These arguments simply had no credibility with the public, which isn't surprising when you consider that our dire predictions in the past rarely came true."[549]

Nexus with gambling

If smoking bans don't stop smokers from going to pubs, and are likely to encourage the return of many non-smokers who stayed away because of the smoke, how do we explain the attitude of bar owners opposing bans? Why would they oppose something that all evidence indicates is of economic benefit? In part it is likely to be simple fear of change, predictable through game theory[550] and mirroring the nervousness of airlines and restaurants, which hesitated unnecessarily for years before taking the painless plunge.

A more complicated answer is that most of the studies about the economic effects of smoking bans have occurred in the USA, where except for Las Vegas, bars do not have gaming machines. The Australian National Institute of Economic and Industry Research has found that smokers spend $A30.29 per capita per session on gambling compared with $A13.93 for non-smokers[551]. Day and night, pub owners observe what a 2003 market research report produced for Victorian gaming interest group, Tattersalls, concluded, namely that "Smoking is a powerful re-inforcement for the trance-inducing rituals associated with gambling"[551]. Smoking gamblers can sit for hours at "their" machine, privately convinced that the next press of the button will change their life. In the worst cases, they can urinate in their seats rather than risk taking a break. To force smoking gamblers to take a break to go outside to smoke would break the gambling trance and trigger many to reconsider their gambling. Fresh air might cool gamblers down, prompting many to consider their gambling and tempting players to "go home rather than play on".

Smoking bans have not closed restaurants, affected international travel volume or caused the end of civilisation as we know it. Tobacco companies oppose smoking bans because they eat away seriously at the number of cigarettes consumed. Their arguments about lost business for others are, by their own internal admissions, absolute nonsense. A hundred years ago, bars had spittoons and often absorbent sawdust on the floor. While one patron was drinking, another would be spitting. Concerns about expectoration spreading tuberculosis saw spitting relegated to bathrooms[2]. Unlike the situation with tobacco, there was no spitting industry fulminating about spitters' rights. Historians of public health are likely to view the present period as a shamefully protracted endgame in the demise of public smoking.

When policy moves beyond evidence: banning smoking outdoors

The movement towards smokefree indoor air has been propelled by the mounting evidence that tobacco smoke concentration inside places where many smokers congregate poses a health risk. Almost all of the studies that have established this risk have examined many years of exposure, by looking at non-smoking spousal exposure to a partner's smoking in residential settings. Collectively, these studies have established that chronic exposure to SHS poses significant health risks. In 2003, the International Agency for Research in Cancer concluded that environmental tobacco smoke was carcinogenic to humans[277]. In 2006, the US Surgeon General concluded:

- Children exposed to secondhand smoke are at an increased risk for sudden infant death syndrome (SIDS), acute respiratory infections, ear problems and more severe asthma. Smoking by parents causes respiratory symptoms and slows lung growth in their children.
- Exposure of adults to secondhand smoke has immediate adverse effects on the cardiovascular system and causes coronary heart disease and lung cancer.
- The scientific evidence indicates that there is no risk-free level of exposure to secondhand smoke[552].

This last summary point, on "no risk-free level of exposure", is supported by evidence of acute cardiovascular and respiratory effects, as well as evidence about DNA damage from exposure to tobacco smoke. The most recent review of this evidence can be found online in the 2006 Surgeon General's report[553]. Jim Repace summarised nicely the transition of acute exposure to chronic risk in a recent post to Globalink:

> The problem with short-term exposures to SHS is that the damage is both immediate and cumulative. A lot of little short-term exposures – in front of

buildings, on sidewalks, at parties, in "non-smoking" sections of restaurants, in a Saturday-night visit to a nightclub, at a wedding – all add up to increased risk. For some people, at some point, it tips over. DNA damage is cumulative and may lead to cancers; blood clotting and arterial wall damage is [sic] cumulative and may lead to thrombosis or ischemia; irritation of the respiratory lining for an asthmatic is immediate and will trigger pain and increase swelling of respiratory epithelium and damage ciliary cleaning and kill macrophages. So although [sic] we all suffer through or ignore these daily insults so we can get about our quotidian existence, it is something to be discouraged, by custom, and by law if necessary.

The evidence has opened up several major policy debates about protecting people from even transitory exposure to tobacco smoke. These include proposals to ban smoking in various outdoor settings such as in alfresco (outdoor) dining settings, sports stadia, beaches and parks, where many people congregate. At the most extreme end of the debate it is proposed that employers are additionally justified in not hiring smokers because their smell, on returning inside a workplace after smoking, allegedly represents a health hazard. This argument has been seriously advanced by several people in an international tobacco control forum, following intense debate about the World Health Organization's 2005 policy announcement that it would no longer hire smokers. The World Health Organization's website states: "Smokers and other tobacco users will not be recruited by WHO as and from 1 December 2005. This policy should be seen in the context of the Organization's credibility in promoting the principle of a tobacco-free environment."

For all the importance of controls on secondhand smoke denormalising smoking and reducing consumption, I strongly believe that some of these developments threaten to undermine public support for rational tobacco control, and below I explore the questions arising from these issues.

Banning smoking outdoors?[i]

Smoking is banned in many outdoor sports stadia, and indeed the 2006 World Cup in Germany attracted controversy because the German government refused to ban smoking in the stadia. Crowd close-ups often showed smoking. The case for banning smoking in stadia is clear-cut. The close proximity of people, seated together for sometimes many hours during long-lasting games like cricket, tennis and baseball, makes exposure to secondhand smoke significant and causes significant reduction in amenity for the majority who don't smoke. A non-smoker cannot move away from a smoker, given seating restrictions, and while unenclosed stadia are outdoors, on still days the presence of smoke is very intrusive.

Smoking in outdoor dining areas of restaurants presents new policy challenges that have arisen following indoor restaurant smoking bans. Smokers now often ask for a table outdoors, thereby concentrating outdoor dining areas with smokers. Particularly in warm climates, outdoor dining areas are in high demand, so the question arises whether it is fair that smokers should be given preferential access to "the best seats" in such restaurants, an unintended consequence of banning smoking indoors. In crowded alfresco situations, people smoking all around you can cause considerable exposure. For this reason, some local authorities are now extending smoking bans in restaurants to embrace outdoor areas. This seems very reasonable to me.

However, proposals to ban smoking in other outdoor settings are far more controversial. Australian hospitals are proposing to extend their indoor smoking bans to outdoor hospital grounds. In 1996, the mayor of Friendship Heights in Maryland, USA, sought to ban smoking in municipal parks and on sidewalks. A leading non-smokers' rights advocate in Sydney attracted publicity for his proposal to take civil action to have his suburban tennis club ban smoking in outdoor spectator areas, typically occupied by a handful of people waiting for courts to become vacant. In Kerala and Goa in India, smoking is banned in public spaces such as beaches, and transgressors face fines[554].

Such proposals "push the envelope" of tobacco control into areas where important questions need to be asked to ensure tobacco control policies are firmly anchored to both scientific evidence and principles of proportionality. According to Mullender, "Proportionality specifies that the state can impose a burden on an individual (or group) if the following two conditions can be satisfied. First, the state must be pursuing a goal that is in the interests of all members of the relevant society. Secondly, the relevant burden must be no greater than is necessary in order for the goal to be effectively pursued[ii]. This description of proportionality reveals it to be a mediating principle. It provides guidance on how to (seek to) accommodate (a) the interests of persons generally and (b) the interests of individuals (or groups) in circumstances where they clash."[555]

The application of the proportionality principle to restrictions on public smoking is most challenging when seeking to ensure that the imposition of restrictions on where smoking can occur is "no greater than is necessary in order for the goal [of doing all that is reasonable to eliminate unwanted exposure to SHS] to be effectively pursued". Moving from the main concern to make non-smoking the norm in all enclosed public spaces (and those like stadia where many people are concentrated in very crowded outdoor areas), some now want the debate to address relatively homeopathic levels of exposures encountered such as when passing a smoker in the street, sunbathing a metre or so away from a smoker on a beach, or standing near a smoker in a park.

Proposals to ban smoking outdoors especially concern those who value the freedom of individuals to do what they please to the extent that this does not harm others[60]. They invite consideration of whether zero tolerance of public exposure to toxic agents is a reasonable policy for civil societies and whether the loudly proclaimed exquisite sensitivities of a small minority should ever drive public policy, which affects everyone.

Further, calls for outdoor bans invite us to reflect on the extent to which these policies risk alienating a large number of people who might otherwise be supportive of efforts to reduce SHS exposure in situations where there is significant risk or reduced amenity. In short, we need to ask whether efforts to prevent people smoking outdoors risk besmirching tobacco control advocates as the embodiment of intolerant, paternalistic busybodies who, not content at protecting their own health, want to force smokers to not smoke even in circumstances where the effects of their smoking on others are immeasurably small. Such alienation may undermine support for other tobacco policies that, if implemented, could bring important public health benefits to communities.

Why should smokers not be allowed to smoke in hospital grounds or other designated outdoor locations, well away from any reasonable prospect of harming (as distinct from visually offending) anyone? Advocates for outdoor bans advance a number of arguments, each of which raise significant ethical concerns. I will now rehearse their arguments, comment on why I believe they are ethically unsustainable, and conclude that there is justification for banning smoking in outdoor settings only in circumstances where exposure is sustained and significant, such as in crowded stadia.

"Any exposure to SHS is harmful"

At the heart of this debate is the question of at what level of acute exposure might SHS reasonably be deemed to be harmful. Exposure to SHS in healthy young adults has been shown to be associated with dose-related impairment of endothelium-dependent dilatation, suggesting early arterial damage[556], which appears to be only partially reversible in those who subsequently avoid exposure to SHS[557]. This study involved healthy young non-smokers who had been exposed to an average of one hour of SHS per day for the previous 3 years. However, the transitory exposure to others' smoking in open outdoor settings is not remotely comparable with that experienced in confined indoor settings such as were involved in the study cited above.

Risk perception research shows that the risks individuals declare unacceptable are not necessarily those that have a high probability of a serious adverse outcome[558]. Equally, people are often prepared to take risks that have high probabilities of negative outcomes. Of all the factors that have been identified as tending to increase public outrage, risks that are imposed rather than voluntary explain much of the variance in public perceptions[559]. SHS represents a quintessential imposed risk and, together with the thought of dreaded outcomes (like lung cancer), often incites public demand for zero exposure. This explains why many get incensed about exposure to a mere whiff of tobacco smoke, but will not hesitate to sit around a romantic smoky campfire where they will, by choice, be exposed to a large range and volume of carcinogenic and toxic particulates and gases.

The question thus remains whether zero tolerance of SHS throughout communities is reasonable public policy. The answer to this question can only be guided by science. Science could attempt to quantify the health consequences of brief outdoor exposures and it would seem certain that for some rare individuals with exquisite sensitivity, an acute exposure at such a level might precipitate an adverse event. Similar claims are sometimes made about a large range of environmental agents, but in general public policy is not based on cocooning such people from exposures that are inconsequential to nearly everyone, by introducing laws that interfere with the liberty of many to protect the very few.

It is correct to say that there is "no safe level of exposure" to tobacco carcinogens, but equally there is "no safe level of exposure" to *any* carcinogen from any source. Social policy rarely proceeds on the basis of zero tolerance, because the cost of totally eliminating every nanogram of exposure would be impossibly high. All smoke (from any source) contains carcinogens, lung irritants, and a whole variety of toxicants. There is nothing magic or unique about tobacco carcinogens that some-how makes them so much worse than carcinogens from all other sources. It is the sheer volume of lifelong dosing/exposure to which smokers and passive smokers are exposed that causes the huge health problem. Societies introduce policies to *minimise* smoke (banning log or coal fires in some cities; emission control – not elimination – devices on cars; fitting exhaust fans over grills in restaurants). These measures greatly reduce, but do not eliminate exposure. The idea that public health policy could ever totally eliminate all exposure to SHS would effectively entail banning smoking. I will explore this further below when I consider the WHO's policy of refusing to employ smokers.

"Outdoor bans send an 'important message' to the community"

Proponents of outdoor bans sometimes argue that such policies send an import-ant "message" to communities that smoking is inconsistent with the sort of healthy environments that health-care facility directors might wish to promote. I've heard it argued that because smoking is not permitted anywhere on school grounds, hospitals ought to set a similar example.

However, schools are different to hospitals. Children do not have the same legal rights or autonomy as adults because they are not regarded as mature enough to make decisions such as choosing not to go to school, to buy alcohol or tobacco, own firearms or drive with safety. School authorities ban smoking by teachers on school grounds because of the important exemplar role teachers have in relation to children. Such rules sometimes apply as conditions of employment in a hospital (such as requiring that health-care staff should not smoke within sight of patients or visitors, just as some employers require, for image reasons, that their staff observe dress standards, do not smoke on duty and so on). I fully support health-care policies that require staff not to smoke while at work and in sight of patients. But outdoor smoking does not harm staff or other patients, and because health-care workers do not employ or somehow control patients and their visitors, there can be no justification for requiring them not to smoke outdoors.

If any message is sent to the community by an outdoor smoking ban, it may well be one that says health policymakers do not care about evidence of harm, but are more concerned to impose standards cut loose from any evidence base and indifferent to a vital ethical principle of respect for autonomy.

"Other freedoms are curtailed in hospitals . . . why not smoking too?"

Some argue that we do not allow patients to go outdoors to drink alcohol or use illicit drugs. All patients already voluntarily forgo many freedoms while in hospital, such as sexual activity. Why then should we allow them to go out to smoke?

When alcohol is restricted in hospitals it is because of the risk of anti-social intoxication. In fact, it is not uncommon to allow patients to drink alcohol with a meal while in hospital. Narcotic-dependent people may be prescribed legal narcotics such as methadone in an attempt to control their cravings and allow treatment for other presenting problems. It is unlikely that there is ever any formal ban on sexual activity in hospitals. That sexual activity does not occur much is due to patients mostly not feeling sexually attuned while ill, and also the lack of privacy. However, the real point here is why "forgoing freedoms" should be construed as virtuous and an argument for adding further restrictions. I would argue that hospitals should rather strive to create an atmosphere that while respecting the rights of others to a healthy and peaceful environment, allows as many normal freedoms as possible for often distressed and dying patients and their visitors. This could include allowing visitors and patients to smoke in outdoor settings, provided these are away from high-traffic hospital entrances or walkways.

"An enforced ban will be good for people's health"

It is argued that patients would benefit by taking a break from smoking as a necessary part of their admission. Even a temporary period of restriction on smoking may improve a patient's prognosis and shorten their length of stay. In a publicly funded health system, there are obligations on patients not unnecessarily to complicate their recovery. They should therefore expect to not to smoke at all while in hospital.

Restrictions on smoking certainly do reduce smoking frequency and may also promote cessation. However, while this is an undoubted positive benefit, it cannot be used as a front end justification to restrict smoking. It is a fortunate by-product of bans introduced because of Millean-based concerns about stopping smokers harming others. The decision to bring benefit to oneself is a decision that should be up to the individual, not for others to impose.

Health-care workers have a duty to offer assistance to those patients who want to quit (and to try to *persuade* them). But there are some smokers who do not want to stop. When they are in hospital, they should not forfeit their rights to smoke if they want to, as long as they are not inflicting their smoking on others. If they are too disabled to get themselves outside to smoke, it would be a callous sort of health care that would say "you might want to smoke, but we so disapprove of it, we will not lift a finger to help you".

"Escorting patients outside can cause staff shortages leading to patient neglect"

If, when there are staff shortages or a generally low staff : patient ratio, staff need to escort incapacitated patients outdoors to smoke, this could cause neglect of patients remaining on wards. Also, if staff were to leave such patients alone while the latter smoked outdoors, liability might arise if, for example, the patient fell or had a coronary event.

This is an argument that should be irrelevant to the smoking status of the patients escorted outdoors. Most hospitals allow, when time permits, staff to escort patients outdoors to get fresh air, sunshine and a change of scenery. Such attention to patient well-being is regarded as compassionate. While such assistance to patients is not a "right", if we exorcised every aspect of patient care down to the level of allowing only those that were "rights", a stay in hospital would be an even more dehumanising experience than it often already is. If such practices endanger patients who remain inside, the issue of absences per se should be addressed and not confounded by arguing that for some patients the reasons for going outdoors with them are somehow more compelling than for others. Similarly, if there are risks in leaving patients unattended outdoors, such risks obviously exist for patients regardless of their smoking status.

"Escort staff will be exposed to patients' SHS"

If staff have to remain near an incapacitated patient who is taken outside to smoke, this may force them to be exposed to SHS, which violates their occupational health and safety rights. The level of SHS exposure a nurse would encounter in an out-door setting while escorting a smoking patient would be minimal. If downwind of the plume, the nurse could move upwind, and so on. Concern about such levels of exposure borders on fumophobia. Nurses would be daily exposed to far greater risks from infectious diseases, despite infection control protocols.

"Any form of air pollution should be stopped"

There have been several attempts to quantify the contribution of cigarette smoke to air pollution. For example, Sanner estimated that a pack-a-day smoker pollutes the air with the same amount of mutagenic substances as when driving 35 km (22 miles) in a car fitted with a catalytic converter[560]. This startling conclusion appears counter-intuitive, not least because the carcinogen benzene has been used to replace lead additives in fuel so that the fuel can be used in catalytic converters. However, former ASH UK director Clive Bates has pointed out that tobacco use is probably carbon neutral on a global level. Whatever carbon is put into the atmosphere from a burn-ing cigarette, equivalent carbon is sequestered during tobacco growing as tobacco leaf fixes carbon from the air through photosynthesis. In a stable market, for each cigarette smoked, there is a tobacco leaf growing to produce the next cigarette. Non-carbon greenhouse emissions from tobacco burning, such as oxides of nitrogen and methane, are likely to be minute in the global scheme of greenhouse emissions.

Conclusions

A minority of people in tobacco control do not like to even *see* people smoking. Australian non-smokers' rights activist Brian McBride wrote to some of his colleagues about outdoor smoking: "We must be prepared to fight the aesthetics and personal standards argument as well as the health argument, and that is what I intend to do. We should not underestimate the public awareness value of having smokers found guilty of negligent actions in all situations indoors or outdoors. The more cases we run the better."

I would argue that the two need to be kept thoroughly apart. Mixing "aesthetics" arguments with health arguments risks infecting tobacco control with the accusation that it is fundamentally the province of people with capricious authoritarian proclivities, caring little for the scientific bedrock on which public health ought to stand.

Health promotion campaigns have often sought to portray smoking in ways different to those typically portrayed in tobacco advertising: smoking has been framed as desperate, disgusting and slovenly. Don't such efforts also appeal to aesthetic rather than health concerns? Yes, but for my own part, I am comfortable with portrayals that seek to counterbalance the distortions of tobacco advertising with alternative definitions of the reality of smoking. If a tobacco company can describe a carcinogenic product as "fresh", I am comfortable in countering that kissing a smoker is like licking an ashtray.

The world is full of people who do not like the "aesthetics" of others of different religions, race, sexual expression, modes of dress or music. Too often these doctrines have found expression in paternalistic or downright oppressive régimes. We do not need authoritarian doctrines in tobacco control.

The "smoker-free" workplace: banning smokers from workplaces

I once taunted the chairman of British American Tobacco Australia in a letter to a newspaper because he had let it be known that he did not smoke. I argued "While the male head of a lingerie company would not be expected to 'choose' to wear women's underwear, smoking is a choice open to all. It is scarcely imaginable that the chairman of Ford would drive a Toyota or the head of the Meat Marketing Board would be a vegetarian. Such lack of personal confidence in their products would probably see them not long in their jobs. The tobacco industry does not seem to mind such an irony."

Some jest that smoking should be compulsory for all tobacco industry executives, but should the reverse ever be made to apply: that employers could choose to insist on smoker-free workplaces? Employers can oblige their staff to wear uniforms and conform to dress codes and address customers with repeated inanities like "not a problem" or sundry company greetings. In an increasing number of nations, workers cannot smoke in indoor work settings. But should employers be able to go further and insist that a worker cannot be a smoker, even if they only smoke after hours? This is exactly what the World Health Organization announced in 2005 as its policy for hiring new staff.

Smokers have been repeatedly shown to have higher workplace absenteeism than non-smokers[561]. In many workplaces, smokers take additional breaks to smoke outside[562], and there is no evidence that these breaks somehow supercharge their subsequent productivity, causing compensatory boosts. Smoking breaks can also cause deep resentment among non-smokers, who see colleagues being "rewarded" for their smoking.

Discriminating against smokers

Against this background, talk of policies to allow employers to discriminate against the hiring of smokers is understandable. But is it justifiable? When running a cancer control agency, Nigel Gray introduced a policy not to hire smokers, reasoning that smoking employees sent an unacceptable message to the community his agency served[563].

Because you can often smell smokers, and see their packs bulging from shirt pockets or peeping from handbags, it is reasonable to assume that a clandestine smoker working for a cancer control agency will sooner or later be revealed as such. Few smokers smoke in total secret. Their friends and families know they smoke, and know where they work. Word gets around. A smoking cancer control advocate walks the thin ice of public hypocrisy that could conceivably undermine the reputation of their agency. Nigel Gray would presumably have the same understandable reservations in hiring a deeply tanned white person to work in skin cancer education, or mammogram and Pap smear refuseniks to spearhead these campaigns.

So I would support Gray in his policy of not hiring smokers in cancer control, as I would if the WHO had wished simply not to hire smokers in its front-line tobacco control section. But I am convinced that to extend such a policy to the wider community – into employment situations where smoking was quite irrelevant – would be unethical.

Gray advances two arguments for such an extension: employers' rights to optimise their selection of staff (smokers are likely to take more sick leave and breaks); and enlightened paternalism ("tough love"). The first argument fails because while it is true that smokers as a class are less productive through their absences, many smokers do not take extra sick leave or smoking breaks. Discriminating against smokers as a group would be like allowing employers not to hire women of child-bearing age because they might get pregnant or take more time off work to look after sick children. This would be grossly unfair to women who did not intend to have children.

But what about paternalism? There are some acts where governments decide that the exercise of free will is so dangerous that individuals should be protected from their poor judgments in their own best interests. Mandatory seat belt and motorcycle crash helmets are good examples. Goodin's famous essay on the ethics of smoking[58] argues that we do not allow someone to knowingly drink a glass of cholera-infected water, assuming such behaviour must indicate mental incapacity. Gray argues that his spectre of "quit or reduce your chances of employment" is founded on similar enlightened paternalism. I think the comparisons are questionable.

Seat belt and helmet laws represent trivial intrusions on liberty and cannot be compared with demands to stop smoking, something that many smokers would wish to continue doing. By the same paternalist precepts, employers might consult insurance company premiums on all dangerous leisure activities, draw up a check list and interrogate employees as to whether they engaged in dangerous sports, rode motorcycles, or even voted for conservative politics[564,565]. Many would find this an odious development that diminished tolerance. There is not much of a step from arguing that smokers should not be employed (in anything but tobacco companies), to arguing that they should be prosecuted for their own good. Smokefree workplaces can act as incentives to cessation. But the quitting effect of smokefree workplaces depends on a choice by those who decide to quit.

WHO's mission is far wider than reducing the health toll from tobacco. Should the WHO bar anyone who is overweight or obese from employment, lest it send the wrong message? Or anyone who has a sedentary lifestyle, for the same reasons? What about someone who is known occasionally to drink excessively? And, why, precisely should a smoker working for WHO in its polio eradication programme be shown the door? The WHO is saying that it doesn't matter if you are the most dedicated, energetic, creative expert control agent for (e.g.) Ebola virus, or the world's best logistical analyst for controlling malaria or fertility: if you smoke, WHO doesn't want you. The late Professor Fred Hollows was an Australian ophthalmologist[566] whose work saved the sight of literally hundreds of thousands of the world's poorest and most illiterate people. He was seldom seen without his pipe. I once asked him to consider quitting and make a statement about the contribution of smoking to macular degeneration, but he declined. The WHO would today refuse to hire a smoker like Professor Hollows.

Some argue that workplace policies do not accommodate alcoholics or narcotics addicts, by allowing them to have drinking or injecting breaks, so nicotine addicts should be no different. The big difference between alcohol/drugs and smoking is intoxication: employers reasonably don't want to employ people who are dangerous on the job, who fall asleep and, in the case of narcotics, are highly likely to be engaged in serious criminal activity to pay for their supplies. I'm not aware of any research showing that smokers are less productive workers than non-smokers (in situations where they are not allowed to take special smoking breaks). Smokers who smoke away from work don't endanger anyone but themselves.

Those who support this policy because they want to stop smokers from harming themselves are presumably benevolently motivated: they feel this policy is for smokers' own good. But such benevolence should extend to all avoidable causes of death, not just those caused by smoking, because if this was not the case, the WHO policy advocates would be nothing but single-issue moralists who cared about a cancer death from smoking, but not one from say, sun exposure.

Exquisite sensitivity

As mentioned earlier, in a protracted debate about the WHO policy on Globalink, some argued that WHO was justified in its actions because smokers after smoking outside would return into the building "off gassing" (as one person called it), the smell of tobacco smoke in their breath and on their clothing. A recent paper measured the "washout time" of exhaled particles measuring 0.3–1.0 μm, finding the mean time to be a mere 59 seconds, after which no exhaled particles could be detected[567].

Besides thus being a largely imaginary phenomenon, the reductio *ad absurdum* of fearing that smoker's breath after smoking is dangerous is that we should not allow smokers to attend cinemas or theatres, travel on buses or trains, stand in queues, attend sporting events, or perhaps even walk past us in the street because some might find the experience of being near them intolerable. Talk of smokers' breath and clothes being endangering will lead the proponents of this position into truly frightening policy obligations. Next they will be asking employees to declare that they will no longer associate with smokers, because they might come to work with trace levels of smoke in their clothing. Perhaps WHO employees should be asked to divorce their smoking wives and agree to hand their smoking children over to state-run de-smoking camps because they might cause their parents to turn up to work smelling of smoke.

By the same argument, people who are allergic to cats should have a similar right to insist that fellow employees who have cats in their homes should be fired from their jobs because they come to work in clothes bearing animal hairs that can cause reactions. Allergic reactions can be very distressing and sometimes deadly serious. The prevalence of allergic reaction to cats is very common (17% of the US population according to one study[568]). So by the same logic that some argue that smokers should be turned away from employment, consistency would demand that cat owners should be sacked.

No one disputes that smokers returning to buildings after smoking outside can smell of tobacco. Equally, non-smokers who live with smokers or who have been with smokers, have plainly detectable smoke in their hair and clothing. So to be consistent, if WHO or any employer wished to ban the hiring of smokers on the grounds that some suggest (toxic emissions from their breath and clothing), then they would need also to screen prospective employees and ask "do you live with any smokers?", "do you associate with any smokers in enclosed spaces?", "do you promise never to do either of these two things, because our policy is that you should not ever come to work off-gassing any detectable volatile organic compounds from tobacco because there are some people who are hypersensitive to it?"

The absurdity of such a policy should be self-evident, and I'm amazed that we have to even debate it. Plainly, there is a scientific debate to be had about what levels of exposure require a protective policy response. At one extreme one might posit almost homeopathic levels of exposure in an office containing a social smoker who smokes only outside work and does not take smoke breaks. Somewhere in between is where the contested area falls: policy predicated on zero exposure is a nonsense because of the traces that almost anyone will have on them from transitory exposure.

Another role for science is in determining the extent to which people claiming sensitivity to the point of nausea and other significant symptoms after being exposed to a smoker's breath or clothing may be exhibiting some form of psychological morbidity. Some of the literature on multiple chemical sensitivity is instructive here.

Multiple chemical sensitivity (MCS), or idiopathic environmental intolerance (IEI), is defined as an acquired disorder with multiple recurrent symptoms associated with environmental chemicals occurring in low concentrations that are well tolerated by the majority of people. Sufferers' symptoms are not explained by any known psychiatric or somatic disorder. One study of 264 patients at an out-patient department for environmental medicine who sought help for MCS or IEI, found that 75% of those presenting "met DSM-IV [*Diagnostic and Statistical Manual of Mental Disorders*, 4th edition] criteria for at least one psychiatric disorder and 35% of all patients suffered from somatoform disorders. Other frequent diagnoses were affective and anxiety disorders, and dependence or substance abuse. In 39% a psychiatric disorder, in 23% a somatic condition and in 19% a combination of the two were considered to provide sufficient explanation of the symptoms. Toxic chemicals were regarded as the most probable cause in only five cases."[569]

The above findings will naturally be passionately contested by people who say they are badly affected by the smallest, fleeting exposure to smoke. They will deeply resent being labelled as having some form of psychological problem. But no frank discussion of this phenomenon can deem such concerns to be off-limits.

Notes

i   This section is an edited adaptation of Chapman S. Banning smoking outdoors is seldom ethically justifiable. *Tob Control* 2000;**9**(1):95–7.

ii For a definition of the proportionality principle, see case 11/70 *Internationale Handelsgesellschaft* (1970) ECR 1125, 1146.

Chapter 7

Vector Control: Controlling the Tobacco Industry and its Promotions

In July 2006, Swiss tobacco control activist Pascal Diethelm sent a congratulatory email to Globalink about the British Parliament having passed clean-sweep indoor air legislation. He wrote: "I trust that the Health Act 2006 will join the ranks of British political achievements and have its place in history right next to Benjamin Disraeli's Public Health Act of 1875, which made drinkable water accessible to all British citizens. It's ironic to think that one had to wait over 130 years before the citizens of the same country could be granted access to breathable air at the work-place and in public establishments. But perhaps this can be explained by the fact that, in 1875, there was no 'fetid water' lobby."

There most certainly is, however, a pro-tobacco lobby. The tobacco industry is the major vector for tobacco-caused disease: the force responsible for getting hundreds of millions of tobacco users each year to want tobacco products and to put them in their mouths. The tobacco industry's fiduciary duty to its shareholders to maximise returns on their investments unavoidably means that the objectives of the industry and of the tobacco control agencies are diametrically opposed. When people stop smoking, reduce consumption or never start, the industry is legally obliged under corporate law to do all it can to reverse the net effect of these trends if they are eroding profitability, the corollary being that if tobacco control succeeds, the tobacco industry's economic health suffers.

A large and vitally important part of contemporary tobacco control practice thus seeks to weaken the tobacco industry, and the organisations and individuals who act for it through what it calls its "third party strategy". This is not some gratuitous undergraduate exercise in striking out at big business and its errand boys in academia, but a broad tactical response to decades of seeing the industry consistently doing all it can to oppose effective tobacco control. Over the years, this has seen the industry working with lawyers, apparently independent technical and professional associations, researchers and academics, educators and many other groups and individuals carefully selected for their willingness strategically to assist the industry. Tobacco control advocacy involves destroying the veneer of independence, by making transparent both these relationships and the "made to order" research reports they produce[570].

Nations with declining smoking prevalence are used to seeing seemingly para-doxical reports about record industry profitability. This is mostly explained by internal efficiencies (more efficient manufacturing processes, vertically integrated marketing innovations, etc.) and by increased population growth and demographic transitions, despite falling smoking prevalence. But company annual reports, while salivating about the potential of less developed nations, invariably contain euphemistically worded allusions to the tobacco industry being on the decline in many industrialised countries.

With some outstanding exceptions (most notably Thailand, South Africa and most recently India), less developed nations have poorly developed tobacco control programmes. But the size of the tobacco-using populations in low- and middle-income nations already far exceeds those in high-income nations. The future of the industry lies in nations with large and growing populations, poorly developed tobacco control policies and a low prevalence of "informed consumers" – the industry's pet notion.

Exporting lessons

The industry is very aware that a domino effect has long operated in global tobacco control. Developments are rapidly shared with other nations through both tobacco control activists and at senior ministerial level. Despite being a relatively small nation, Australia has long been in the vanguard of international tobacco control, as internal industry documents often make plain:

- "Australia has one of the best organised, best financed, most politically savvy and well connected anti-smoking movements in the world. They are aggressive and have been able to use the levers of power very effectively to propose and pass draconian legislation . . . The implications of Australian anti-smoking activity are significant outside Australia because Australia serves as a seedbed for anti-smoking programs around the world."[571]
- "In Australasia . . . we have perhaps the most virulent and nasty-edged anti-tobacco lobbies to be found anywhere in the world. There is nothing less than a battle raging in Australia and New Zealand, and all the guns are out, on both sides . . . they have seen it all down there, and there is more of that to come. It is a bear garden. It is a zoo, and aggression, political in-fighting, dirty tricks by the opposition, and all manner of hassle and public argument is a feature of the business in Australasia."[572]

In 1994, British American Tobacco (BAT) named Australia as one of six nations that were "driving tobacco control"[404] and in 1997 R.J. Reynolds referred to likely regulatory developments in the USA as "an outgrowth of what was put in place in other countries", naming Australia[573]. In 2001, I was leaked a BAT Australia staff training DVD. The marketing director, David Crowe, intoned: "Australia is one of the darkest markets in the world . . . it probably is the darkest . . . ourselves and Canada fight every month for who's got the darkest conditions to do tobacco manufacturing and marketing. And one of the things we can offer the world is what we do best, which is how to work, maximize, proactively drive our market position in a market that's completely dark. Now that takes a different skill set . . . a different type of learning. We need to export that . . . we know we have a lot of expatriates who come down to Australia for learning . . . they can come here and learn these techniques and take them back to Europe or Latin America or to the United States or to Africa."

Advertising bans

Article 13 of the WHO's Framework Convention on Tobacco Control (FCTC) requires each nation ratifying the Convention to "in accordance with its constitution or constitutional principles, undertake a comprehensive ban of all tobacco advertising, promotion and sponsorship". This needs to occur within 5 years after entry into force of this Convention.

Nations whose constitutional principles preclude such bans (this mostly means the USA, which at the time of writing has not ratified the FCTC) "shall apply restrictions on all tobacco advertising, promotion and sponsorship". As a minimum, each party shall "prohibit all forms of tobacco advertising, promotion and sponsorship that promote a tobacco product by any means that are false, misleading or deceptive or likely to create an erroneous impression about its characteristics, health effects, hazards or emissions; restrict the use of direct or indirect incentives that encourage the purchase of tobacco products by the public"[347].

In this chapter, after briefly describing the size of the global tobacco industry, I will examine how it continues to promote its products to consumers in nations with comprehensive advertising bans. Over the next few years, because many other nations will become "dark markets" like Australia and Canada because of the above provisions of the FCTC, the tobacco industry will move increasingly into what is referred to as "guerrilla", "dark", "stealth" or "below the line" marketing, all devious, ambiguously legal means of promoting smoking. These unorthodox forms of marketing need to be anticipated, monitored and above all challenged. The tobacco industry is like the Black Knight in the Monty Python movie *Monty Python and the Holy Grail*. The famous scene where the Black Knight loses one arm, then another, then a leg and then another, only to fight on calling out "It's only a flesh wound!", mirrors the indefatigable efforts of the industry to keep promoting its products after advertising bans.

I will give particular attention to nascent moves to ban or restrict scenes of smoking in movies, as I regard this as a dangerous development that threatens the credibility of tobacco control in civil society. I will also consider the ways in which the industry has engaged in global efforts at "rebirthing" – attempting to redefine itself as an ethical, responsible industry unfairly deserving of stringent controls and its pariah reputation as a "merchant of death". This activity is calculated as a cynical exercise in slowing effective tobacco control. Finally, I will turn to the volatile issue of the importance of keeping the tobacco industry away from the academic community, which it prizes as among its most important scalps.

Dimensions of the tobacco industry

The global tobacco industry is a major economic force, although it is only a fraction of the size of industries like oil, mining, retail, tourism, banking and automobiles.

Table 7.1   2005 cigarette volume, global share and market capitalisation

Company	Cigarette volume (billion)	Global share	Market capitalisation ($US billion)	Operating income ($US billion)[a]	Fortune 500 rank in 2006
Chinese National Tobacco Corporation (China)	1933	35.8	Not traded	NA	–
Philip Morris (USA)[b]	1003	18.6	100.6	11.9	62 (Altria)
Larger BAT (UK)[c]	910	16.9	64.3	6.6	390
BAT (UK)[c]	678	12.6	46.8	4.2	–
Reynolds American (USA)[c]	110	2.0	8.2	1.5	–
Imperial & Virginia Sultan Tobacco[c]	93	1.7	8.2	0.7	–
Japan Tobacco (Japan/USA)	415	7.7	27.9	2.6	365
Imperial Tobacco (UK)	175	3.2	21.5	2.1	–
Gallaher	174	3.2	9.8	1.1	–
Altadis (Spain)	129	2.4	12.0	1.3	429
Korea Tobacco & Ginseng Corp (Korea)	89	1.6	7.2	0.7	–
Gudang Garam (Indonesia)	60	1.1	2.3	0.3	–
Eastern Tobacco (Egypt)	59	1.1	1.4	0.1	–
United States Tobacco	–	–	6.7	0.9	
Swedish Match	–	–	3.6	0.4	
Total	5400	100	257.4	27.9	

All data provided by Jonathan Fell, tobacco analyst, Deutsche Bank, London. Volume is for calendar year 2005. Market capitalisation (MC) as at 31 December 2005.

[a]Operating income data are before tax and before interest. For Philip Morris, the figure is just the tobacco figure. BAT operating income does not include any associate income.
[b]Philip Morris data are only for tobacco, not other Altria products (total Altria MC was $154.6 billion, less $46.2 billion for stake in Kraft and $7.8 billion for holding in SABMiller).
[c]The $46.8 billion BAT MC is the core BAT MC, including its stakes in its affiliates. The portions of MCs in these associates that BAT does not own have been added to calculate a "Larger BAT" MC, which is BAT's own MC plus the additional value of the associates not already included in BAT's own MC.

Table 7.1 shows its major players in 2005. In terms of cigarette volume, the Chinese National Tobacco Corporation (CNTC) is almost double the size of the runner-up, Philip Morris, the tobacco division of Altria. In December 2005, The CNTC entered into a joint venture with Philip Morris International (PMI) involving PMI distributing *Marlboro* in China and the CNTC offering consumers "a comprehensive portfolio of Chinese heritage brands globally, [and] expand[ing] the export of tobacco products and tobacco materials from China"[574].

Promoting tobacco use after advertising bans

Historically, the standard advertising media used to promote smoking have been TV, radio, cinema, print, billboards and other outdoor media (e.g. shopfronts, taxis and other mobile media). With the advent of tobacco control, the typical pattern of erosion sees either voluntary industry withdrawal or government legislation banning advertising, first via radio and television, followed by incremental bites into the remaining media, typically lasting at least a decade. Extensive sponsorship of mass appeal sport and strategically selected cultural events designed to garner influence among politically influential groups also occurs during this time.

While this incremental erosion of "above the line" advertising is happening, the industry accommodates by radically increasing its ad-spend in the remaining advertising media, in what has been described as "like squeezing a balloon. You can shut down one medium, but the problem just moves somewhere else"[575]. Today, in-store promotions have become the key site for industry advertising expenditure, amounting to 85% of ad-spend in the USA. Point-of-sale dollars go towards painting and decorating shops, installing displays, merchant incentives and paying shopkeepers to keep particular brands at carefully researched eyelines, often near confectionery displays[119]. As discussed below, efforts to end retail tobacco displays, consigning them to under-the-counter status, therefore strike at the heart of post ad-ban promotions.

While the tobacco industry takes great pains to emphasise that different brands are very distinctive, its internal research has long shown that many smokers cannot differentiate brands: "one of every two smokers is not able to distinguish in blind (masked) tests between similar cigarettes. I do not wish to underrate the importance of smoking characteristics but for most smokers, and for the decisive group of new, younger smokers, the consumer's choice is dictated by psychological, image factors than by relatively minor differences in product characteristics"[576]. Product image or branding, created through advertising and packaging, is thus crucial in efforts to command greater market share and to position brands as appealing to the "the decisive group of new, younger smokers" (i.e. mostly children).

The pack as advertising

The industry invests heavily in pack design and in the development of appealing brand names[577]. Brands smoked by the poorest socioeconomic groups in Australia, for example, include *Holiday*, *Horizon* and *Longbeach* – all names suggestive of escape. In the Philippine slums, a leading brand is called *Hope*, and in Taiwan, *Long Life* sells well. *World Tobacco*, an industry trade journal, stated in 1992 that "limitations on advertising will inevitably mean that increasing use will be made of tobacco packs themselves to get messages across"[578]. Systematic and extensive research is carried out by tobacco companies to ensure that cigarette packaging appeals to selected target groups, including young adults and women[65]. Down-market brands are promoted as vicarious escape tickets for people trapped in unemployment, poverty and dead-end jobs. Aspirational brands target insecure image-conscious young people seeking a conspicuous pack-as-badge that can display an at-a-glance code about personal identity. A cigarette package designer explained it this way: "A cigarette package is unique because the consumer carries it around with him all day . . . it's a part of a smoker's clothing, and when he saunters into a bar and plunks it down, he makes a statement about himself."[579]

The recent desecration of packs with full-colour photos of suppurating diseases has dealt a devastating blow to tobacco branding. Now that an unstoppable

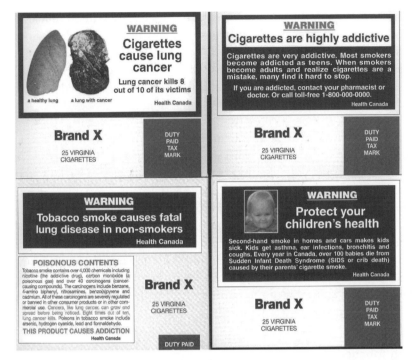

Fig. 7.1 Generic pack showing Canadian warning. Used with permission of Garfield Mahood, Canadian Non-Smokers' Movement.

momentum has commenced toward graphic pack warnings[i], the next battle the industry will face will be over generic packs (see Fig. 7.1). Generic policy allows only brand names to differentiate brands, removing all pack and cigarette colours except for those in the graphic health warning. Companies have even used cigarettes to differentiate brands, as recently occurred with a Dutch brand being marketed with a coloured filter in the national football team's orange.

In 1994, the Canadian government subjected a proposal for generic packs to unprecedented scrutiny, and was heavily and successfully lobbied by the tobacco and the packaging industries to abandon the plan. Cunningham and Kyle's review of the limited experimental evidence advanced in favour of generic packs and their rebuttal of the arguments that are ranged against the proposal should be essential reading for anyone about to rekindle the idea[580].

Their arguments for generic packs include:

- Ugly, unappealing packs diminish positive smoking imagery and substitute negative imagery. Brand "badging" is greatly diminished.
- After advertising bans, manufacturers rely on "brand memory" to maintain loyalty. Generic packs radically disrupt consumer associations of brands with past advertising appeals.
- Generic packs reduce the impact of foreign advertising that enters ad ban nations.
- Lack of brand colours ruins sponsorship opportunities. Racing cars, for example, could no longer be painted in cigarette brand colours that no longer applied.

- Generic packs send an important message that cigarettes are so different in risk to all other consumer goods, that governments decree that they should only be sold in unattractive packs.
- Consumers may feel that cigarettes sold in generic packs are "inferior" goods (research has shown that when identical cigarettes are smoked from different packs, some consumers find them less appealing).

In the USA and Canada, generic brand packs have not gained significant market share despite being much cheaper than premium brands, and are strongly identified as "down-market" brands. This lack of appeal is precisely why they should be introduced. The argument that needs to be central here is exactly that which has been used successfully to end tobacco advertising: that companies use packs as a key part of the overall promotion of their tobacco products. In ratifying the FCTC, governments now have carte blanche to eliminate all promotion. The ball is in the court of the tobacco industry to demonstrate that packaging is not a key ingredient in its promotional efforts. With abundant internal documentation explicitly referring to packs as central to the promotional mix, this will herald a whole new era of amusing argumentative duplicity.

Banning tobacco displays

Two nations (Iceland and Thailand) and seven Canadian provinces have adopted denormalising laws to prohibit the visible display of tobacco products at point of purchase. Ireland has passed legislation but not set a commencement date. In Tasmania, such a law is under active consideration. The industry fiercely resists such proposals, but shoots itself in the foot by basing its concerns around the very point that underscores the argument *for* banning displays: that the bans will reduce sales. By the time debate moves to calling for display bans, governments have typically enshrined high-level policy statements that commit to reducing tobacco use in communities. So when the industry bases its opposition to display bans on the threat to sales volume, the response is simply to say "precisely! That's the whole idea!"

There is an important precedent for consumer products being banned from display in retail environments. Prescription-only pharmaceuticals, designed to *improve* health, are kept out of sight of pharmacy customers in dispensaries. The pharmacist processes the prescription, and hands the wrapped drugs, packaged in plain packaging, to the customer. No one argues that this is anything but appropriate for products that cannot be purchased by anyone but the bearer of a doctor's prescription. By the same reasoning, tobacco products, being legally available only to adults, should not be on open display to children in stores.

Below-the-line marketing

Stacy Carter has produced some of the most comprehensive work reviewing below-the-line approaches to tobacco marketing in "dark markets" where tobacco companies are unable to use traditional promotional media[581–583]. She writes:

. . . "buzz", "viral" or "guerrilla" marketing that is "intended to create a word-of-mouth "buzz" and thus spread like a "virus". It is characterised by subversion of the transparency of commercial messages to make a consumer think that they are discovering something for themselves (thus "guerrilla") – a phenomenon which is also central to coercions such as pyramid selling and cult recruitment. Guerrilla marketers may, for example, pay teens to talk to their friends about a product, commission footpath graffiti, or create an event or a website which, rather than containing overt brand imagery, is consistent with the image of the product and "coincidentally" contains it, without overtly delivering a selling message.[582]

Guerrilla event marketing for tobacco is well developed and documented in Australia. There are many examples. A leading fashion designers' after-show party, bankrolled by a cigarette manufacturer, featured cigarette-bearing models[584]. A 1950s-themed room in a club was visited, with much fanfare, by young models who stacked a strategically placed retro refrigerator with cigarettes. A dance party featuring a wide range of "feminine" products, including cigarettes, was promoted via the street press and followed up with questionnaires to party-goers about their smoking. Philip Morris (Australia) Limited (PML) has pleaded guilty to the charge that the latter event was cigarette advertising.[585,586]

In 2002, when BAT relaunched *Lucky Strike* in South Africa (a country that has an advertising ban) it used the viral marketing strategy of "friend get friend" and employing stylish young "brand amplifiers" who would "represent the embodiment of the brand in all they do or say". They were given branded cars and "encouraged to 'live' the brand lifestyle" as they promoted the brand[587]. The brand amplifiers spread rumours about events featuring international DJ Paul Okenfold and the Violent Femmes band, whose website at the time stated "for the most part the audience remains the same high school and college kids who have always been the core of the Femmes crowd"[588].

Tobacco control advocates need routinely to immerse themselves in environments like bars[589,590], music festivals, the alternative music press, and teenage-oriented fashion and gossip websites to gather intelligence about below-the-line promotions where the line between selling and promotion is being blurred.

It is also important to keep a close eye on tobacco retail environments where occasional gift horses can land and provide powerful, shaming ammunition. The best example I have seen of this was a key ring with an attached vial that teenagers judged to be a party drug concealment capsule, which was being marketed with Philip Morris's *Alpine* cigarettes in Melbourne, Australia, with the company claiming it was to be used to store perfume (Fig. 7.2)!

Banning "mobile sellers" is of critical importance, as has been done in the state of Western Australia. When advertising is banned, tobacco companies accelerate the use of attractive young sellers who move from bar to bar in cities, selling cigarettes. The practice is extremely widespread in Asia, where it extends to the distribution of free samples, a practice that should always be outlawed in comprehensive tobacco advertising bans. My own athletic, good-looking stepson was recruited outside a

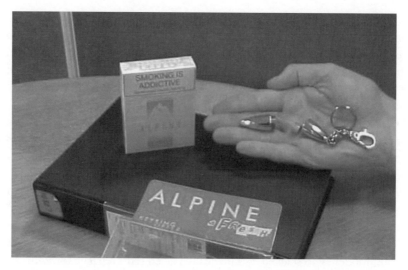

Fig. 7.2   Alpine cigarettes marketed with a "perfume container", Melbourne.

sporting venue to attend a Philip Morris training session for mobile sellers to sell *Marlboro* at strategically selected nightspots in Sydney. He took detailed notes about how the hand-picked young men and women were instructed to respond if challenged about whether they were "promoting" cigarettes and what sort of people to approach most. All were drilled by the industry staff to reply to any enquiries that they were *selling*, not promoting. Heavily price-discounted offers can be made in such promotional operations without breaking laws forbidding the distribution of free samples. Bars are key environments where a significant number of young people first start serious smoking[548].

Should we control smoking in movies?

One of the most important ways in which the tobacco industry can continue to promote smoking after advertising bans is to arrange for tobacco products and smoking to be "placed" in movies. Internal documents have provided many examples of how the tobacco industry nurtured its relationship with Hollywood[591] to ensure that its products were seen often and advantageously in movies.

In 1983, Philip Morris chief executive Hamish Maxwell wrote: "I do feel heartened at the increasing number of occasions when I go to a movie and see a pack of cigarettes in the hands of the leading lady . . . We must continue to exploit new opportunities to get cigarettes on screen . . . the PMI Corporate Affairs Department is helping. The Department is working with Dr Sherwin Feinhandler from Harvard University and Michael Dowling of Ogilvy and Mather to develop an international approach to the problem."[592]

The American Tobacco Company was in on it too: "For the last four years we have had a contractual arrangement with Unique Product Placement (UPP) to place our advertising and products in major motion pictures. For the past four years UPP has exceeded their original estimate of the number of films in which we would be placed. We have averaged approximately 30 major motion pictures for each of the last four years. [these included the] spectacular opening in *Beverly Hills Cop* . . . which provides us exposure for our *Lucky* and *Pall Mall* brands."[593]

If you think you've been seeing smoking more and more in films, you are correct. There is now considerable evidence that tobacco products and smoking scenes are not only prevalent in many movies today, but that the frequency of such scenes has returned to levels not seen for several decades[594,595]. We can all recall scenes in movies where smoking has been portrayed very positively, choreographed into scenes and character identity to show it as attractive, sensual and iconic.

Various studies claim to demonstrate causal associations between viewing of smoking in films and subsequent smoking[596,597]. If rampant tobacco advertising can culturally "normalise" smoking and play an important role in influencing young people to smoke, it is obviously very sensible to assume that carefully directed smoking scenes in movies, particularly those with broad appeal to young people, should also be seen as important vehicles capable of promoting smoking too. Because banning tobacco advertising has been a basic platform of every comprehensive tobacco control policy in the past 30 years, some argue that it is reasonable that such policies should now also address the control of smoking in movies and on television.

In 2005 I received an email from a colleague who had just seen *Little Fish*, starring Cate Blanchett, someone certain to win a suitcase full of Oscars in the years to come. My colleague noticed smoking throughout the film and implored "why can't you do something about all the smoking in films!" I had seen and enjoyed the low-budget film, in which Blanchett stars as a young woman living in an impoverished Sydney outer suburb awash with narcotics, crime and hopelessness. This is the sort of suburb where smoking rates among such young women are the highest in Australia[598]. So predictably and realistically, she smoked. It would have been almost remarkable if she had not. The film follows her futile efforts to lift herself out of the crime and poverty spiral. Given the optimistic ending, we walk from the cinema depressed, but feeling hopeful that even against the odds, people with spirit can see a better life for themselves. Her smoking was the least of her problems. Only a person truly obsessed about smoking would see the smoking as anything more than a faithfully observed part of her life, along with the poverty, the poor judgment, and the difficulties faced by anyone living in such environments.

I reflected on my colleague's email that he had said nothing about other scenes in the movie: the murders, the betrayals, the misogyny, the injustice of government policy that allows such ghettos to flourish. All this was apparently OK . . . but smoking! Something needed to be done!

My email correspondent asked me to "do something" about smoking in movies. But what should be "done"? There are four main proposals being advocated, and in two nations these are actually or about to be implemented. I will summarise each of these, and then argue why I believe efforts to try to ban or restrict smoking in movies are fraught with problems and need extremely careful consideration before the international tobacco control community embraces such proposals.

Professor Stan Glantz from the University of California in San Francisco is the most prominent world voice calling for action on smoking in movies. His project, SmokeFree movies[599] has attracted support from many key public health agencies and calls for four basic reforms (Box 7.1).

Box 7.1   Proposed smoking reforms for movies

- **Rate new smoking movies "R":** Any film that shows or implies tobacco should be rated "R". The only exceptions should be when the presentation of tobacco clearly and unambiguously reflects the dangers and consequences of tobacco use or is necessary to represent the smoking of a real historical figure.
- **Certify no pay-offs:** The producers should post a certificate in the closing credits declaring that nobody on the production received anything of value (cash, free cigarettes or other gifts, free publicity, interest-free loans or anything else) from anyone in exchange for using or displaying tobacco.
- **Require strong anti-smoking ads:** Studios and theatres should require a genuinely strong anti-smoking ad (not one produced by a tobacco company) to run before any film with any tobacco presence, in any distribution channel, regardless of its MPAA rating (the US system for rating suitability of films for different age groups).
- **Stop identifying tobacco brands:** There should be no tobacco brand identification or presence of tobacco brand imagery (such as billboards) in the background of any movie scene.

Two of these proposals (banning the identification of tobacco brands, and requiring film producers to certify that they have not received any form of payment for displaying tobacco) are eminently sensible and uncontroversial. Only the most diehard of movie fans stay to read the credits at the end of a movie, but the main purpose of posting such a declaration (or failing to, where such transaction had occurred) would be its evidential value in legal challenges to the use of product placement as paid advertising, in breach of national laws. So this is important too.

The other two – rating films with depictions of smoking as R (in the USA meaning that anyone aged under 17 can only see the film with an adult; in some other nations it means no person under 18 can legally see the film) and the requirement to show a warning message before every such film – are far more contentious and will be discussed below. But neither of these is as controversial as the laws that now apply in Thailand and, at the time of writing, are about to be implemented in India.

India. The Indian government's Cigarette and other Tobacco Products (Prohibition of Advertisement and Regulation of Trade and Commerce, Production, Supply and Distribution) Act, 2003, implemented from 2 October 2006, requires that:

> No individual or a person or a character in cinema and television programmes shall display tobacco products or their use. Where, however, cinema and television programmes which have been produced prior to this notification have scenes with smoking situations and use of other forms of tobacco, it shall be mandatory to place a health warning as a prominent scroll at the bottom of

the television or cinema screen . . . in the same language(s) as used in the cinema or the television programme.

Thailand. Thai law requires that any films that are broadcast on television showing cigarettes or smoking must have the cigarettes pixilated. The reasoning here would appear to be that as long as you don't actually see the cigarette, somehow the normative message won't get through. Bungon Ritthiphakdee, a Thai tobacco control expert, says that television movie and drama producers seldom show scenes of people smoking since the law was introduced, because the required pixilation adds an extra production cost and more importantly, annoys viewers. Foreign-produced movies shown on television continue to show pixilated smoking.

Pixilation is common practice on television news crime reports: we see arrested felons' faces pixilated as they enter court before a trial. But is there anyone who doesn't think "there's the felon!" just as a pixilated cigarette would not immediately tell viewers that here was someone smoking. It is difficult to imagine what the Thai authorities think that not actually *seeing* the cigarette will achieve. At best, the pixilation "makes strange" smoking, perhaps causing people to reflect on why this censorship has been put in place. But at worst, it may generate a forbidden fruit effect. In the 1960s when I was a boy, my local newsagent had naturist magazines where the nipples and genitals of naked volley-ball players and barbeque cooks cavorting at nudist camps were pixilated or airbrushed out. Reflecting on how my friends and I furtively turned the pages, keeping an eye peeled for the newsagent's accusatory gaze, I am certain that this pixilation generated intense anticipation in us about one day seeing the real thing. It was a hopelessly ill-conceived policy. Must we really feel obliged to regard such policies as the admirable exercise of comprehensive tobacco control policy? The Thais are among the world's best at tobacco control, but on this issue I must demur.

Banning and regulating smoking scenes: censorship

Most – perhaps all – nations have systems of film censorship and classification, the latter designed to "triage" gradations of violence, sexual conduct and illicit drug use against an overarching concern to protect impressionable children from frank exposures that may disturb them. Many nations have panels of citizens (or state officials) that view all new films and assign ratings. Children are able to watch the cartoon character Road Runner inflict unlimited catastrophic violence on the Coyote, but would be shielded from realistic depictions of the same thing. A sustained scene of a gang kicking to death a disabled person, a graphic scene of someone injecting narcotics and euphorically lying back to enjoy the rush, or a sustained, explicit sexual act are examples of three scenes that most reasonable people would agree could confuse or disturb immature children and adolescents. Such scenes typically result in a restricted classification so that only adults can legally see the movie in a cinema or rent it.

Proponents of classifying as "R" any movie with a smoking scene (except ones overtly proselytising against smoking) argue that there are complete parallels with smoking and the sorts of scenes I have just described. These parallels are fatuous. The scenes of violent, explicit sex or of characters injecting drugs that see movies rated R or occasionally banned, are scenes that are judged as shocking, grossly offensive, emotionally disturbing or in the case of frank sex scenes, disturbing cultural taboos against displays of full-on sexuality to children. By contrast, many children see smoking every day, many times. Smoking is not a "strange", disturbing or frightening behaviour, however much we might wish to denormalise it.

When the Indian government received the Luther Terry Medal at the 13th World Conference on Tobacco or Health in Washington in 2006 for its exemplary leadership, the citation included its action to ban smoking in movies. I was on the selection committee and voted for India because of its outstanding recent record of political action. But I wished I could have somehow protested its ban on smoking in movies.

I have three principal objections to this policy. In general, I oppose government appropriation of the entertainment or literary industries for state-sanctioned purposes of any sort. I also believe it is grossly inconsistent and indefensible to single out particular "unhealthy" depictions for censorship while ignoring others. Also, I regard approaches to classifying smoking scenes as "acceptable" and "unacceptable", as in the SmokeFree Movies proposal to certify most scenes as "R", as being simplistic to the point of opening up tobacco control to deserved ridicule. Moreover, I believe the research literature that has been advanced in support of arguments that smoking in movies is hugely influential in causing children to smoke is open to serious challenge. I will now examine each of these concerns.

The state should not control artistic freedom to depict smoking

There are many examples of prohibited items and proscribed behaviours, and often there are sound ethical reasons for advancing these controls. For example, some nations ban explosive fireworks because of the unacceptably high incidence of severe injuries they cause[600]. In general, I support bans and strong restrictions on products and activities that harm others. Plastic bags harm the environment and they can readily be replaced with other less environmentally damaging forms of packaging, so I am sympathetic to policies like plastic bag taxes, which seek to discourage their use. I support bans on smoking in situations where it harms others. But I do not support bans on smoking per se in situations where it is only harming the smoker, just as I don't support bans on many highly dangerous personal behaviours (e.g. motorcycle riding, mountain climbing, skiing, lone ocean sailing). I'd prefer to live in a world where the personal freedom to take risks that do not harm others is respected.

I sense that those who are trigger happy for banning smoking in movies are sometimes those who would sign up to banning smoking itself. The Indian health minister Dr Anbumani Ramadoss is one such person, having stated "I will be happy if the sale of tobacco products is totally banned in the country, as has been done in Bhutan. And, let me tell you it is a matter of time before Parliament takes a decision on it. It is inevitable"[601]. Historical depictions of smoking, such as Winston

Churchill with his cigar or Sigmund Freud with his pipe, are spared in the Indian legislation as presumably being a step too far in protecting Indians from those realities. But in India today, after October 2006, no new film showing smoking by mere mortals can be made.

The core objections to R-ratings (or bans) for "positive depictions" of smoking are more fundamental than a concern to jump in whatever direction "the evidence" might suggest which, as I will argue later, is debatable. My assumption is that many people's support for banning or restricting smoking in movies develops independently of the available evidence, and proceeds from views that it is "wrong" to show smoking. The gallant purpose of denormalising smoking is seen as noble enough to sweep all before it.

After spending 30 years of my life trying to denormalise smoking within a framework of ethically sustainable principles, I nonetheless cannot support a proposition that would see (e.g.) a movie set today in Java, Indonesia, where 84% of men smoke[602], showing a nation of non-smokers; or a film about homeless men showing them to be all health aesthetes sipping herbal tea, eschewing alcohol and not smoking; or a film about a self-destructive character being allowed to show such a person engaged in every conceivable form of self-absorbed, anti-social behaviour, except smoking. If we were considering literature instead of film, we would have no hesitation to call it censorship or book burning, and see this as a sign of an immature or authoritarian society. Film is the modern extension of literature. Both must be allowed to be true to whatever creative (including realist) depictions their authors want.

I completely support bans on tobacco advertising, but commercial speech is not the same as free speech. This is reflected by whole areas of law that apply to regulating commercial speech because of its essentially different status.

Many people in tobacco control see a cigarette in a movie and immediately think "tobacco industry!" Sometimes it will be, but often it is not, anymore than every time we see a car in a movie we should feel obliged to think "automobile industry!" People drive. People smoke. Life is filled with undesirable people doing often unspeakable things. Film makers reflect these diverse realities in seeking to portray the world as it is within their creative vision, not necessarily as it should be in the eyes of health promoters. Basically, state proscriptions on depictions of smoking are saying: "just pretend it doesn't happen".

The wider concern in all this is the assumption that film makers should be obliged to carry the flag for public health: that literature and film are fundamentally vehicles for state-sanctioned views of the life that we should all be encouraged to lead. I do not go to the cinema expecting to see versions of life that conform to some state committee's view of what it thinks appropriate I should see. The Japanese government has been criticised for many years for refusing to allow references to World War II war crimes in Japanese school textbooks[603]. This was presumably driven by well-meaning nationalism. But many saw the deliberate effort artificially to censor an uncomfortable reality as unacceptable. North Korean state-controlled television is the apotheosis of such a mentality.

Some argue that "artistic freedom" is an overdone argument, but I believe there are fewer more important signs of a healthy society than one that allows freedom of expression. There are many people in the world who want all manner of things banned from film: nudity, sexuality, profanity, blasphemy, unpatriotic sentiments, anything that might conceivably inspire terrorism, illicit drug use, left-wing values that are critical of big business, suicide and abortion. Some religious-minded people are intent on closing down just about everything other than behaviours and attitudes conforming to their wholesome, doctrinaire views of the world. One only has to watch television in some of the world's more authoritarian nations to appreciate the utterly bleak world that we would live in if greater power was wielded by those with a taste for banning depictions of things they don't like.

Banning pernicious scenes from movies, one by one until all the world's single-issue health advocates were satisfied that going to a movie was not "dangerous", is a very slippery slope. A long list of potentially influential scenes that could cause impressionable youth to deviate in different ways from an entirely wholesome life path could easily be made. Motivated by the same concerns, what should be done about eradicating all scenes of violence from movies? Dangerous driving and car chases? Risk taking of any sort that might be copied by impressionable youth? Speaking angrily to others? Gluttony or contented obesity? Drunkeness? Cruelty? Laughing at others' misfortunes? Licentious music that may cause young people to "loosen their morals"? It is important to ask "why stop with smoking?" Advocates for censoring smoking in films reply that they have no intention of moving onto other areas. This misses the point, that others will take inspiration from the smoking example, and that once the precedent is established, the door opens.

In India, every film maker must now pull every scene of smoking. But imagine if next year "conclusive evidence" is published in a leading research journal showing that young people who prefer to watch movies with gun violence, are ten times more likely to get into fights as those who don't; the next year more research appears showing that people who enjoy movies featuring car chase scenes have higher rates of dangerous driving offences. Do you get the picture? Actually, we won't get the picture. If we were consistent in applying film censorship to each and every issue for which a case could be made, we would soon get a Mary Poppins view of the world where imaginary communities are shown, air-brushed clean of any pernicious influences.

It would be tragic if tobacco control, in the single-minded pursuit of its goals, alienated millions of supportive people who would be appalled that we would not hesitate to sanitise reality and that we would not draw breath before assuming that we had the right to appropriate film and literature in the service of health. These concerns reflect core values that should not be surrendered.

There is a well-established association between parental smoking and adolescent smoking[604]. If evidence was all that was relevant here, it might not be long before someone starts labelling parental smoking as "child abuse" because of its pernicious influence on children. Shortly afterwards, someone would go the next step and propose ways of fining parents who smoke or sending them to mandatory correctional classes, and that neighbours be encouraged to report them to authorities.

To anyone seeing health in its wider context, the price of such actions would be far too high, even if "evidence" could be produced to show that such steps reduced parental smoking.

R-rating?

SmokeFree Movies, and the CEOs of a galaxy of US health and medical agencies, have called for all films showing or "implying" smoking to be R-rated except "when the presentation of tobacco clearly and unambiguously reflects the dangers and consequences of tobacco use"[599]. The website of SmokeFree Movies hints at ways that this exception could be operationalised, asking "Is smoking on screen realistic? Does it kill half the characters?" This suggests that films where smoking features as an overt health education message (actor smokes, is profoundly regretful, perhaps dies horribly) could be screened unrestricted.

This narrow approach to defining an "acceptable" depiction of smoking is hopelessly naive about the complexity and richness of the ways that film communicates meaning. There are innumerable ways in which smoking can be made to communicate different meanings to the many different demographic target groups that movie producers are seeking to attract as audiences: what appears sensual and attractive to a 50-year-old person may appear laughably corny or washed-up to a 16-year-old. Equally, the 50-year-old may look at a scene showing a teenager smoking and see as pathetic the "try hard" antics of gauche adolescents trying to look sophisticated. The polysemic nature of smoking – the many ways that an act of smoking can signify different things to different people – presents a core challenge to anyone seeking to argue that any single cinematic act of smoking "means" something in particular. Responding to this by simply saying that "*any* scene of smoking (other than a blatantly down-your-throat, negative one) is a bad influence and must be kept away from children's eyes" would not withstand any empirical test conducted by a cross-section of the general population (as opposed to a panel of public health researchers with track records of making the same point). Moreover, some movies that show "positive" smoking scenes also show scenes where smokers are depicted as total losers. Would adolescents be allowed to see a movie where a non-smoking hero taunted and ridiculed a bunch of heavy smoking losers? If not, why not? The spectre of a panel earnestly adjudicating the dominance of negative over positive depictions to the net meaning of smoking in a film is fascinating.

Anyone who asserts that it is easy to allocate a simple yes or no to whether a complex narrative in a movie promotes smoking or not is almost certainly taking some cavalier methodological liberties. The world is infinitely more complex than such an "in" or "out" dichotomy would suggest. Unlike swearing or sex, where formulae like "more than one four-letter word means R" or "no frontal nudity or sex scenes" can be applied, the notion that you can look at a smoking character and unproblematically rate the scene "bad" or "OK" is utterly simplistic and would invite gales of ridicule from anyone with a minute's experience in cinema, literary criticism or education.

As one critic wrote of Julia Roberts' smoking in *My Best Friend's Wedding*, "The Roberts character is deeply flawed, and smokes as a manifestation of being highly strung and nervous. That's a legitimate use of artistic shorthand to tell us something about a character. And it's hardly a positive portrayal of smoking." There are dozens of movies where smoking is presented in complex ways. Certainly there are overtly positive depictions where smoking is made to look unambiguously good. But there are many instances where people smoke who are wholly unattractive. Apparently, unless they turn to camera and deliver a message in the style of Yul Brynner – "whatever you do, don't smoke" – they are to be relegated to R box-office classification, where reduced returns are guaranteed.

Jenny Foreit of the Campaign for Tobacco Free Kids (in Washington DC) lists examples of movies in which smoking is shown in ways that are more complex than simply "OK" or "not OK" (Box 7.2).

Box 7.2 Mixed smoking "messages" in the movies

- *Constantine* (2005), starring Keanu Reeves. A major plot point is that he has lung cancer from smoking.
- *Cat's Eye* (1985), a movie made up of a series of short Steven King stories, and featuring Quitters Inc, which highlights the difficulties of quitting smoking.
- *Rounders* (1998), starring Ed Norton. At the start of the movie, Norton's character is playing poker in prison for cigarettes. He wins, refuses to share any with the other players, saying something along the lines of "these will kill you". On his way out of prison, he purposefully throws them all in a trash can.
- *The Italian Job* (2003), when Handsome Rob (Jason Statham) is stuck in traffic during a timing exercise, he sees a "scorecard" billboard proclaiming how many people have died of smoking-related illnesses. He looks at his cigarette, and flicks it into the street.
- *Thank You For Smoking* (2005), a biting satire about the tobacco industry in which plenty of people smoke and get their comeuppance.
- *The Insider* (1999), the powerful story of tobacco industry whistleblower Jeff Wigand's efforts to relate what goes on in the tobacco industry.
- *Cube* (1997), featuring a conversation that illustrates the difficulty of quitting and the effects of nicotine dependence.
- *Jennifer 8* (1992), in which there are two friends trying to help each other through quitting.
- *Wild at Heart* (1990), includes a conversation about how many people in a family have died of smoke-related illness.
- *El Mariachi* (1992), in which Antonio Banderas tells a bartender he doesn't drink or smoke because his voice is his life. Plenty of others smoke in the film.
- *Mrs Doubtfire* (1993), has Robin Williams quitting his job because he doesn't think it's morally right to promote smoking to children.

It may be significant that proposals to ban smoking in movies are most advanced in India, which until recently banned on-screen kissing, and the USA, which went into national apoplexy in 2004 at singer Janet Jackson's "wardrobe malfunction", which inadvertently exposed her breast to a national audience.

How strong is the evidence that smoking scenes influence smoking?

Strong claims are being made about the effect of smoking scenes in movies. They don't come stronger than this statement in an Indian newspaper: "Smoking in the movies is the most powerful pro-tobacco influence and stronger amongst non-smokers. Research has shown that smoking in movies helps cigarette sales, as 52 per cent of kids start smoking after watching movie stars light up."[605]

How strong is the evidence for such astonishing claims? Probably the strongest paper yet published is that by Jim Sargent and colleagues[597], which concluded that there is a dose–response relationship between seeing movies containing scenes of smoking and initiation of smoking: the more smoking scenes children see, the more likely they are to take up smoking. The paper goes further than others in its efforts to consider a good range of intuitively plausible confounders and covariates in adolescent viewers. But in trying hard to explore these, the paper shows the limitations of trying to push complexity into quantifiable categories. For example, "sensation seeking" was assessed using a scale that included items such as "I like to do scary things" and "I like to listen to loud music". Faith that such crude measures adequately capture the richness of what is going on in teenagers who might be more likely to smoke is not very reassuring.

Is smoking a covariate for other factors that attract children who will go on to smoke?

Sargent and colleagues have only done half the job. Neither their paper, nor any others I have seen, considers the possibility that smoking scenes might be confounded by a constellation of factors that could be more influential than actual depictions of smoking in attracting the sort of children who will go on to take up smoking. Smoking may well be a covariate for other factors in movies that attract children who are likely to smoke.

Many writers and directors presumably direct actors to smoke in movies because smoking is seen to be an easily decoded symbol of a wide range of characterisations they wish to convey. Let's assume that there is a cinematic tendency to depict "bad attitude" characters smoking, or particular types of seducers, or intense march-to-the-beat-of-a-different drum, romantic, alienated types, or rebellious adolescents, or generally socially irreverent people.

It may be that young people at risk of smoking initiation are attracted to certain types of films populated by such characters. They do not consciously seek films where there will be smoking ("you should see Movie X! Lots of people smoke in it!" but rather "You should see Movie X – about a bunch of guys who do all sorts of cool stuff, with a great gangsta rap soundtrack!"). Young people at risk for smoking may have strong tastes in films with a range of features of which smoking is but one, perhaps very minor, element: a covariate rather than the decisive variable. If we managed to succeed in getting smoking removed from such characterisations (in order to escape a ban or an R rating), the question arises whether the overall meaning and appeal of such movies would change significantly. The children at risk for smoking would in all probability still select such movies.

As I stated earlier, if tobacco advertising imagery can promote smoking, it would be remarkable if smoking imagery in movies could not also influence the way that smoking is seen. No one questions the broad proposition that smoking in movies may often be influential in forging smoking-positive associations. This common-sense assumption is done a great disservice by research that tries to drill into the huge complexity of all the ways that young people develop their sense of what smoking signifies and emerge holding the villain of movies as being "directly" responsible for "52%" of children starting to smoke[605].

Shaming and raising awareness

In all this, it remains clear that paid efforts by the tobacco industry to place product in movies are very legitimate and important targets for tobacco control. Efforts to find evidence of product placement and legally prosecute it when those responsible break laws should be given high priority. If the practice is as widespread as is assumed, it will presumably be possible to unearth whistle-blowers who will burst industry assurances that they don't do it today. There are many disaffected employees in the world of movies.

Similarly, critiques of lazy, gratuitous cinematic direction that equates smouldering character intensity, artistic temperament or sexual allure with smoking need to lift their pace. There has been very little effort to research the ways in which smoking does come to be scripted into films so much[606]. Gratuitous smoking is insidious, and the way to change this without sacrificing important principles of artistic expression is to expose where this is happening, and to draw film directors' attentions to the consequences of their actions through greater effort at dialogue with the film industry, bringing on board industry leaders and continuing the research that monitors the incidence of smoking. Stan Glantz has done vital, pioneering work in raising these issues but I believe has gone too quickly to the wrong solution, which as I have argued, threatens important values in open societies. Glantz points to evidence of widespread community support for his proposals[607], but history is full of widespread support for all manner of dubious proposals. The principles involved will always be more important.

Corporate responsibility and the tobacco industry

In the late 1990s, the US tobacco industry's world was turned upside down by a series of five court cases brought against them by the states of Mississippi, Florida, Texas and Minnesota to recover the costs of treating uninsured smokers in the public health system. Each of these was settled before judgment. The Minnesota case in part required the companies to make public millions of pages of previously internal documents in a repository. When the state of Washington then sued, the industry saw a potential conga line of similar trials forming, and struck the historic Master Settlement Agreement with US states in November 1998. The Agreement provided for $206 billion to be paid by the companies to the states, and significantly, that all documents "discovered" in any trial up until 2010 be placed on the worldwide web. Today, some 60 million pages of previously private memos, faxes, reports and letters are available to anyone with a computer[ii].

Faced with this deluge of embarrassing revelations, including many thousands from its highest officials, the international industry was forced to change strategy. It embarked on the world's most public corporate rebirthing exercise, asking to be appreciated henceforth as an ethical industry devoted to providing tobacco products to sentient adults, all supposedly fully informed of the risks they take. No longer was the relationship between smoking and illness merely a dubious "statistical association"; the new tobacco industry now admits in carefully weasel worded statements that tobacco use is a highly risky practice. As BAT carefully put it in its 2003/4 Social Report: "Our main role is to recognise the relevant health authorities as the prime public voice on the health risks of tobacco consumption, while at the same time making our views clear."[608] Translated, this can be read as meaning: "Like everyone else, we can see it is a fact that health authorities are the main voice on smoking and health. We 'recognise' this, but we also have 'our views' on smoking and health and we'll take every opportunity to make them clear to governments trying to do heinous things like place graphic photos of tobacco diseases on our packs." In 2004, BAT Australia, for example, fresh from gushing about its dedication to informing smokers about risk, lobbied hard but unsuccessfully to persuade the government to shelve plans for these warnings, including unacknowledged funding of smoker petitions in retailers[609].

For the rebirthed industry, no longer is nicotine a simple "habit" akin to chewing gum, eating chocolate or watching television; the industry now concedes that the common understanding is that nicotine is addictive. Translated, this means: "We concede that everyone says nicotine is addictive . . . but we don't necessarily agree. And if someone claims in court they were addicted to our products, we'll probably keep on doing what we have been doing for years and challenge that, pointing to all the ex-smokers in the community, as a way of trivialising the idea that nicotine is addictive."

Philip Morris has been engaging in a global programme of spending vast sums of money to publicise its support for projects like domestic violence awareness. Who could attack anyone who is helping to reduce domestic violence or feeding and sheltering the homeless? In Australia Philip Morris even funded an Aboriginal health promotion campaign, knowing well that the indigenous population has among the highest smoking rates in the country.

A 1988 Philip Morris memo set out the rationale for its public relations strategy of engaging in socially responsible activities. Far from engaging in these pursuits for altruistic purposes, the memo advises that "Benefits PM-USA may realize from a program of this type include . . . access to political decision makers" and that these programmes could "Enhance PM-USA's position with legislative bodies who might be considering marketing sanctions, advertising bans and public smoking restrictions"[610].

A lesson that most of us learned as children is that the purpose of charitable giving is to help those in need, not self-aggrandisement. In one year Philip Morris gave $115 million to people in need, but spent $150 million on public advertising telling Americans about its corporate good work such as charitable giving and youth smoking prevention. At the time, Philip Morris's Peggy Roberts said the company spent so much on the ad campaign because it thinks "it's an important thing that people know in a fuller sense who Philip Morris is"[611].

When the tobacco industry succeeds in positioning itself as just another ordinary industry, it is halfway home in its normalisation strategy designed to soften government and community attitudes to its contribution to the world. Corporate Social Responsibility (CSR) programmes also benefit the marketing ambitions of tobacco companies. In May 2006, a report from Korea on BAT's plans for expanding its market share noted "BAT has managed to raise its brand awareness through what some experts have described as 'imaginative' ways. They include sponsoring world-class motor sports events and social programs such as youth smoking prevention and environmental causes".[612]

There is wholesale cynicism and disgust in health and medical circles about this exercise, and it holds great potential to add to the industry's low trust rating throughout communities[11,135]. Critics point out that contrary to the most elementary procedures for wrongdoers seeking public absolution, the industry has made no public apology about its years of misleading conduct. Doubtless mindful of the legal ramifications of doing so, it has made no admissions that it lied to smokers for decades, and that it engaged in a globally orchestrated campaign falsely to reassure smokers about the alleged risks of smoking[100]. It has made no gestures to compensate those it has harmed. It remains implacable in its refusal to acknowledge that intriguing children about smoking is intrinsic to its continuing economic welfare, despite oceans of internal documents affirming this[613]. Indeed, it is so sincere in not wanting children to smoke that it has so far forgotten to hand back its annual massive earnings from underage smokers, who it says *ad nauseum* it doesn't want to smoke. In Australia, the industry take in 2002–03 from the underage market was estimated to be $A18.7 million[533], about nine times more than the Federal government spends each year on tobacco control campaigns.

There can be few more instructive documents illustrating the "business as usual" approach of tobacco companies who publicly embrace CSR than a 2006 submission made by BAT to the New South Wales Parliament[414], which contained the following gems:

- "It is unreasonable for regulators [to pursue] . . . an objective of reaching an impossible 'zero smoking incidence' target" [*my interpretation*: enough is enough, please stop policies that see smoking falling every year].
- "The costs associated with smoking must be matched against an assessment of those positive features of a local tobacco growing, manufacturing and retailing industry which outweigh those costs" [*my interpretation*: the economic benefits of tobacco are more important than its health impacts. So please let the industry continue to reap those benefits!].
- "the efficacy of tobacco control strategies must be measured in terms of the unintended consequences of regulation, including . . . the ability to undermine

youth smoking prevention . . . and the disproportionate commercial impacts on small business" [*my interpretation*: tobacco control encourages children to smoke and causes commercial losses in tobacco retailers, so governments should take their feet off tobacco control accelerators].

- "Lower Ignition Propensity Cigarettes have not been found to work in the real world; have been rejected by a number of jurisdictions; and may encourage irresponsible disposal" [*my interpretation*: They want to be allowed to keep selling higher ignition propensity cigarettes, which cause many fires and deaths each year].

- "product 'shrouding' [storing cigarettes under the counter] may in fact *encourage* youth smoking" [*my comment*: if hiding cigarettes caused more sales to youth, tobacco companies would have made it mandatory years ago].

- "BATA would support a *reallocation* of [tobacco control] funding to . . . inform adults that they can continue to smoke in non-enclosed areas at NSW hotels" [*my comment*: in all seriousness, BAT is here suggesting that cancer authorities spend their campaign budgets to encourage smokers to keep smoking].

In 2005, it was revealed that BAT had for four years been operating a joint venture cigarette factory with a state-owned corporation in North Korea, a nation denounced by US president George Bush as a member of the "axis of evil", and having an appalling human rights record. BAT's annual reports make no mention of the factory[614].

Denormalisation in action[iii]

Emboldened in their fetching new sheepskins, and barely finished gagging from being publicly force-fed truth serum via their embarrassing public documents, tobacco industry wolves are doing the rounds of the world's CSR conferences where corporate spin doctors meet to swap war stories about clothing naked emperors and turning frogs into princes. Tobacco companies are also entering the corporate world's equivalent to the plastic surgery gawp TV show *Extreme Makeover* – the Corporate Responsibility Index (CRI). In 2006, remarkably, the CRI ranked British American Tobacco as the eighth most responsible company in Australia.

On 26 May 2004, corporate responsibility watcher Bert Hirschhorn[615] noticed that BAT and Philip Morris had home page billing as speakers and gold sponsors at a conference to be held in Hong Kong in October 2004 run by *Ethical Corporation* magazine. Email alerts saw tobacco control activists contact Asian delegates listed as speaking at the conference. One also protested to his University Chancellor over the involvement of his university's business school in the event.

An online petition was set up on Globalink for professional ethicists to condemn the industry's involvement[616]. Within days, 86 ethicists had signed, including bioethics heavyweights Peter Singer from Princeton University and Arthur Kaplan from the University of Pennsylvania.

The petition stated in part "We, the undersigned ethicists and philosophers, condemn the cynical appropriation of 'ethics' by tobacco companies. We call on all businesses genuinely committed to the promotion of more ethical corporate practices to dissociate themselves from all forums and conferences that give a stage from which the tobacco industry can continue its assault on society."

The two tobacco companies disappeared from the conference website within a week of the campaign commencing. *Ethical Corporation* advised that they had received heated complaints about tobacco industry involvement and that they had advised Philip Morris that their sponsorship was cancelled and were considering whether to cancel BAT's speaking role, writing: "This furore made us realise that there are some companies who we cannot take sponsorship money from, this list of industry sectors, along with tobacco, includes defence, nuclear and biotechnology." Two speakers withdrew from the conference in protest and the conference went ahead without tobacco involvement.

A second opportunity to test this strategy arose in July 2004 in Sydney when a website advertising the "Australian Public Relations and Corporate Communications Summit 2004" showed Philip Morris on the programme. All speakers were emailed a letter signed by myself and the head of the Cancer Council New South Wales, Andrew Penman, in which we urged them to reconsider their participation alongside a tobacco company. At least two prominent business speakers contacted the organisers, threatening to withdraw should Philip Morris remain on the programme. The organisers promptly "de-invited" Philip Morris from the programme.

Why so easy?

The speed with which the organisers of both conferences showed their already invited tobacco industry participants the back door was remarkable. Despite Philip Morris being a "gold sponsor", a simple show of protest consisting of a few emails and phone calls was sufficient to abort their involvement.

The tobacco industry has had many doors closed in its face over the years. The 2004 BAT Social Report shows that no UK public health or tobacco control groups chose to participate in its consultations. Similar refusal to buy into the industry's oleaginous talk about dialogue with stakeholders has occurred in other nations, with groups and individuals refusing to risk being appropriated into the industry's public relations ambitions. With vigilance, tobacco control advocates can easily foment similar distaste in many areas of the business community. Our actions sought to denormalise the tobacco industry by disrupting its efforts to take its place alongside other industries – often with considerable social credit – in the hope that it might gain by association.

Tobacco industry posturing about its corporate responsibility can never hide the ugly consequences of its ongoing efforts to "work with all relevant stakeholders for the preservation of opportunities for informed adults to consume tobacco products" (*translation*: "we will build alliances with others who want to profit from tobacco use, to do all we can to counteract effective tobacco control"). In 2005, BAT had 16.9% and Philip Morris 18.6% of the global cigarette market. With 4.9 million smokers currently dying from tobacco use each year this leaves BAT to explain its role in the annual deaths of some 828 100 smokers, and Philip Morris in the deaths of some 911 400.

Like the mafia boss who ostentatiously deposits $5000 in the church plate on Sunday, tobacco companies have the temerity to enter corporate responsibility contests. BAT's Michael Prideaux briefed his Board in 2000 that indices like the Corporate Responsibility Index "will not only help BAT achieve a position of recognised responsibility but also provide 'air cover' from criticism while improvements are being made. Essentially it provides a degree of publicly endorsed amnesty"[617].

An ethical tobacco company is an oxymoron. The Hong Kong conference promised to help companies "profit" from CSR, but illness and death for millions are the *sine qua non* of the industry's "business as usual". The latest incarnation of their harm reduction strategy is highly unlikely to be any different from past performance, because tobacco companies can only act responsibly by meaningfully discouraging consumption and taking the road to financial ruin. That will never happen.

Academic denormalisation

Engagement with universities and research institutes is highly prized by the tobacco industry as a means of producing apparently independent research in policy-relevant areas central to the industry's corporate interests. In this respect, it is little different to any commercial entity and all universities actively encourage their staff to engage with industry, establishing protocols to ensure the integrity of the research produced. A growing body of research shows that commercial research patronage is often predictive of research results that are commercially advantageous to the research sponsor[618]. In the area of pharmaceutical drug trials in particular, this tendency has become so pronounced that the editors of the world's leading medical journals have expressed great concern over the implications for public confidence in pharmaceutical industry-sponsored research and have insisted on the establishment of a publicly accessible clinical trial register[619].

Universities rarely have explicit policies about sources of research support that are unacceptable. Significantly, the one exception is the tobacco industry. In several nations (USA, UK, Canada and Australia) there is a momentum building to exclude tobacco companies from supporting university-based research. As at December 2004, 17 universities in the USA had schools, departments or centres that prohibit the acceptance of tobacco industry funding for research. The 17 universities include 22 academic units: 13 Schools of Public Health (Arizona, Columbia, Harvard, Johns Hopkins, Iowa, Loma Linda, North Carolina, Puerto Rico, South Carolina, UC Berkeley, UCLA, University of Medicine and Dentistry of New Jersey, and Washington); three Schools of Medicine (Emory, Harvard and Johns Hopkins); one School of Nursing (UCLA); one Department of Medicine (UC San Francisco) and one Department of Family and Preventive Medicine (UC San Diego); and three Comprehensive Cancer Centers (Ohio State, UC San Diego and UC San Francisco).

In the UK, a BAT-commissioned report from 2000[620] shows there were 18 universities with restrictive policies on the acceptance of tobacco industry research money. The report noted that in over 87% of cases, the policy had been influenced by the work of the Cancer Research Council in urging that these policies be established. In Australia, 15 universities have explicit policies that forbid staff from accepting tobacco money[621].

Why has this exceptional momentum developed, applied uniquely to just one industry? There is now a well-documented history of the tobacco industry's effort to recruit scientists for lawyer-managed strategic purposes[622], particularly in the case of secondhand smoke (SHS) issues[136,202,546]. This programme of research has produced documented conduct such as failure to disclose competing interests[623], "unprecedented scientific fraud"[624] and data fabrication[177]. In the notable words of one internal industry document, consultants retained by the industry were said to be "prepared to do the kinds of things they were recruited to do"[139]. Most recently, Judge Gladys Kessler of the US Court of Appeals, in finding that tobacco companies had engaged in "racketeering", described the tobacco industry thus: "It is . . . an industry, and in particular these Defendants, that survives, and profits, from selling a highly addictive product which causes diseases that lead to a staggering number of deaths per year, an immeasurable amount of human suffering and economic loss, and a profound burden on our national health care system. Defendants have known many of these facts for at least 50 years or more. Despite that knowledge, they have consistently, repeatedly and with enormous skill and sophistication, denied these facts to the public, to the Government, and to the public health community."[625]

Barnes and Bero[626] have shown that the only variable explaining the difference in findings of studies on the health risks of SHS is author affiliation to the tobacco industry. Knowing this about the industry-supported research on SHS, why should we imagine the situation will be any different with regard to its research support for other branches of tobacco-related research?

Those who work for the tobacco industry are committed by contract of employment to defend and promote its interests. In the words of the Geneva Court of Appeal in the infamous case concerning industry consultant Ragner Rylander[627]: "Rylander's infringements of scientific integrity take on their full significance only when viewed within the framework of a strategy devised and conducted by the tobacco industry to cast doubt on the toxicity of tobacco smoke, particularly for non-smokers. The case of one person should not make us forget that the most unforgivable fault lies with an institutional and commercial force, the tobacco industry, whose objectives and interests run counter to both public health and medical science."[628]

The tobacco industry does not subscribe to the independent research ethos of transparent enquiry that is at the heart of scholarship. While the scientific community strives to be ever more open about its research methods, data sources and ethical governance, the tobacco industry has shredded documents it anticipated might be incriminating or embarrassing. The primary purpose of any research the industry undertakes or commissions is to advance its commercial objectives. Despite what we know from its internal documents[629], we will never see a public domain paper from a tobacco industry or industry-sponsored scientist demonstrating that tobacco advertising is highly influential with children, or that new forms of undeclared nicotine analogues[83] might be even more addictive than nicotine itself. Publication of such inflammatory material would see the industry scientists not long in their jobs, and the grant recipients would not be funded again. Only the profoundly naïve would believe that the tobacco industry would continue to support research that might potentially harm its bottom line.

Notes

i   Implemented by Australia, Belgium, Brazil, Canada, Jordan, Singapore, Thailand, Uruguay and Venezuela. Countries in the 25-member European Community have the option of requiring picture-based warnings, choosing from among 42 picture messages prepared by the European Commission. The governments of Bangladesh, Czech Republic, Hong Kong, India, Ireland, Malaysia, New Zealand, South Africa, Taiwan and United Kingdom have all said publicly that picture-based warnings are under consideration.

ii See the Legacy Tobacco Documents Library (http://legacy.library.ucsf.edu/).

iii This section is an edited version of Chapman S. Advocacy in action: extreme corporate makeover interruptus: denormalising tobacco industry corporate schmoozing. *Tob Control* 2004;**13**:445–7.

Chapter 8

Making Smoking History:
How Low Can We Go?

How low might we be able to reduce smoking prevalence in whole communities? An uncritical view of the global league table[i] today can give a misleading picture of apparent progress. The nations that have the lowest smoking prevalence for both sexes combined are all nations that have strong cultural proscriptions against smoking by women. The NationMaster website[ii], sourcing data from the World Health Organization, shows there are 44 nations where reported female smoking prevalence is under 10%, 28 where it is under 5%, and 12 that are under 2% (Qatar reports that 0.5% of women smoke). Ultra-low female smoking rates, which generally owe nothing to public health-based policies, lower the combined rate to levels sometimes far below those in nations where female smoking prevalence has been high but has fallen. There are few, if any, lessons for public health in examining most nations with an ultra-low prevalence of female smoking.

Greatest reductions in national prevalence

From a smoking control policy perspective, it is nations that have experienced large *falls* in smoking that invite informed speculation about how far the decline in tobacco use might continue. There are three frontrunners for the title of world's most successful smoking control nation: Canada, Australia and Sweden. At the state level, California and British Columbia stand out. Sweden, where a major shift has occurred from cigarettes to snus, has been discussed at length in Chapter 4. In Sweden in 2002, 13% of adult men and 19% of women smoked daily, giving a 16% daily smoking prevalence. Another 20% of men and 2% of women use snus daily but do not smoke[266], and Sweden has one of the lowest rates of tobacco-caused disease in the world.

In Canada in 2005, 15% of people aged 15 and over smoked daily (18% men, 12% women), with another 4% smoking less than daily (19% total). The province of British Columbia has 11% of people smoking daily. Just 7% of Canadian university graduates smoked daily[630]. In 2004, Australia had the same prevalence as Canada (19%) for daily plus weekly smoking, and had 17.4% of people aged 14 years and up smoking daily (18.6% men, 16.3% women). The state of Western Australia had 15.5% of people smoking daily[5].

As discussed in Chapter 5, for several years California hosted the world's best-funded tobacco control programme and pioneered smokefree public places, factors that have driven down both smoking frequency and prevalence. Today daily smoking prevalence in California is 9.8% with a further 5.3% smoking less than daily, giving a state prevalence of 15.2%. Puerto Rico's daily prevalence is 7.9%, with less than daily smokers adding another 5.2% for a total of 13.1% smoking. Latino populations in the USA generally have a lower smoking prevalence. Utah, with a strong Mormon population, has 11.5% smoking, but there are few practical implications in this for other populations[631].

How reliable are the data?

There are important concerns about the reliability of survey methods in determining true rates of smoking in communities. Some subpopulations with high smoking rates are never included in national survey-based estimates of smoking. These include prisoners (in mid-2005 there were 2 186 230 people in US jails – about 1% of the entire US adult population – and comprising an estimated 12% of all Black males, 3.7% of all Hispanic males and 1.7% of White males in their late twenties[632]. Seventy-nine percent of prisoners in New South Wales jails smoke[633]. Other groups generally excluded from surveys of smoking include: the homeless[634]; illegal immigrants; people in mental health institutions; people who do not speak the language of the country in which surveys are being conducted; and poor people living in remote areas with no phone.

Another concern is that rates are increasingly likely to be under-reported as response rates to telephone surveys decline. Technological advances (increased use of mobile phones and the use of answering machines to screen unwanted callers) have caused increases in under-reporting. In the California Tobacco Surveys, for example, response rates fell from 70% in 1992–93 to 51.1% in 1998–99[635]. However, one study comparing estimates obtained from the US Current Population Survey, which uses expensive door-to-door interviewing and obtains significantly higher response rates than phone surveys, showed that "under or over-representation of population sub-groups has not changed as response rates have declined"[635].

Together, these considerations combine to suggest an underclass of hidden smokers who may collectively add several percentage points onto "official" smoking prevalence rates in communities.

Projections for Australia

Survey-measured smoking prevalence has been falling in males almost continuously since the 1960s, when it was just below 60%. In women the fall has been from a lesser height (a maximum of 33% in 1976), but it has also fallen[636]. Between 1991 and 2004, smoking prevalence (daily + weekly) fell from 27.1% to 19.0%, a fall of 8.1% in absolute terms, averaging 0.58% a year and representing a 29.9% fall in relative terms from the 1991 level. In the 5 years 1991–1995, smoking prevalence fell on average by 0.34% per year, but in the most recent seven years (1998–2004), when mass-reach campaigning was resuscitated (see Chapter 7), the decline nearly doubled to 0.66% a year[5]. If this later rate continued, smoking would theoretically reach zero prevalence in 29 years, in 2034.

Is this realistic? Will smoking ever disappear or occupy the eccentric status enjoyed today by (e.g.) the tiny number of powdered snuff takers reliving the custom of the Victorian era? Or will it reach some low level below 10% and remain there? Optimists would argue that there are sound grounds for suggesting that the decline we are now seeing in nations addressing the problem will accelerate even faster. One 1998 US projection built on reducing youth smoking initiation from 30% to 20%, forecast that eventually no more than one-eighth of the US population (12.5%) would smoke, even if cessation rates did not decrease[637].

The current Californian "gold standard" of 9.8% smoking prevalence might be one benchmark. But why not strive for the levels reached by various subpopulations as an "art of the possible" reference point? Physicians in the USA and Australia have long had self-reported smoking prevalence rates of below 3%[535,638], driven presumably by peer and community expectations and their constant encounters with the harms of smoking. Warner and Burns argue "whether the hard core is best represented by the 2.1% of pregnant college graduates who continue to smoke, 3% of physicians, 6.4% of college-educated Californians, or 8.5% of Americans with postgraduate degrees, the majority of the 36.4% of blue-collar workers who smoke cannot reasonably be categorized as hard core" and that there is a long way to go before standard tried-and-true tobacco control strategies fail to deliver more ex-smokers[422].

In Australia, with 17.4% smoking daily, we have yet to see the impact of the introduction in 2007 of smokefree bars; pictorial pack warnings were only introduced in 2006; and recent sustained declines in youth smoking[518] will see smaller cohorts of new smokers entering smoking prevalence calculations in the next decade. Trends in home smoking bans are heading south, with 34% of Australian smokers living in smokefree homes[539]. Tasmania looks like implementing retail display bans, and several states are now dedicating unprecedented budgets to quit campaigns. There would appear to be no coherent case for forecasting any slowing of the current cessation rate.

When less than one in ten of the community smoke, and these continue to express almost universal regret about having started[536], the dynamics of smoking may change considerably from those operating today when nations "doing well" have more like one in five smoking. The increasing denormalisation of public smoking is likely to infect politicians as well, making them more receptive to "finishing the job" on tobacco control by mopping up remaining inconsistencies in overall policy and less anxious about offending ever-diminishing portions of the electorate.

Subpopulations with high smoking rates

As is the case for almost every disease and risk factor, smoking rates in all but the most impoverished nations are highest among those who have had the least formal education and are in the lowest socioeconomic groups. While many *countries* might be doing well by international standards, smoking in subpopulations of low socio-economic status typically shows a very different picture. For example in Australia, compared with the highest quintile for education and income, those in the lowest quintile have odds ratios for smoking of 1.69 (for education) and 1.43 (for income)[639]. Smoking duration from onset to cessation is 38% longer for those earning under $300 per week compared with those earning over $800. Those with less than 10 years of education smoked for 13% longer than those with more than 12 years of education[640]. Indigenous Australians have a smoking prevalence of 54%[641]. Australian lone mothers are more than twice as likely to smoke as mothers with partners[598]. People with current mental health problems are about twice as likely to smoke as those without any history of mental health problems. However, a substantial number of people with mental health problems (30.5%) have successfully quit smoking[642].

There are two broad analyses of what might be done about these disparities. The first argues that disparities in smoking prevalence mirror broad societal socio-economic disparities and that the differential between high and low socioeconomic segments of the population will not narrow until societies become more egalitarian on wider indices like income distribution and educational opportunity. In such analyses, particularly when they apply to subpopulations with multiple social and health disadvantages, smoking is seen as unlikely to yield much to "single risk factor" interventions. Qualitative research has often shown that smoking is used by people living in poverty to relieve stress and as a sort of "holiday" from hopelessness[643].

The second analysis emphasises that while smoking is much more prevalent in low-income groups and other disadvantaged populations, in many nations it remains the case that a minority of the very poor *don't* smoke, and that characterising the poverty/low education nexus with smoking as a kind of inevitability is not only inaccurate, but underestimates such groups' responsiveness to the same factors that have reduced smoking in all social strata.

To illustrate, Fig. 8.1 shows 20 years of smoking prevalence data from Victoria, Australia, for three levels of education. While the lowest educated group have always had a greater smoking prevalence than more educated groups, all three groups shown are tracking down in broadly parallel "tram tracks". This demonstrates that the major reason for smoking differentials is not different degrees of responsiveness to smoking cessation policies and programmes, but the higher initial prevalence from which less educated groups have had to reduce. If one looks at three groups (ever smokers, ex-smokers and current smokers) across the range of socioeconomic status, disadvantaged groups typically have higher ever and current smoking rates, but often identical ex-smoking rates, suggesting that the criticism that "orthodox" mass-reach policies and programmes "don't work" for them is misinformed.

More precision targeting?

Subpopulation disparities often produce calls for campaign money to be fractured into a series of different "targeted" campaigns designed to appeal better to differ-ent genders, age groups, sexual orientations, and (most often) socioeconomic, racial and ethnic groups. The argument runs that important cultural differences in each

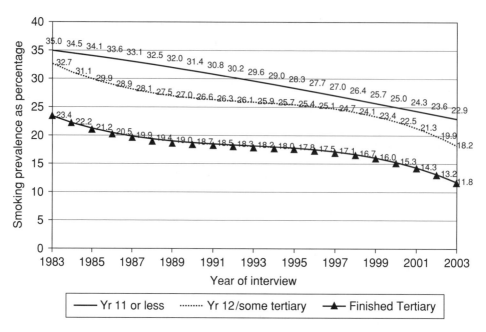

Fig. 8.1   Smoking prevalence trends of people aged 18 and over in Victoria, Australia, for three levels of education. Source: Centre for Behavioural Research in Cancer, Carlton.

of these groups cause smoking to be phenomenologically different from its role and meaning in other groups. "One size fits all" standard approaches to motivating cessation are therefore said to be insensitive, ill-conceived and bound not to work.

It is worth reflecting on whether the tobacco industry – in trying to promote smoking – conceives of the challenge in the same way. While the tobacco industry certainly does nuance many of its promotional efforts to make them more appealing to particular subpopulations[644,645], it rarely develops or succeeds in selling major brands exclusively to such groups. Major brand advertising and packaging is largely and increasingly globalised, suggesting that industry marketing intelligence believes that appeals are universal. We don't see *Marlboro*, *Camel* or *Mild Seven* packaged differently in different nations. Where advertising continues, it too is largely uniform and not fractured into major promotions for each of the many different cultural groups that make up multicultural societies today.

Moreover, research shows that different racial and socioeconomic groups respond equally well to quit campaigns. A recent analysis showed that declines in smoking prevalence among African-Americans from 1992 to 2002 showed no differences across US states, despite differing degrees of targeted smoking cessation activity between states[646]. Efforts to fracture limited campaign budgets into multiple smaller, targeted campaigns have many supporters in the professional health promotion community, but the cost will inevitably be a greatly diluted ability to mount the necessary large campaigns directed at the whole smoker population.

Smoking by doctors

In many nations today, smoking by doctors, medical students and other primary health-care workers remains outrageously high (see Box 8.1 for examples). When professionals at the coalface of health are known by their patients and the wider community to smoke, an obvious problem arises for efforts to convince communities that smoking is a serious health issue. Smoking by doctors may be a key indicator of a nation's overall standing in tobacco control: it seems unlikely that serious inroads can ever be made into a nation's smoking while its doctors smoke at levels that shout to the community "don't worry about this!"

Box 8.1   Incidence of smoking among doctors

- Armenia (Yerevan state medical university): 87.8% (A. Tadevosyan, personal communication)
- Australia: 2%[535]
- Czech Republic: 28% males, 17% females (E. Kralikova, personal communication)
- France: 28.8%[647]
- Germany: 10%[648]
- Italy: 28–33%[649]
- Moldova: 31.6% males, 9.2% females (I. Zatushevski, personal communication)
- New Zealand: 5%[650]
- Syria: 40.7% men, 11.4% women[651]
- Uruguay: 27%[652]
- USA: 3.3%[638]

The future

Today's tobacco control landscape in nations with advanced tobacco control would be almost unrecognisable to someone waking up from a 30-year sleep. So what changes are likely in the future? The momentum towards pictorial pack warnings, smokefree indoor air (including in bars), subsidised cessation and an overall denormalisation of smoking appears unstoppable. The Framework Convention on Tobacco Control will see many governments stimulated to implement laws and low-cost initiatives that will give tobacco control an unprecedented international boost.

Large public awareness campaigns to inform and motivate millions of smokers about quitting seem destined to remain a feature of everyday life in wealthier nations. However, very few poorer nations can afford to get even to the starting line with such campaigns, and try in vain to inform their communities through valiant, low-budget publicity efforts on World No Tobacco Day. A sustained international initiative to fund major public awareness campaigns in nations that could never afford to run such campaigns would make a huge difference to nations in which awareness remains rudimentary. The profligacy of certain areas of tobacco control expenditure in some industrialised nations is embarrassing when there are now many more smokers and smoking-caused deaths in less developed nations.

Items on a more radical agenda that I expect to see emerge in cutting edge nations at the vanguard of tobacco control include:

- laws that would require tobacco companies to pay for any cost incurred in smokers trying to quit;
- mandatory repatriation of all earnings from underage smokers to a central fund to be used to fund prevention campaigns;
- regulation of the industry that would see an international network of national nicotine regulatory authorities stipulate and enforce standards for maximum emissions;
- quality assurance accreditation procedures, validated by pseudo-patient methods, that would see doctors who failed to offer smokers advice to quit deemed medically incompetent.

Licensing smokers?

There is one possibility that today seems utterly radical, but may develop some momentum among those concerned to reduce smoking dramatically while safe-guarding inviolate ethical concerns for the protection of fully sentient individuals to harm themselves with tobacco if they choose to do so.

The tobacco industry commonly asserts that it wishes to sell its products only to informed adults: smoking is a highly risky choice, undertaken, it says, by people who know the risks they are taking. In Chapter 1, I cited examples of research demonstrating that large proportions of adult smokers are in fact poorly informed about these risks and that the tobacco industry currently does little to try to rectify this. However, the industry accepts, at least as a matter of public rhetoric, that it is not legitimate to sell to the uninformed. Further, it is inconceivable that it would try to make a virtue out of selling to the ill-informed, so opposing the principle of the adequately informed smoker would present it with considerable difficulties.

What if we took the industry at its word and introduced a system of smoker licensing that required all smokers to pass a knowledge test showing that they were adequately informed of the risks they took. Licensed smokers might be given a photo ID smart card, which would be used on each occasion of purchase. This would record all purchases and not permit sales unless recorded against a licence. Purchasing limits in the smart card (say two packets per day maximum) could prevent large-scale purchasing of cigarettes by licensed smokers for on-selling to unlicensed smokers (particularly young people). Further, governments could experiment with financial incentives to encourage licensed smokers to surrender their cards. This would place a major obstacle in the way of relapse because with-out a smart card, former smokers would find it much more difficult to obtain a regular supply of cigarettes without re-obtaining a licence.

Objections about restrictions on civil liberties arising from purchasing limits could be countered by analogies with other restricted products such as prescription drugs, where users are only permitted to purchase defined quantities with a form of licence (a doctor's prescription) because of concerns about potential abuse and harm. And where harm is suffered not only by individuals but also by the community through transferred social costs, the justification is not only protecting people from themselves, but also protecting the community against incurring preventable costs. Concerns about the privacy of one's smoking status being potentially abused could be countered by pointing out that life insurance companies already require clients to declare their smoking status.

A licensing scheme could be funded either by smokers themselves, just as driving tests and licence renewal are paid for by drivers, or perhaps more appropriately by industry. Given the uniqueness of tobacco in terms of harm and addictiveness, why should the industry, which profits from its use, not be responsible for the costs of ensuring that use is limited to those deemed sufficiently informed? This seems a very small price to pay to be allowed to profit from the sale of this anomalous product and to avoid being sued by smokers, who in being licensed, would have given their documented informed consent.

Two further matters of cardinal importance need to be addressed in considering any potential test of whether or not smokers are adequately informed: addiction and equity. The foregoing argument is greatly complicated by the occurrence of (often rapid) nicotine addiction, and the fact that most smokers begin smoking in childhood when they are legally incapable of making informed decisions on important matters. The importance of adequate information presupposes that people are able to make free, self-regarding decisions based on relevant facts. But as the tobacco industry knows "the entire matter of addiction is the most potent weapon a prosecuting attorney can have in a lung cancer/cigarette case. We can't defend continued smoking as 'free choice' if the person was 'addicted' "[85].

As discussed in Chapter 1, the notion of voluntarily taking on the risks of having one's capacity for future voluntary activity impaired is highly problematic. An addicted smoker who passed a smokers' licence knowledge test could hardly be said to be "freely" choosing to smoke, despite their tested awareness of the risks involved. Adding to the difficulty, most would have become addicted as children, when by legal definition they could not be said to be capable of making an informed choice.

Requiring a personalised smart card that would be extremely difficult to forge and would allow an agreed daily limit of supply to each licensed smoker would almost certainly reduce opportunities for non-licensed children to gain open access to cigarettes, so the concept may be worth exploring for that additional advantage.

Finally, important issues of equity are relevant. While smoking is less common among people with intellectual disability than in the general population[653] there are still many such people who smoke. In designing any policy or regulatory responses to the problems of being adequately informed, it would be important to pay proper regard to the different levels of education that exist within the populations targeted, and to tailor responses where appropriate. Passing a test of adequate comprehension of the risks of smoking would present greater difficulties to less educated people and those with disabilities, yet tailoring such a test to a level that made passing require only rudimentary knowledge would defeat the purpose of trying to ensure truly adequate understanding among smokers. This issue is likely to be the most problematic associated with establishing any common standard of being "adequately informed".

Notes

i   Latest data in 2003 for 196 nations are given at Globalink (http://www. globalink.org/tccp/).

ii See NationMaster (http://www.nationmaster.com).

Part II

An A–Z of Tobacco Control Advocacy Strategy

Introduction

I've been involved in public health advocacy since the late 1970s, when the success I and colleagues had in removing the actor Paul Hogan from Winfield cigarette advertising because of his appeal to children[9] caused me to reflect that there was in fact a great deal of method in the day-to-day of rat-cunning, street-wise, opportunistic efforts that characterize advocacy practice.

At the time, *The Australian* newspaper headlined our victory with "MOP UP's slingshot cuts down the advertising ogre" – an allusion to the most clichéd and *disabling* metaphor in public health advocacy – David's single-handed victory over Goliath. For many years, it has been common to use the metaphor to describe advocacy struggles. Its essence is the victory of the small and good over the big and evil: about contests between adroit, strategic little groups and the lumbering, all-powerful ogres like the tobacco industry. In this respect the metaphor has always been apt. However, advocacy victories are rarely won with the casting of a single stone that hits its mark in one celebrated action. Accounts of the passage of public health victories that focus exclusively on these final acts do huge injustice to the protracted social and political processes that invariably precede victories in the more publicised endgames of these fights.

A more instructive metaphor is one attributed to the 18th century French satirist Voltaire, and once picked up by a former head of the US Tobacco Institute, who said that working for his industry was like being slowly pecked to death by ducks. Pecks from single ducks are merely irritating, but resolute ducks persistently foraging over the years will distract, humiliate, weaken, ostracise and enfeeble even the most robust of foes.

Michael Pertschuk, a founder of the Advocacy Institute in Washington DC, counsels that "Media advocacy requires art, imagination, and creativity; any effort to reduce it to a series of rigid and prescribed steps is doomed to mediocrity or failure. But practitioners tend to agree on the soundness of certain basic operating principles or practices". This statement summarises well the scope, spirit and intent of this second part of the book. I hope to present a comprehensive selection of what most experienced public health advocates would regard as core strategies, tactics and general guiding principles that should underlie advocacy work. Case studies are included to better enliven the text.

I have taught classes in public health advocacy since 1992. One of the most challenging tasks I always face is how to make students comfortable with the notion that a two-hour session on, say, "dealing with your opposition" or "interview strategies", can only scrape the surface of the range of possibilities that any public health advocate will encounter. Some students sit expectantly hoping to take down a sure-fire blueprint for catapulting any health issue onto the front page or for blasting any anti-public health interest group out of the water. They are often disillusioned to find that even when very experienced and successful public health advocates describe their work, their accounts frequently include vast tracts of untheorised and on-the-run tactics that, of necessity, have been developed or adapted to fit new, unique or changing circumstances. This is very much the reality of the day-to-day of advocacy, and one of the most cardinal sections in this part of the book is that dealing with "Opportunism".

Nonetheless, most experienced advocates also know that there is considerable preparation, analysis and strategic planning involved, and I hope I have captured much of this. The section is updated from my 1994 book *The Fight for Public Health: Principles and Practice of Media Advocacy*[1]. Some of the material has been adapted from my 1983 book *The Lung Goodbye*[654]. Parts of the sections on "Columnists", "Editorials", "Interview strategies", "Letters to the editor", "Media etiquette", "Op-Ed page access", "Reporters and journalists", and "Targeting or narrowcasting" have been borrowed and adapted from two publications from the Washington DC Advocacy Institute[655,656] with their kind permission.

Not losing sight of the big picture

Before considering specific strategies, it is important to place advocacy in the wider perspective of the goals it is designed to achieve. Anyone engaging in advocacy needs to be clear about the overall public health aims and objectives of the advocacy work in which they are engaged. Failure to understand and constantly to reflect on these objectives can mean embarking on strategies that consume much unproductive energy and contribute little to advancing the real public health goals with which advocates should be ultimately concerned. Advocacy is a *strategy* within public health, and like the adoption of any strategy, decisions about advocacy should result from a disciplined analysis of the problem being addressed. Advocacy is not an end in itself. Failure to understand this can lead to situations where advocacy objectives override the public health objectives that they were originally designed to meet.

The Advocacy Institute in Washington DC advises:

> From the beginning, you should have a good idea of what your media advocacy strategies are trying to accomplish. Review those goals as your messages develop into the framing stages: Are your goals still being met by the way you have framed your issue? Are the goals still appropriate? Finally, when the message has been spread and the results can be seen, take time to evaluate the process you went through. Did anything go wrong and, if so, how can you frame your message differently the next time? What worked especially well? *Throughout the goals and message process, always keep in mind media advocacy's ultimate aim: to use media to advance your group's public policy goals.* [my emphasis][2]

The main, broad strategies of public health advocacy – media advocacy, political lobbying, coalition and network building – can each exert a mesmerising effect on advocates and blind them to the real goals and objectives that these strategies are intended to address. In the case of media advocacy, perhaps the most common confusion of objectives with strategy lies with the mistaking of mere *coverage* in the media with the *purpose* of being covered in the media. The phenomenon of "column inches envy" is widely encountered in the advocacy arena, with many being impressed by the volume of coverage certain issues or spokespeople attract, when the far more important issue is whether this volume actually advances the cause that it is supposed to serve.

With most issues, the media have a very short attention span. They may think your issue is fine and newsworthy and give it an avalanche of prominent coverage, lulling you into the belief that you have done all the right things, satisfied the news values and so on. But a day or two later, there will be not a trace of the story: the media will have "consumed" your issue to its satisfaction and moved onto other issues in the never-ending chase for what the very word *news* implies – newness and difference.

A good example of this was the introduction of a new brand of flavoured cigarettes, *DJ Mix*, to the Australian market in 2005. The cigarettes were packed in fluoro-coloured packs and available in several artificial fruit flavours. The total package, from the brand name, the pack and the sickly-sweet flavouring, was nakedly and unmistakably directed at teenagers. The cigarettes were the tobacco equivalent of alco-pops. Australian tobacco control agencies purchased packs and opportunistically placed these with various journalists and politicians. A few days of positive news publicity followed but, months on, the packs remained on sale in all but two states. Some agencies failed to see beyond the initial potential for outrage and did not seem to have any plan beyond simply saying "Look at this! Please do something!"

Providing a sumptuous feast to feed the media's appetite for commentary, perspective and "angles" on any particular massacre or incident should *not* be seen as the main objective of public health advocacy. Merely playing out the role of outraged health group against the evil empire of the tobacco lobby may make good television, but may do relatively little tangibly to advance policy. The objective should be to harness this appetite in the service of objectives that will lead to reduced tobacco death in the community. The power of the media in capturing a nation's attention about an issue should be exploited in the strategic service of objectives like transforming public concern into public pressure, causing political decision-makers to move closer to introducing legislation or laying the foundations that will establish an enduring structure or movement that will assist these processes in the future.

Ten basic questions for planning advocacy strategy[i]

For those wanting a quick, nutshell view of the most important questions I believe all advocates should consider before embarking on an advocacy campaign, the following ten questions may be helpful.

1. What are your public health objectives with this issue?

Put simply, what do you want to change or preserve? All proposed advocacy strategies need then to be interrogated for their relevancy to achieving these objectives.

2. Can a "win-win" outcome be first engineered with decision-makers?

Politicians and other key decision-makers are naturally keen to avoid being seen to be pressured into making decisions, and would much prefer to be seen to be leading initiatives. Wherever possible, advocates should try first to work with government to effect a marriage of interests. When obdurate government intransigence is the root problem, criticism is generally unavoidable but will often close doors. In such circumstances, divide your advocacy voices into the moderates, who will continue to work the "inside route" with government, and the vanguards, who will take a critical public role in the media, setting the public agenda (see "Criticising government" and "Inside and outside the tent" below).

3. Who do the key decision-makers answer to, and how can these people be influenced?

In all democracies, key health decision-makers remain answerable to those who appoint or elect them. Political parties hang onto power by virtue of winning marginal seats in elections. If those marginal electorates vote differently at the next election, governments can fall (see "Marginal seats"). Health ministers are answerable to political cabinets, and health bureaucrats are answerable to health ministers, who will not relish their portfolio being criticised. Business executives are answerable to boards of directors. Advocates therefore need to study ways of accessing and influencing those whom key decision-makers worry about or who endorse their policies.

4. What are the strengths and weaknesses of your and your opposition's position?

You, your opposition and the positions both are advocating require ruthless auditing for the ways in which they are perceived by those whose support and influence is being courted. What you learn here will be critical both to your own presentation and to the tack you take in discrediting your opponents. Know your opposition inside out and keep all manner of antennae alert for feedback about your own organisation's public reception. Rehearse the worst questions you could face, and practice putting forward your own most compelling points. Go to every interview with a maximum of three points you want to make, regardless of what you are asked (see "Know your opposition" and "Interview strategies").

5. What are your media advocacy objectives?

Your advocacy objectives must always serve your agreed public health objectives, and not be confused as ends in themselves (such as relentlessly pursuing media exposure with dubious connection to your agreed goals). Media advocacy objectives can include: causing a neglected issue to become discussed or a much discussed issue to be discussed *differently*; discrediting one's opponents; introducing pivotally compelling facts and perspectives into a debate; or introducing different voices in ways calculated to enhance the authenticity or power of an argument.

6. How will you frame what is at issue?

Political debate is largely about multiple definitions of the same events and, accordingly, advocates need to ensure that the way they define what is at issue in a health debate becomes the dominant definition circulating in the community. As discussed in Chapters 2 and 3, framing strategy is the core skill of media advocacy. For example, the tobacco industry seeks to frame tobacco advertising as freedom of speech, whereas tobacco control advocates try to reframe it as the highly researched effort at attracting children to smoking that will lead many of them into years of addiction and eventual disease. If the industry's definition dominates, controls on advertising are unlikely.

7. What symbols or word pictures can be brought into this frame?

The news media's demands for brevity require that we maximise every opportunity to leave a lasting impression with media audiences. Many public health issues appear arcane, technical and impenetrable to ordinary people and unlikely to excite public or political interest. To gain their attention and to locate public health issues in shared value frameworks, the perspicacious and evocative use of analogy and metaphor is important. Think of how the change you want has parallels and precedents in other widely embraced areas of public life. Associate your cause with the same values that underlie these accepted issues.

Advocates also need to appreciate the dramaturgical dimension to news gathering. Significantly, journalists refer to those appearing in the news as "talent" and audiences often assess news "performance" through criteria like believability, trustworthiness and how likeable those in the news were. Decide which "role" you want to play and how you will seek to cast your opposition (see "Talent").

8. What sound bites can be used to convey 6 and 7?

The length of time given to newsmakers to speak in the media continues to shrink[657,658]. Often, these "sound bites" are the only statements reported and so they assume crucial importance. The larger the audience for a news bulletin, the more truncated is the time devoted to each item. Those who disdain and eschew such news media should be disqualified as serious advocates. Every interview with a journalist should plan to inject at least one sound bite into the conversation. These are pithy, memorable and repeatable summations that can come to epitomise a debate. A memorable example: "a non-smoking section of a restaurant is like a non-urinating section of a swimming pool". See "Interview strategies".

9. Can the issue be personalised?

A senior Sydney journalist once told me, unforgettably, that "experts are fine, but they are not actually a living thing". Journalists hunger for ways to locate health stories within stories about real people who are affected by a health problem. Experts are typically stock embellishments to the "real" human story that is crafted to address the concerns and interests of ordinary readers. If journalists will try to ground the story through an ordinary citizen's perspective, involving consumers in advocacy will be important because you will be seen as having both expertise and authenticity.

10. How can large numbers of people quickly be organised to express their concerns?

Statements from "the usual suspects" who always speak up for an issue risk being marginalised by politicians as predictable and unimportant. Efforts to build vocal constituencies who are willing to speak out for issues at strategically important times should therefore be given high priority. Newspapers' letters pages are seen as key barometers of community concern. All politicians talk of the impression they gain from the reaction (or lack of it) of their electorate to issues in the news. Internet tools such as distribution lists, list servers and chat rooms permit instant mass dissemination of "action alerts": email templates that describe a problem, provide key pieces of information, outline suggested courses of action, and equip recipients with relevant facts and data. Within minutes, thousands of people can be mobilised to write letters to politicians and newspapers, call radio stations, vote in online opinion polls, or petition decision-makers. See "Action alerts", "Internet", "Letters to the editor".

Further reading

- A large bibliography on health, advocacy and the mass media compiled by me (http://www.health.usyd.edu.au/current/coursework/media.php).
- Two recent guides on tobacco control advocacy and movement building; see Tobacco Control Strategy Planning (http://strategyguides.globalink.org/).
- The National Coalition Building Institute (http://www.ncbi.org/).
- Jim Shultz's Strategy Development: Key Questions for Developing an Advocacy Strategy (http://www.democracyctr.org/resources/strategy.html) (plus a link to his book *The Democracy Owner's Manual*).

AN A–Z OF STRATEGY

Accuracy

Accuracy is the bedrock of responsible advocacy. Inaccurate data or facts are one of the quickest ways of seeing your credibility walk out the door with journalists and influential people, perhaps permanently. Always check and double-check statements and data before releasing them, and surround yourself with trusted, responsive people with specialised skills who understand the importance of accuracy and who can help with checking statements and calculations. Some advocates, though, are overly preoccupied with the supposed inaccuracy of press reports. However, a survey of first authors of scientific papers appearing in the *New England Journal of Medicine* found that only 3% of the authors believed that the press coverage of their articles had been "inaccurate". Importantly, most felt positive about the role of the media in reporting medical and health issues to the public[121]. Despite such studies, many health workers who are wary of dealing with the media cite as their main concern past experiences of inaccuracy in reporting. Often, such statements reflect a wholesale misunderstanding of the nature of news reporting. There is often an unreasonable expectation that a newspaper report should be almost like a truncated version of a scientific paper, replete with the same emphases and detached language that are conventional in scientific reports. In the eyes of the media, the big news about your study may be perceived quite differently from the emphasis that you as an author would want to see stressed. Such differences in interest or emphasis can create tensions that are not easily resolved. However, if you are concerned that you might be misquoted or that the issue under discussion runs a high risk of being reported in a technically incorrect or misleading way, it is perfectly sensible to ask press journalists to send you their copy before it goes to press. Do this in a spirit of cooperation and friendliness, not of obvious mistrust. Journalists will also be concerned that their reports are accurate, because glaring inaccuracies that attract corrections or retractions can make journalists look unprofessional (see also "Media etiquette").

When you get the draft text of the article, it is imperative that you respect the journalist's need to observe any deadlines that they have specified and return any corrections to them quickly. If the journalist has put a critical or unkind interpretation or slant on your issue, but has not transgressed any matters of accuracy, your position regarding corrections is rather different than when there are simple factual errors in the report. Remember that the journalist has not extended the courtesy of allowing you to check the report in order that you might engage him or her in debate about contentious issues or your differing perceptions of the key news angle.

Acronyms

If you are forming a public health advocacy group, it will need a name. Journalists generally cannot cope with a negative answer to "who do you represent?" The name of your group does not have to be acronymic, but acronymic names for advocacy groups can be useful in capturing the interest of journalists and the public. An acronym should ideally be a real word or a play on a word that is somehow apposite to or suggestive of the issue that a group is addressing, or the actions they are intending to perform (see examples below). Acronyms that spell words that do not exist (e.g. FCA – the Framework Convention Alliance), or allude to nothing meaningful require people not only to inquire about what the letters in the words stand for, but also to remember a vocabulary of new names that do not trigger apposite associations.

When should an acronymic name be used? Most groups that decide to use acronyms tend to be fringe groups with confrontational agendas and that operate outside the more established non-governmental organisations (NGOs). Establishment NGOs have a more sober, serious sense of themselves, often bound up with needing to appeal to the broad and conservative public for donations and bequests. Acronyms, especially those that are strident or irreverent, do not sit well with such bodies. This can often mean that establishment organisations will be reluctant to be seen to associate with acronymic groups, even when they are working towards the same cause. Conservative groups fear that association with radical groups may be perceived by the public as meaning that they share all aspects of the radical groups' agenda and strategies. But the fact that they often do not share these, goes a long way to explaining why radical groups may decide to form (see "Radicalism").

Acronymic names have historically connoted radicalism, irreverence and mocking, a "gloves-off" approach to campaigning and a more ephemeral existence for the group. They are seldom listed in a telephone directory, for example. Such objectives and the strategies that are consistent with them often have an important role in public health advocacy. Therefore before deciding to name your group with an acronym you should consider whether this is the sort of profile and set of expectations you wish to foster.

Examples of reader-friendly acronyms

ACT UP (AIDS Coalition to Unleash Power)
AGHAST (Action Groups to Halt Advertising and Sponsorship of Tobacco)
ASH (Action on Smoking and Health)
BUGA UP (Billboard Utilising Graffitists Against Unhealthy Promotions)
DOC (Doctors Ought to Care)
MADD (Mothers Against Drunk Drivers)
MOP UP (Movement Opposed to the Promotion of Unhealthy Products)

Action alerts

These are succinct emailed calls to action, sent out to members of coalitions and networks, or to advocacy email groups of people willing to take action on an advocacy initiative (see also "Networks and coalitions", "Internet", "Letters to politicians"). They are built around a template with the following headings, which I have illustrated with a hypothetical (although realistic) example.

Headline

A bold, attention-getting title for the alert.

Summary

Here, summarise what has happened, is about to happen or, in the case of your advocacy taking the lead on an issue, what you are wanting to see happen.

Example: The Acme Tobacco Company (ATC) has produced a glossy educational package for schools on "making healthy choices" about drugs, including tobacco. ATC is distributing this to schools. It includes a schoolchildren's essay competition with prizes of educational equipment for 50 schools and university fee scholarships for ten outstanding students. The package has been designed by a retired high-school principal with an outstanding reputation. This person is seen on national television meeting with the national parliamentary secretary for education who enthuses about the new package and urges schools to use it.

Objectives

Here, you say what you want to see happen as a result of the advocacy campaign described in this action alert.

Example:

- To discredit the ATC kit as a cynical public relations exercise designed to distract attention from the company's lucrative earnings from teenage smoking and as a possible means of accessing school students for market research purposes.
- To use the incident as a trigger to call on the tobacco industry to hand all its earnings from youth smoking to a truly independent tobacco control trust, which would run effective interventions.

Useful facts

A set of facts and statistics that can be highlighted in recipients' actions (see below).

Example:

- More than 85% of smokers commence smoking as teenagers.
- Tobacco industry internal documents repeatedly refer to the vital commercial importance of capturing teenage smokers. See industry quotes below.
- The value of the teenage market to the tobacco industry in Australia is $18.7 million[533].
- The ATC's market share of the teenage market is 60%, therefore they earn $11.22 million from youth smoking each year.
- The estimated cost of the ATC education kit is $50 000 – 0.44% of the company's earnings from youth.
- If all companies were obliged to return their teenage earnings to an independent tobacco control agency, $18.7 million a year would provide a massive boost to the limited funds now available for prevention efforts.

Analysis of problem

Here, succinctly outline why the episode is a problem that needs addressing.

Example: Tobacco companies derive major income from underage smoking. Their internal documents repeatedly reveal that they invest small, token sums in teenage smoking prevention campaigns as a way of feigning social responsibility and distracting government from regulation that will affect consumption. The embrace of the ATC kit by the education minister illustrates that this cynical public relations exercise can work. Tobacco companies have no role in smoking prevention. In allowing "the fox into the henhouse" there is a risk that under the guise of "educational research" the company may seek to learn more about how better to market cigarettes to youth. Government should consider imposing a tax on tobacco companies based on an audited assessment of the income flowing to each company from illegal underage sales. This tax should be hypothecated to a national independent tobacco control trust fund, with no input from tobacco companies, and used to run evidence-based interventions known to decrease tobacco use.

Suggested actions

Here, say what you want recipients of the action alert to actually do (other than be outraged!)

Example:

- Email your local political representative (here the action alert should electronically link to a directory of all politicians' email addresses to allow recipients of the alert to compose and send an email with just a few mouse clicks. Such directories can often be found on government websites).
- Write to or visit your local high-school principal, urging that he or she refuses to use the kit and to make a public statement about why they have done this. (Suggest recipients write the letter citing the information provided in this action alert.)
- Write a letter to a newspaper; call up a talk-back radio programme and express your concerns.
- Write a letter to the renowned educational expert, politely suggesting that they reconsider their involvement in this exercise.

You might also consider providing a set of Frequently Asked Questions/Responses that may be thrown back at critics of this exercise.

Sources of information

Here, list a limited number of relevant background readings, accessible to anyone with internet access, which will give your recipients relevant information.

Example:

- White V, Scollo M. What are underage smokers worth to Australian tobacco companies? *Aust NZ J Pub Health* 2003;**27**:360–1 (with an online link to the paper).
- *Danger in the Playground*. ASH UK's detailed analysis of why tobacco companies run youth prevention programmes (http://www.ash.org.uk/html/advspo/html/playground.html#_edn5).

Relevant tobacco industry quotes

Here are several industry quotes that would be relevant to our example under discussion:

- "This is one of the proposals we shall initiate to show that we as an industry are doing something about discouraging young people to smoke. This of course is a phony way of showing sincerity as we all know."[528]
- "If younger adults turn away from smoking, the industry will decline, just as a population which does not give birth will eventually dwindle."[659]
- "As we discussed, the ultimate means for determining the success of this program will be: 1) A reduction in legislation introduced and passed restricting or banning our sales and marketing activities; 2) Passage of legislation favorable to the industry; 3) greater support from business, parent, and teacher groups."[660]

Advertising in advocacy

This is the purchasing of space or broadcast time to have your issue publicised in a fully controlled, unedited way. Because the advertiser controls the text, script and layout, nothing needs to be left to chance, with no reliance on journalists to put the desired inflection in your message. However, advertising costs money, with the greater the size of the audience or readership, the greater the cost. Unless your agency is well funded or you have a philanthropic benefactor, such advertising will generally be out of reach and you will need to rely on news making and publicity to get your messages out. This is the situation for the overwhelming majority of advocacy groups working in the public health field.

There are hundreds of books, courses, consultants and advertising agencies offering advice on how to achieve optimal results through advertising. Such advice lies beyond the scope of this book, save for mention of one potentially inexpensive way that poorly funded advocacy groups can get to use this medium.

Signature "petition" advertising

Statements and "open letters" (see "Open letters") to politicians, regulatory authorities or industries can be published as paid advertisements with a long list of signatories below the statement text. The cost of the advertisement can be shared by having each signatory contribute. Many individuals and agencies like to see their name in print and, moreover, may feel concerned about their name being absent from a long published list of prominent people supporting an issue. If you have a network of agencies that support your cause, the text of the letter should be circulated with a request that those wishing to sign should notify their approval to the organisers. Payment should quickly follow as most newspapers will insist on pre-payment for large advertisements placed by groups without regular advertising accounts.

Once you know the price of the size and placement of advertisement required, you can calculate how many signatories are needed if you are to request contributions that are within the means of your supporters. When a minimum number of signatories have been gathered, you can then decide on whether to gather more and turn the exercise into a fund-raising venture.

If your list of signatories includes celebrities (see "Celebrities"), ask if they can suggest other celebrities who might sign. Celebrities tend to associate with other celebrities and may have access to their unlisted phone numbers, saving you much time. Celebrity signatures will add news value and the media may want to interview some. By going public, signatories must accept responsibility for their views, but it is likely that some of the signatories will not have up-to-date or accurate information and may become a liability if they are interviewed without proper briefing. You should follow up with information kits or fact sheets, and offer to assist with briefings if media follow-up occurs.

Analogies, metaphors, similes and word pictures

These can be powerful ways of efficiently and memorably translating your issue into concepts and comparisons that will mean more to people. Analogies are a time-honoured way of constructing *sound bites* (see below). Some examples:

- When former British Prime Minister Margaret Thatcher gave an export award to a tobacco company, David Simpson, then director of Great Britain's Action on Smoking and Health, described the award as being "like a rabid dog winning Cruft's Dog Show".

- The appointment of an industry representative to a role where their vested interests are likely to be safeguarded or promoted can evoke the time-honoured "it's like putting Dracula in charge of the blood bank" or "giving the fox the keys to the henhouse".

- Greg Connolly of Harvard's School of Public Health has argued that the public health principle that you do not "flavour rancid meat" should also apply to the flavouring of cigarettes with delectable ingredients designed to cool the mouth and throat, and make smoking easier for children starting to experiment.

- Canadian Heather Crowe who, despite being gravely ill, energetically campaigned about secondhand smoke before dying in May 2006, aged 61, was quoted in *The Ottawa Citizen*: "You wouldn't put your dog in the garage, turn the car on, and walk away. And neither should governments allow people to work in what pretty much amounts to gas chambers. It's too late for me, but it's the next generation I've been doing this for."

Anniversaries

Many public health issues are mile-posted by significant events such as catastrophes, deaths of significant people who died from particular diseases, the publication of expert reports or inquiries, and government decisions or back-offs. Journalists will sometimes flag such events and on their anniversaries will prepare "re-visit" stories. These typically ask "what has progressed?" questions, and explore whether the same problems are still happening.

Advocates know these milestones more than others, but too seldom plan to exploit them, opting instead simply to react to approaches from journalists. Anniversaries that could give rise to large and positive media coverage are often completely overlooked. Here are some actions that you should take:

- Note all significant anniversaries on planning charts; enter them into electronic diaries so that they are flagged automatically for you some weeks earlier.
- Contact journalists in advance, suggesting angles that they may wish to pursue.
- Brief appropriate spokespeople who could give expert or personal commentary.
- Undertake any creative calculations relating to the passage of time since the anniversary (e.g. number of tobacco deaths since publication of a major report on smoking and health in your country).
- Consider if there is scope for sending a very public and poignant anniversary present to friends or foes of public health.
- Plan media events or stunts that might break through media indifference to the anniversary.

Be there! The first rule of advocacy

There are critical political decision-making forums in every society, whether these are parliamentary, religious, local governmental or even particular golf clubs! Public health advocates need to understand the way these forums operate. Who is known to have influence with a key health minister or politician? With their political peers? With their marginal seat colleagues? With members of their families? With their church leaders? With someone in their tennis groups or ski lodge? Where is the real business of a political party forged? This sort of information needs to be gathered and exploited through all the other principles of opportunism and networking discussed in this section of the book.

The core "being there" principle needs translation into the multitude of opportunities that can be important in public health advocacy. For example, if you work in an institution like a large hospital or university where a tobacco policy is being debated, and know that certain administrative committees are where the relevant decisions could be taken, try and get yourself or a trusted representative appointed to that committee. If you succeed, this may involve many hours of attending to matters that are very distant from public health – valuable time that you might consider wasted. However, if your committee membership leads to the passage of important policies that would be unlikely to have been raised in your absence, what more is there to say? Personal friendships with key decision-makers and politicians can also be critical avenues of influence.

Bluff

In advocacy, as in poker, bluff can be an important tactic that can cause your opponents to act unwisely. Saul Alinsky wrote that "Power is not only what you have but what the enemy thinks you have"[661]. This principle can have special meaning to small, unfunded community groups engaged in public health advocacy against formidably powerful foes. Bluff in advocacy can mean anything from cultivating a deliberate ambiguity about the size of your group to allusions about the extent of your contacts within your opponents' ranks (see "Infiltration"). Your opponents may well be adept bluffers as well. So again, as in poker, calling the bluff of your opponents can sometimes precipitate ill-advised moves by them that may advantage your cause.

Boycotts

The call for the boycott of a service, institution or product, formidable as it can sound, is probably the most over-used and ineffective strategy in public health advocacy. This is because there is a world of difference between simply *calling* for a boycott and successfully *organising* a boycott. And mostly, boycotts are simply called for, rather than organised in a sustained way that enables them to achieve their intended objectives. It is not difficult to recall many examples of outraged health workers or consumers calling for concerned people to boycott products made by a company that has in some way offended. But there are few examples of boycotts that have actually worked, hurting their targets and causing changes to occur in the factors that inspired the boycott[662,663].

The call for a boycott carries the powerful subtext that the product or company is in some way morally reprehensible. Consequently, a highly publicised call for a boycott may lend a degree of negative publicity to the object of the boycott. But because so much news is transitory and ephemeral, a mere call for a boycott will probably gain publicity once or twice, whereas the boycott process and its results will be a different matter. In summary then, don't abuse the potential power of a boycott by merely hurling the word into the media ether if you do not make an extensive commitment to following through with the threat.

Successful boycotts are most easily organised at a local level, where loss of trade or customers by, for example, a hospital canteen that insists on stocking cigarettes, can be realistically organised. A boycott in such circumstances should be a last resort, following representations to the offending outlet, then publicity about its inaction and perhaps other lobbying strategies such as customer petitions and picketing.

Bureaucratic constraints

Many working in public health are employed by government departments, or by non-governmental organisations with conservative political agendas. Bureaucrats are often frustrated by the political constraints under which they are obliged to work. Often they report conflict between their professional assessment of what should be done to advance government policy and their knowledge that certain important actions are politically unacceptable in the wider context of government, perhaps conflicting with other portfolios like agriculture, labour and industry. For example, government may be underfunding public health campaigns or refusing to implement policy or legislation that is vital to a public health objective. Such situations can create tensions between the professional views of those ostensibly employed by government to reduce the tobacco toll and the sense of duty they are supposed to feel towards the policies of the government that employs them. Their own ideals become compromised and their roles are reduced to appearing to protect politicians' careers. This frustration can often breed a willingness to help outsiders by precipitating courses of action that they themselves cannot be seen to participate in, but that once placed on the government agenda, they may be able to manipulate to advantage.

The classic ways of bureaucrats helping are by leaking documents and by fore-warning of events, meetings and impending announcements, thus enabling anticipatory action by public health groups in the community. Bureaucrats will be the best judge of what is potentially useful and of their own security in leaking particular pieces of information. They may be able to suggest prudent times for writing certain letters, or provide valuable background information that might assist the content and timing of your submissions to politicians.

One view of government bureaucracy is that the duty of those working in it is to provide unquestioning support for policies of the government of the day. If the government is going soft on the tobacco industry, the duty of a health bureaucrat, according to this view, is not to take any actions that might provoke a change in government policy or practice. Rather, the bureaucrat is expected to offer or suppress advice and information in ways that will best serve the government policy of the day. I am not writing this book for those who subscribe to this view, but rather for public health workers (including government bureaucrats) dedicated to improving public health outcomes. This section offers some advice about how to circumvent such bureaucratic constraints and oil the wheels of public health advocacy from inside government or conservative organisations.

A note of caution: it is wise to be on guard about your relationship with bureaucrats. Situations can arise where your independence can be severely compromised through "past favours owed". In a situation of conflicting wishes – of bureaucrats wanting to tone you down for fear you will embarrass their department over inactivity or suchlike – awkward decisions must sometimes be made. The following are some of the more usual ways in which bureaucrats can be useful.

Leaks

Leaking is anonymous whistle-blowing (see "Whistle-blowers"). Leaked documents are a veritable media institution as old as the newspaper scoop itself. Leaked documents are generally headlined as such, lending them an aura of secretiveness, suggesting cover-ups and intrigue within the leaking organisation. Secrets, by their nature, are beguiling. A journalist who receives a leak will often feel more privileged than colleagues for having received the leak. This may translate into more sympathetic and detailed coverage than would be the case with a routine press release sent to all media.

Leakers should think hard about the consequences that will flow both to their issue and to themselves and their colleagues. You need to consider whether you wish potentially to martyr yourself as a whistle-blower or how to best cover your tracks and give the leaked information the momentum that you might hope for it.

Issues to consider include:

- Take care to ensure that you do not commit a criminal offence.
- How easily might the leak be traced?
- How many other people have access to the information?
- Are there identifying marks on the leaked copy that can be traced?
- If you are sending material by fax, is the sender's number going to be printed on the faxed copy?
- If you are sending electronic files via email, each file has identifying information on it showing who produced the file (to remove this, in Microsoft® Word, go to File then Properties, then delete all identifying information). Similarly if you send email from an identifiable computer, this can be easily traced. De-identified files sent from a pseudonymous account on a public account email provider, sent from a public computer at an internet café, will be safe.

Consumer participation

Many governments subscribe, at least in their rhetoric, to the principles and values of consumer participation. "Consumer participation" can sound like a benign and harmless process where relatively small amounts of money are siphoned into community groups to enable them to do politically innocuous things like advise on community services or sit on committees. However, the consumer participation process can often foment groups of citizens who can become key players in advocacy. There are many examples in the contemporary public health scene where consumer advocacy has been critical to advancing public health goals. These are particularly issues where government employees' hands are tied by being unable to criticise, lobby and generally advocate for health issues where government policy is not in the best interests of health. In such circumstances, consumer and community groups quickly become the leading edge of advocacy.

Such groups can usually be relied on to shoot from the hip about public health issues in contrast to the guarded equivocations of establishment agency or government representatives. Independent groups can decide for themselves far more flexibly than their established counterparts, not only what should be said and done about public health issues, but the style in which these actions might be executed.

An active climate of consumer advocacy can act as a safeguard against syco-phantic *Yes, Minister!* decision-making environments, and can force high-profile public consideration of issues that will often be critical of government policy. If policy, programmes and resource allocations are made by people only mindful of the political acceptability of particular positions, there will be very many instances of the health agenda being emasculated or wholly neglected.

If you work for government and anticipate that a political era is approaching where there will be many conflicts between government policy and public health, try to use the rhetoric of consumer participation as a Trojan horse to ensure that strong, uncompromised, independent voices from the community will be put in place and heard during the lean times ahead. The same principle applies to allowing academics, traditionally the other main source of independent views, to play an active part in the advocacy process. Using the seemingly benign rhetoric of consumer participation or sponsoring academically independent assessments, try to set up enduring structures for consultation, funding and participation in plan-ning, organisation and evaluation that require community members and academics to be involved.

Fostering such involvement will often be seen by politicians as entirely posi-tive when expressed in the abstract, rather than in specific terms of introducing "loose cannons" into policy debates. If you can be astute in establishing and safe-guarding such structures, consultation processes and funding arrangements in ways that make them genuinely open to the community (and not just to nominal "community" political stooges or yea-sayers), then you will find policy forums invigorated with public health perspectives that will often be challenging to government policies inimical to public health.

Celebrities

Celebrities are, by definition, newsworthy. If Margaret Russell (who?) has lung cancer, there is probably no news value in this unless she is receiving some new treatment, has been subjected to some form of negligence or neglect, or fulfils any of the other news criteria described in Chapter 2. But when George Harrison, the former Beatle, died from lung cancer, the media gave immense coverage to his condition. Celebrity illnesses, or even those of their families, fascinate the media and can provide valuable vehicles for sympathetic coverage of health issues.

Public health advocates need to plan how to respond to news of a celebrity death or illness. This requires a great deal of sensitivity, particularly if there is any potential for the interpretation that you are in any way "dancing on the grave" or exploiting the misfortune of the celebrity. If the celebrity is still alive, it goes without saying that you must make contact before making any statement to the media, and determine whether the celebrity is likely to be supportive of any comments you may be making. If you intend making comments about the preventability of a disease affecting a celebrity, a subtext that may be problematic is one that says "Celebrity X has lung cancer. Most lung cancer is preventable if people didn't smoke. X smoked and now has lung cancer. Therefore we are suggesting that X has been rather foolish". If the celebrity has died, careful thought should also be given to the way in which you couch your comments on the death.

Contacting celebrities

Celebrities, in voicing their views on health issues, can also be valuable advocates for public health. Advocates can do much better than simply waiting for a celebrity to announce their views and then contacting them. Hints and clues that a celebrity may be sympathetic to your issue can be gleaned from reported comments they make on similar areas. If you suspect that a celebrity is on-side, contact them and ask directly if they can help. It is interesting just how many people know a celebrity, or know someone well who knows a celebrity. Ask around. This may turn up someone who will be in a good position to contact them and get a more favourable outcome. There are many ways in which this can happen.

Failing this, all celebrities have agents who look after their bookings and protect them from the public. A phone call to any of the big management agencies will quickly give you the name and contact details of the agency that handles the celebrity you are after. Working through an agent can sometimes be a disadvantage, because you will be obliged to deal through an intermediary who may be unsympathetic to your issue and will not present it well to the celebrity.

Untrained cannons?

There are also problems associated with using celebrities. It may be that a celebrity agrees with your policies only on a limited basis or in a very superficial way, and that when unleashed before an inquiring media, embarrassing differences may emerge. If you are going to use a celebrity, you must feel entirely comfortable that they are thoroughly briefed about the issue and the likely line of questioning from both supportive and hostile media. Before committing a celebrity to any particular role in your advocacy campaign, it is wise to develop a good understanding of their strengths and weaknesses and to tailor their role accordingly.

The issue of sincerity is also a problem. Audiences have become accustomed to celebrities giving paid testimonials for all manner of products through advertising. To avoid the suspicion that celebrities are being paid for their involvement it is important that they are personally committed to the issue and not simply taking the role to enhance their public image[217]. Finally, you should be on guard against the media becoming infatuated with the human interest angle provided by the celebrity if this angle threatens to overwhelm other essential but possibly less "interesting" facets of your campaign.

Columnists

Most newspapers print columns by regular contributors such as social commentators, retired politicians or celebrities. Some syndicated columnists are published in several papers. Most papers also have their own columnists who write on a variety of local and national issues. Developing a relationship with a columnist is similar to developing a relationship with a reporter. You will be better off if you develop long-term relationships with the columnists who publish in your local paper. Once they know and trust you, it will be much easier for you to influence what they write.

Start by knowing which columnists write in the newspapers you want to see cover your issue. Even if they are nationally syndicated and headquartered elsewhere, if they write about subjects relevant to your area of interest, it is important to make contact. Columnists, like all reporters, are always hungry for new ideas and good information. I wrote a column every 6 weeks in the *British Medical Journal* between 1994 and 1996, and briefly in 1999 in *The Weekend Australian* newspaper. Writing the columns was never a problem, but deciding on a good idea for a story was sometimes agonising. Columnists can be hungrier than reporters because they don't have editors telling them what to write and they know that they must produce their column on a regular basis (ordinary journalists can often afford to have low news days – their bylines will not be missed by readers as much as a columnist).

Know columnists' styles and predilections: what are the themes that often appear in their writing? Making an inappropriate suggestion for a column will waste your time and that of the columnist. Some, for example, will have no interest in the geopolitics of tobacco control. Others will probably not want to hear about your evidence of ineptitude in the local bureaucracy. If they want a specific type of story idea or information from you, get it to them as soon as possible. A continuing relationship with a columnist is a very valuable resource that should be nurtured. Columnists, because of their prominence, will want exclusives.

Creative epidemiology

Creative epidemiology marries the science of the researcher with the creativity of the media advocate. The term, originally coined by Australian public health advocate Mike Daube, describes the process of translating often complicated epidemiological data into terms more easily understood by the media and general public. It is particularly concerned with placing unfamiliar or complicated data in perspective against more familiar data. Creative epidemiology can assist in translating the important aspects of research findings to inexpert audiences who may well be mistrustful of data and who are likely to glaze over when statistics are mentioned.

Here are several common ways of expressing epidemiological data in more meaningful or powerful ways:

- If your annual mortality, disease or smoking incidence numbers seem relatively small and unimpressive, consider aggregating them over a longer period. How many have died in a decade, or since a key date? How many will die by the end of the century? For example, Sir Richard Peto has calculated that one billion people will die from tobacco by the end of the present century[664].

- The incidence of seemingly unremarkable or inconsequential behaviours or exposures can be made to appear much more startling. For example, the tobacco industry may try to hint that urban pollution is of far more consequence to respiratory health than smoking. Many people might find this argument appealing. Using creative epidemiology, you can argue that 20-a-day smokers, inhaling an average of 12 times per cigarette, will pull a carcinogenic smoke cocktail into their lungs at point blank range some 87 600 times a year (20 × 12 × 365 days) or 1 752 000 times in 20 years. Such a figure places the vague claims about ambient, dissipated urban pollution in greater perspective. For example, similar back-of-an-envelope calculations can be done on things like lifetime expenditure on tobacco products (and what this might have earned if invested) or on the weight of tar inhaled by a smoker in a lifetime of smoking.

- Conversely, if the numbers you are dealing with are mind-bogglingly large, these can sometimes be expressed more dramatically if they are placed in perspective against short time-frames. For example, world population control advocates frequently make statements such as "Every day, about 382 650 babies are born worldwide and 144 902 people die. So on average, 237 748 more people inhabit the Earth each day – 86 778 020 each year. That's like adding the population of an entire United States to the world every three years!"[ii], with the last sentence added to try to make the hazy implications of world population blow-out appear more meaningful. Another example: Sir Patrick Sheehy, former head of transnational tobacco giant BAT, was described in Great Britain's *Daily Telegraph* as earning "£19 000 a day" rather than in the harder-to-relate-to annual salary and benefits sum of £6 935 000 from which this figure must have been calculated[665].

- When trying to give some sense of meaning to extremely large sums of money (e.g. the annual public cost of tobacco-caused disease), consider translating this sum into how many socially beneficial alternatives this sum could buy (e.g. how many schools, how many public housing units, how many shelters for the homeless, etc.).

- People today are so used to seeing the numbers "million" and "billion" that they lose their impact, especially when used to describe national or international problems. One strategy for overcoming this tendency is to *localise* statistics, calculating, for example, how many people in your area alone are affected by (e.g.) emphysema, or how much community-wide health problems will cost each citizen. Such calculations often present a new and engaging angle on a seemingly remote story. Making a story local and personal involves your community in a way that global or national stories rarely can. Even within a good national campaign, much can be done to add local content and perspective

– and help create support for local initiatives. To ordinary people, 19 000 Australian deaths a year from smoking is less involving than ten deaths a day in their own large town. Local statistics, local role models (such as a local shopkeeper who won't sell cigarettes), or local efforts to change public health policies can seem more relevant to your fellow citizens and community leaders than more remote national stories.

- The newly emerging field of decision aids[666–668], where consumers are presented with visual representations of probabilistic information in an effort to have them more easily understand comparative risks, is highly recommended as an area to be further explored.

- Try to give some *relativity* to numbers by contrasting the new and unfamiliar with the old and familiar. Time-honoured examples here compare losses from particular diseases with losses during wars or major catastrophes. The lives lost in the September 11 terrorist attacks were, after a time, sensitively compared with annual tobacco-caused deaths in the USA[44]. In April 2006, the International Agency for Research in Cancer (IARC) in Lyon, France, issued a press release to accompany what was always going to be a huge cancer story: the forecast cancer burden in Europe arising from the 1986 Chernobyl disaster[29]. The report concluded that about 16 000 cases of thyroid cancer and 25 000 cases of other cancers may be expected due to radiation from the accident and that about 16 000 deaths from these cancers may occur. The IARC's director, Peter Boyle, concluded the release by saying: "To put it in perspective, tobacco smoking will cause several thousand times more cancers in the same population."

Case study: ill-gotten gains

Tobacco control in Australia is very underfunded relative to many other more politically "fashionable" public health problems[108]. In an effort to present political parties with a compelling case to allocate more funding, in 1998 a number of health groups in Australia decided to calculate the money earned by governments in tobacco excise tax from illegal, under-age smokers. The sum – which turned out to be $A64 million – became the theme of a campaign called the $64 Million Question, which simply asked all political parties to commit to earmarking this sum for tobacco control campaigns.

Calculating the amount was relatively simple. We used publicly available data on the prevalence of 12–17-year-old smokers, how much they smoked per week, and on the population of 12–17-year-olds in each political electorate. Using the sales-weighted average price of a cigarette, we then calculated the national expenditure of this age group on cigarettes. We then divided this amount into the component that went to government (65%), to tobacco manufacturers (18%) and to tobacco retailers (16%). Finally, we published, electorate by electorate, how much children who smoked in each electorate were contributing to the government in excise tax. We then asked all politicians to commit to giving it back to a national campaign.

This campaign caused huge waves (see "Criticising governments"), but put an unanswerable case to all political parties that here was money that was ill-gotten and should be handed back.

Criticising government

While counteracting the tobacco industry and its acolytes will be a principal objective of advocacy efforts, government neglect of tobacco control is often a key and sensitive problem too. Derisory funding for public education, failure to legislate and regulate, and acceptance of political donations from the tobacco industry are three broad areas that demand response from tobacco control advocates. However, many people are anxious about being critical of government, fearing backlash and being shut out of future consultation. The result is that many tobacco control groups can appear timid and politically inconsequential.

A former Australian health minister who was personally highly committed to tobacco control but consistently failed to persuade his cabinet colleagues to commit significant funding to the area, was renowned as highly sensitive to any criticism about his government's performance. When I and a few others voiced these criticisms about his government, he wrote an angry broadside about public health advocates, his core message being that we should be content with whatever governments are willing to deliver and not "lie on the ground kicking and screaming" when governments "deliver seven out of ten things [advocates have] been fighting for, for twenty years . . . It's pointless aggravating someone who's there to help you."[669]

I replied that "Politicians generally prefer political lap dogs, not Rottweilers. In liking people who don't criticise them, they of course express a perfectly human preference. But surrounding oneself with brow-soothing sycophants and lashing out at those who dare to do an Oliver Twist and ask for more, shows little insight into the way power can mute those around it: few are willing to bite the hand that might feed them, which is not to say that many were not hungry to so do. The question for the public health community is whether being cowed into silence in deference to a minister's thin skin has wider consequences that should be resisted."[670]

Two questions arise: is criticism of governments counterproductive, and even if it is, is that reason for advocates to keep quiet? It is unarguable that squeaky wheels very often get greased. The proposition that criticism of governments never leverages change is flagrantly contradicted by countless examples across all areas of politics.

So are there virtues in advocacy groups keeping their heads down in the face of public health concerns that would ordinarily merit tenacious advocacy efforts? When advocacy groups have respect from the community, the media and decision-makers it is because of their expertise, integrity and consistency over the years. There is moral force, evidence and credibility in what they say. So when we are conspicuous by our failure to criticise people or political parties whose actions or inactions are inimical to public health, people notice. Any politician knows that interest groups who are unwilling to voice criticism of governments are political cream-puffs who can be safely ignored.

Successive summits of the Australian tobacco control community had placed the area's abject funding as top priority for advocacy. Detailed evidence-based, value-for-money cases for funding had been placed in the hands of the government for years. In the previous two federal budgets, zero dollars had been allocated to tobacco control, despite the very first line of a document distributed with the Ministerial Council on Drug Strategy's *National Tobacco Strategy 1999 to 2002–03*, stating: "Tobacco smoking is the single largest preventable cause of premature death and disease in Australia." In the face of this neglect, the Minister argued that public health advocates should remain silent and grateful for the funding crumbs that can be swept from the table of departmental internal budgets.

Those advocates who are in tobacco control for the long haul, consider being out of favour with a given minister or a government to be a battle lost, not a war gone wrong. Gains are counted across decades, rather than in ministerial terms of office. Advocates would do well not to be intimidated by arguments that their role is only to support government (see also "Inside and outside the tent").

Demonstrations

Well-attended demonstrations and street marches nearly always attract media attention by virtue of their sheer size. However, tobacco control is not an issue that is likely to get tens of thousands of people onto the streets because its threats to public health are chronic and not acute. Small demonstrations can also be newsworthy if they are dramatic or if they involve the participation of people who disturb usual expectations of who takes part in demonstrations. Counter-demonstrations can also be newsworthy (see "Gatecrashing") and importantly, can cut deeply into the news time being obtained by the principal demonstration.

There is a genre of demonstration reporting that includes the following elements: a statement of the grievance or purpose causing the demonstration; an estimate of the size of the crowd; shots of placards or banners that have caught the camera operator's eye (usually witty or bordering on the slanderous); close-ups of any famous or bizarrely dressed people marching or involved in the demonstration; excerpts from speeches made at the demonstration or from interviews with its organisers; comments from the opponents of the demonstration; and comments from passers-by witnessing the demonstration.

Most of these elements can inspire some planning by advocates. Rather than just hoping to leave the positive reporting of a demonstration to luck, thought should be put into the "tone" that you would like to set. For example, if you sense that your issue is often negatively characterised by the media as one driven by neopuritans and health zealots, think of ways to project images that belie such assumptions (risqué placards, celebrities as spokespeople, etc.). During the anti-Vietnam war demonstrations in the 1960s and 1970s in Australia, efforts were made to encourage marchers who were middle-aged and elderly to join in: students were urged to coax their parents into marching, and to wear suits. This was an attempt to counter community feelings that anti-war demonstrators were mostly young anarchists who did not represent mainstream Australian society.

If you feel your issue is one that will attract very angry people (either on your side or as interjectors from your opposition) give strong consideration to whether this aspect of the demonstration has the potential to become the main news angle, replacing the reasons for the demonstration in the way it is reported. If this happens, your demonstration will probably be counterproductive, despite making prime time news (see "Introduction" above).

Keep the following tips in mind when planning demonstrations:

- Inform the media about what your group intends doing in regard to the planned demonstration.
- Demonstrations can sometimes be short-lived if officials require you to leave the scene. It is therefore important that whatever you do occurs when cameras and journalists are present and ready.
- Produce pamphlets, bumper stickers, T-shirts with slogans, banners and placards.
- Distribute pamphlets explaining your protest and giving suggestions for action by those who share your concerns.
- Create an alternative prize to display to those queuing to enter the arena.

At the Adelaide Grand Prix in 1986 a suitably worded banner ("Tobacco companies – corporate drug pushers") was tied to the roof of a college of nursing that happened to be by the track. The TV station broadcasting the race ignored the banner, but stations that did not have rights to cover the race were delighted to cover the protest as a different news angle on what would have otherwise been standard reportage. This was opportunism in full flight.

For some years, the makers of *John Player Special* cigarettes have sponsored an exhibition for portraiture at London's National Portrait Gallery. In 1984 Bristol AGHAST entered the competition with a portrait by a sympathetic Bristol artist, William Guilding, of a wasted, emaciated man in his early 30s propped up in a hospital bed with an oxygen cylinder. In his hand he held a cigarette. The painting was entitled *The early death of Jack Filbert*. The painting was sent for first round judging by the gallery's staff and short-listed for the second round of judging, when it failed to go further. For reasons known only to the judges, they decided that this portrait of a smoker dying from lung cancer would not be hung in their tobacco-sponsored exhibition.

Like all good campaigners, AGHAST were aware that failures must be turned into successes and so decided to hold an alternative exhibition, titled the Lung Slayer Portrait Award. The footpath outside the National Portrait Gallery seemed as good a place as any to stage the exhibition, and the morning of the announcement of the John Player award, when art critics and journalists would be turning up, seemed a suitable time. About eight people staffed the alternative exhibition. A suitable pamphlet was produced, the rejected painting made up into a poster for sale to passers-by, and some appropriate banners displayed ("John Slayer Portraits: In your local cancer ward now!"; "The real sponsors are dying in cancer wards"; "Who put the 'art' in heart disease?"). Good press coverage of the alternative award was achieved, with the *Guardian* newspaper running a photo of the alternative award but not the tobacco award winner.

Divide and rule

The British colonial empire principle of "divide and rule" has application in advocacy. If your opposition is somehow disunited on any aspect of the tobacco control issue in question, try to prise open this disunity causing them to become sidetracked into squabbling among themselves rather than being more powerfully united in their opposition to your goals. This has been most memorably accomplished by dividing the hospitality industry over the issue of secondhand smoke. The restaurant sector is typically far more progressive than the pub and bar sector in seeing the potential for improved trade when banning smoking indoors. Such disunity can be exploited. Future moves to limit sites where tobacco products can be sold promise to see some retail sectors (such as dedicated tobacconists or supermarkets able to offer adults-only entry to closed-off tobacco sections) fighting against other retail sectors like corner stores and petrol stations, whose appalling sales-to-minors track record might make them vulnerable to losing the ability to sell tobacco when this argument gathers more momentum.

Case study: rock bottom

In 1986, the Philip Morris tobacco company launched a promotional exercise throughout Australia known as the Peter Jackson Rock Circuit. It signed up dozens of local rock bands and heavily promoted the concerts and venues where the Rock Circuit would be playing. The exercise was an obvious attempt to associate smoking and the Peter Jackson brand of cigarettes with rock culture.

A colleague and I decided to try to use the divide-and-rule principle to throw the promotion into chaos by fanning the already glowing embers of a divided rock music industry. We contacted several leading rock bands who were not involved in the tobacco circuit and asked them if they were prepared to sign a statement condemning the use of rock musicians to promote tobacco. We had no difficulty in getting support and decided then to publish an advertisement incorporating the signed statement in the national press. Because the rock bands supporting us included "stars" who were speaking out on a social issue (i.e. doing something other than playing music), the media went into a feeding frenzy of interviews where the rock stars expressed their views on the issue.

For reasons that were never disclosed, the tobacco promotion simply folded. We strongly suspect that the amount of criticism it attracted was judged as being too counterproductive to Philip Morris's wider marketing objectives, and hence a decision was made to cut its losses early and abandon the promotion. No tobacco-sponsored rock promotions have been held in Australia since.

Beware also of the "divide-and-rule" principle being used by your opposition to weaken *your* efforts. In the context of discussing resource allocations by government to health issues, Wachter warns that "disease-specific activist groups may find themselves pitted against one another as they advocate their own interests".[671] If you can be sensitive enough to see that such divide-and-rule equivalents are happening, try to stand back from the foreground conflicts and ask yourself if the issues involved in these are as important as the bigger picture issues that are being neglected because of petty conflicts.

Doctors

There is a long-established historical reluctance among doctors to become involved in any activity that might be construed as publicity. Ever since the time of Hippocrates, the medical profession has considered that its professionalism has little in common with ventures in the public arena. Hippocrates exhorted physicians to avoid activities that "savour of fuss or show"[672], and in 1905 William Osler advised doctors not to "dally with the Delilah of the press"[673]. DeVries reports that until the late 1970s, some medical students were taught that a doctor's name should appear in the press only at birth, death and marriage[674]. Many doctors today remain highly suspicious of the media and are reluctant actively to court their attention in the ways advocated in this book.

Doctors can play very powerful roles in media advocacy. Those who break out of the sanctum of the doctor–patient relationship and into public health advocacy can fascinate the media. Their relationship to patients lends them an authenticity of concern for prevention that is unique and rarely challenged. The subtext of a clinician speaking out in the media is "here is a person who knows first hand the consequences of the neglect of this public health issue". It is difficult to refute or obfuscate the here-and-now clinical experience of a clinician. If a politician talks about the need to rationalise health services or the waste of taxpayers' money going into duplication of a service, many of the public will acknowledge that this framing of budget cuts to health services makes sense: who could agree with waste and duplication? Statements against such cuts by the political opposition to the government will be dismissed by many as just plain politicking, but if hospital surgeons speak out about the human face of surgical waiting lists, the frame is invariably a more powerful one of "people at the coal-face speaking out about the realities". Getting doctors to speak out about prevention can be similarly compelling. The medical profession has been among those in the vanguard of smoking control, and the clinical, pathological and epidemiological assessment of tobacco's role in ill health continues to be the main reference point in the arguments for smoking control.

Saul Alinsky advised: "Wherever possible go outside of the experience of the enemy."[661] Doctors do this whenever they evoke their clinical experience of people afflicted with disease or injuries. If you are a doctor and work in a clinical situation, emphasise, in debates with your opposition, how distressing it is to hear your opponent trying to downplay the significance of the public health problem. For example, publicly invite a member of a hotel association opposing smoking bans to meet with bar staff affected by secondhand smoke.

Doctors are also prized scalps for many of the opponents of public health. There is an old saying that "a doubting or smoking doctor is worth millions of dollars in free advertising" to the tobacco industry. In the early 1980s, the tobacco industry in Australia actively encouraged an eccentric, pipe-smoking doctor who wrote a book called *Smoking is Good for You* to get training for media appearances[675]. The tobacco industry's "Project Whitecoat" and other efforts to recruit doctors to speak out publicly in the globally coordinated, multi-company "smoker reassurance" campaign, and efforts to denigrate concern about secondhand smoke[100], provide major evidence of the perceived power of having doctors speak out.

Any doctor who overtly or inadvertently supports your opposition should either be quickly confronted privately (if it seems to have been done in ignorance or innocence) or publicly challenged by his or her peers in the medical profession if the support is plainly deliberate. The public must be left in no doubt that the doctor is unrepresentative of the overwhelming consensus in the profession.

One of the major obstacles to tobacco control in many countries is the high prevalence of smoking by doctors. Efforts to convince the public that smoking is a serious health problem are seriously undermined by public awareness that many doctors smoke themselves. In such countries, it is difficult to think of any higher strategic priority for tobacco control than to try to reduce smoking by doctors and other health-care workers. In China, an estimated 57% of physicians smoke, as do more than 41% in Turkey. In Albania, 65% of male medical students and 36% of female students smoke. In Croatia, the corresponding figures are 36% and 37%; in Argentina, 33% and 37%[676]. There is a very scant research literature, beyond that simply measuring the problem, on how any country has reduced the rate of smoking among health care workers.

Editorials

All major newspapers print daily editorials. These usually concern major current news stories although editorials about on-going or seasonal issues are also published. Forthcoming important dates (World No Tobacco Day, pre-budget periods, etc.) can serve as good pretexts to raise particular issues with the press in the hope of attracting an editorial or feature.

Editorials are written by editorial staff employed by a newspaper. These staff may be totally dedicated to editorial writing, or reporters who have been asked to write an editorial based on their recent reporting of an issue. In either case, those writing editorials will be looking for inspiration and material in much the same way that ordinary news reporting occurs. Special interest groups can approach newspapers with requests that editorials be written.

Before you make such an approach, make sure you know what the paper has written on your subject in the past. If you are going to ask a newspaper to take a particular stand on an issue, you should know what the paper has already said about it. It will also help you tailor your case to the special interests of your target audience. Some organisations keep ongoing files on what their local papers have written on issues of importance to them. Such a filing system can be very useful in preparing for discussions with representatives of the papers.

Editorial memoranda

An editorial memorandum is a detailed explanation of a particular position on a particular issue that can be sent to an editor. The tone of an editorial memorandum should be thoughtful and reasoned. Although an editorial memo takes an unapologetically partisan approach to a topic, it should not be as strident as a piece of political propaganda, such as a leaflet or partisan speech.

An editorial memo should be sent out with a cover letter clearly stating the position the memo advocates. The memo can be several pages long and should spell out all of the major arguments supporting the stated position. Significant supporting evidence, such as articles or studies, can be attached as appendices. The memo should also anticipate major counterarguments to your position and provide adequate responses.

A good editorial memo should serve as a primary resource for the journalist allocated to write an editorial endorsing your position. Therefore, editorial memos are best produced by a peak policy body, national organisation or other reputable group of people. Newspapers receiving a memo will want to know without doubt that the information contained within it is current and accurate. An editorial memo should never be thought of as a replacement for personal contact. Even if your editorial memo contains every good argument that exists in favour of your position, a personal meeting with editorial representatives will greatly enhance your chances for success.

Élitism

Many public health workers are middle-class, well-educated people whose own high-brow media habits place them in stark contrast with those of the great majority of the population. I know a senior public health figure in Australia who proudly boasts that he does not own a television. It is not uncommon to hear people in public health being disdainful of the quality of populist media and averse to watching, listening to and reading it. Such attitudes can sometimes translate into an ill-advised neglect of the importance of populist media as vehicles for media advocacy discourses.

Advocates should reflect on whether their own media preferences are biasing their objective assessment of how best to target particular media. If populist media are considered important to your campaign, you may need to swallow your pride and get into the habit of regularly reading populist newspapers and listening to tedious and irritating radio programmes to enable you better to judge how to pitch an upcoming interview. If you are going to be interviewed for a particular radio or TV programme, it is imperative that you familiarise yourself with it before you do the interview. Assess the style of the interviewer; the length of the interviews; the length of the "bites" or "grabs" if it is an edited programme; whether it is a "serious" or light programme and so on (see "Interview strategies").

Engaging communities

A doctrine that has gained considerable support in health promotion circles is that if advocacy is to succeed and for its gains to be sustained, it must emanate from and be driven by communities as a "bottom–up" expression of their concerns and priorities. In summary, this doctrine is suspicious of "top–down" policy change as being imposed by public health elites who have not consulted their communities and who have not worked to empower community members to become effective advocates for change. It argues that without the support of communities, the fruits of such top-down advocacy are unlikely to be supported.

How does this doctrine fit with the tobacco control advocacy experience? In short, not very well. The popular view is that smoking is a voluntary activity and therefore categorically different from many of the "imposed" health problems that public health advocacy typically addresses (e.g. violent communities; environmental health concerns such as leaded petrol; lack of access to health facilities; unsafe public utilities and poor infrastructure). Advocacy also is often undertaken on behalf of groups unable to speak up for their own interests, such as children. These two considerations would suggest that tobacco control advocacy is likely to attract community involvement only with regard to environmental tobacco smoke (because of the way it is imposed on others) and on behalf of children (such as actions to stop shopkeepers selling tobacco to children). Additionally, because tobacco-caused diseases typically manifest themselves decades after individuals commence smoking, tobacco control attracts far less grass-roots attention than public health issues about acute health problems for which solutions promise immediate benefit.

This analysis has been broadly confirmed by the recent history of tobacco control in Australia. Only in three cases have leading tobacco control advocacy groups been located predominantly in the Australian lay community: the Non Smokers' Movement, BUGA UP and individual litigants. On all other issues advocacy has been driven by professionals within NGOs and dedicated advocacy offices set up explicitly to pursue these objectives. As these groups began to set the agenda for tobacco control reform, indices of community support for tobacco control showed rapid signs of positive growth. While professionals were most often newsmakers, letters pages in newspapers and callers to talk-back radio have increasingly featured the expressions of ordinary citizens' concerns about the same range of issues. In several celebrated cases, citizens played key roles in litigation, although in all cases these were supported by professional advocates who assisted with expert information, publicity and general support.

Hence, tobacco control advocacy in Australia did not emerge spontaneously out of the community except in some small but important instances. Rather, it has mostly been initiated by professional advocates who took the recommendations of the early expert reports on reducing the tobacco epidemic and the results of relevant local policy-relevant research and advocated for changes to be adopted. Whereas today there are countless examples of citizens joining in this advocacy (by complaining to management in smoky bars; declaring their homes smokefree; etc.), the leading edge of contemporary advocacy for tobacco control (e.g. to secure strengthened pack warnings or regulation of tobacco as a product) is still being almost wholly driven by health NGOs and policy-oriented researchers.

In 2004, the NSW Cancer Council took up the challenge of turning all this on its head by trying to tap into the widespread community anger about smoking continuing to be allowed in pubs and bars. It utilised its community outreach functions in the areas of fundraising and public education to sign up over 25 000 people into its Tobacco Action Group, which has since been used to send post-cards and emails to local politicians about smokefree legislation; more information is available from the website of the Cancer Council of New South Wales (http://www.cancercouncil.com.au/editorial.asp?pageid=4). Opportunities can arise to use such people in local area monitoring of the implementation of tobacco con-trol policies, allowing rapid assessment of what is going on in communities.

The Washington-based Campaign for Tobacco free Kids has an online "E-champions" sign-on facility – see the E-Champions Action Center (http://tfk.grassroots.com/act/) – which builds a database of people wanting to take action against tobacco. Those signing up receive occasional action alerts (see "Action alerts") and newsletters and can petition their local governor for action. Internet tech-nology empowers citizens more easily to get involved in advocacy.

Fact sheets

Succinct, comprehensive and journalist-friendly fact sheets are an invaluable part of advocacy work. Most journalists have educational backgrounds in the human-ities, not the sciences, and consequently can be awed or intimidated by health and medical issues[30]. Succinct summaries and demystified background material on public health issues will often be gratefully snapped up by journalists who feel a little at sea about your issue. Fact sheets should be written with particular readers in mind: for example, students, politicians, journalists, volunteers and fund-raisers, or the general public. The content, style and comprehensiveness of the sheets will vary according to what you understand to be the typical information needs and existing awareness of your target audience.

It is often a good idea to set out fact sheets in question-and-answer format, anti-cipating the top-of-mind issues with which your target group may be preoccupied. The questions you select can be a mixture of the questions that you know are the most commonly asked by (say) journalists; those that address the main arguments put forward by your opposition (remember that journalists seeking "balance" will often want to see where you stand in relation to your opposition's main arguments); and those questions that frame your position best, allowing you to position par-ticular perspectives that may not have received wide coverage. Include references to the facts and claims made in such material to give the sheets more of an appear-ance of authority and credibility.

Gate-crashing

Your opposition will almost certainly hold functions, ceremonies, press conferences, public meetings, prize-givings and sponsored events where your group's presence will be most unwelcome. These events will often attract huge media coverage and be attended by people you seek to influence or wish to draw out on an issue. Your presence at the event may cause a valuable split in the media coverage given to it. Instead of one-sided reports focusing on your opposition's claims or activities at their meeting, media stories on the event will cover your presence and arguments too, often halving the media coverage obtained by your opposition. The party the organisers meant to hold may not turn out to be the party that they get.

Case study: smarting with shame

One year, BAT Australia held its Annual General Meeting at a city hotel. ASH Australia contacted the local laryngectomy association, who found three ex-smokers with laryngectomies who were willing to form a "Laryngectomy Choir" and come to the AGM to serenade the BAT board as it entered the meeting room. They wrote new, biting words to the standard "Smoke gets in your eyes", and with news cameras rolling, sang to a glum line of board members as they entered through the hotel lobby. Mr Siggi Butts (a person inside a giant cigarette costume) slipped into the hotel foyer toilets unnoticed and donned the costume, emerging only to be asked to leave by hotel security, who were unprepared to demand that the choir leave. Alerted news media gave the board coverage it didn't want.

Infiltration

If your group poses a serious threat to the tobacco industry they will attempt to gain as much intelligence about you as possible (see "Know your opposition"). They will endeavour to obtain any newsletters or publications you produce (see "Mailing lists"), attend all public meetings you call and may even infiltrate your organisation using interested citizens or students preparing essays.

Community groups that operate with volunteers and accordingly do not run reference checks or other authenticating procedures on their staff may be vulnerable to such infiltration. Similarly, if you are organising meetings or conferences where you hope and expect open discussion of strategy and planning among like-minded colleagues, attendance at such events will be very tempting to your opposition. World Conferences on Tobacco or Health have tried to exclude any representatives from the tobacco or allied industries. These have failed, with tobacco industry spies sitting in on sessions that promise even a whiff of revelation about strategy[677].

If you wish to exclude your opposition from public meetings or conferences, you should indicate this on any announcements or registration brochures and require people to indicate their affiliation when they register. Suspicious-looking registrants can then be scrutinised in advance. Door registrations can leave you more vulnerable, especially in the busy, chaotic periods when registration staff do not have the time to check details. If you suspect that someone in a seminar or meeting is a spy, you can ask everyone to introduce themselves and say where they are from. If someone sounds doubtful, your next step may be politely to confront the person with your suspicions, explaining the sensitive nature of the meeting, and that "no one else here seems to know you, so you'll understand that we are concerned".

Case study: a fifth column?

In the early 1980s, BUGA UP, the Australian anti-tobacco billboard graffiti group, was infiltrated by a man, John, who posed as someone who had long admired their work and wanted to assist. He assisted in driving BUGA UP members around to billboards and was very keen to do whatever he could. After a television programme had run a major item on the anti-smoking movement in Australia, four activists' houses were spray-painted the next day. A BUGA UP meeting was called to discuss tactics in dealing with the issue. John attended and offered to drive around to each house that had been defaced, and to photograph the damage. As the details of this were being discussed and John was being given all the addresses of the houses, another BUGA UP member joined the meeting saying that her neighbour had taken the details of a car driving slowly up her street and photographing the sprayed fence. The licence plate had been noted and the car turned out to be John's. He was confronted, and admitted he was an infiltrator, although he refused to say for whom he worked.

There are also ways in which you can infiltrate your opposition. Students regularly call or visit businesses and community organisations involved in topical issues in an attempt to gather information or interviews for assignments. In my academic work, I have set assignments for students to analyse public health issues from the perspective of both public health advocates and their oppositions. This has sometimes inspired students to try to interview (e.g.) tobacco industry executives, and sometimes they have succeeded, returning assignments that include most interesting material full of candid information.

One way of making contact with lapsed industry workers or with current disillusioned ones willing to help your efforts is simply to advertise for them. Place an ad in a magazine, journal or newspaper that is likely to be read by your opposition inviting confidential contact. I've advertised like this twice to the tobacco industry and got one big fish on the line. He was an advertising executive who worked at a senior level on a tobacco account. He spoke about how many people who worked on such accounts were often plagued by guilt. The subject was always being raised in conversation by their friends, putting them on the spot and causing them to utter limp, self-justifying arguments that they could scarcely believe they were saying. He said the advantages of a tobacco account were legion – a virtual licence to print money for the agency – but that the costs to integrity were high. He said he was sure there was a sort of fragile conspiracy between some people who worked on tobacco accounts to put on a bold face and make out they were unaffected by the issue, but that chinks could be seen in the character armour everywhere.

He said he had watched the smoking control debate for some years and thought that tactically we had got one thing quite wrong. People in the tobacco industry, he suggested, were self-selecting in their total indifference or contempt both for what we represented and our arguments. Water off ducks' backs. But people in the advertising industry, like him, were much more vulnerable targets for persuasion. His advice was to target a campaign at advertising agencies handling tobacco accounts. This would be unlikely to cause any of them suddenly to abandon their accounts but it might well further undermine morale, which in turn might affect the enthusiasm and drive of their work. The more certain effect would be to make those on the outside more determined to keep their agencies "tobacco free".

Inside and outside the tent

Advocacy, by its nature, involves contested debates: there are always losers when change occurs, and so often they are determined to resist change and are angry when it happens. Public health advocacy often requires pushing governments to act and being critical of inaction. This can brand advocates as troublemakers, with all that can go along with that. I have known David Hill, the director of the Cancer Council Victoria, since 1978 and count him as a close friend. A few years ago when I was feeling mildly disconsolate at being excluded from some key national committees appointed by the then Australian health minister Michael Wooldridge, David counselled me to consider that every cause needs different people to "work inside and outside the political tent". He said that those inside greatly appreciated that someone like me was outside helping to keep policy agendas alive that risked being neglected by being largely off-limits for those working with government committees.

There have been many times in my career when I have negotiated with colleagues inside the government tent to take particular actions calculated to influence agendas when those colleagues felt they could not effectively raise the concerns themselves. Advocacy movements should always develop capacity to have people who are warmly welcomed by government as well as those who remain capable of being highly critical. If advocates are all totally cosy with government, they will be impotent whenever government has other priorities. Equally, if all advocates are seen by government as constantly critical, the entire movement can be marginalised. Weigh your actions and role and decide whether you want to be mostly inside, or mostly outside. Things can change dramatically with changes of government.

Internet

In the last 15 years, the internet has utterly changed the fundamentals of day-to-day advocacy. Its principal legacy has been to allow advocates to communicate with thousands of like-minded people instantly, and to locate and exchange information in nanoseconds. Its impact has been particularly profound for residents in less-developed nations where libraries are typically impoverished. This is not the place to explain the virtues of the internet, other than to mention the importance of listservers. These are email lists that allow members to post to one, several or all other members, and for recipients to exercise the same reply options. Globalink is the principal international listserver to the tobacco control community. New members are vetted, and require several existing members to vouch for them being involved in some aspect of tobacco control. Anyone with a connection to the tobacco industry is ineligible to join. Almost daily, Globalink members seek and find assistance with strategic matters from over 5000 members.

There are now thousands of tobacco-control related websites. My top ten are:

- My site, the Tobacco Control Supersite (http://tobacco.health.usyd.edu.au/), which incorporates annotated links to over 10 000 selected tobacco industry documents from Australasia and Asia, plus hundreds of useful subject-indexed links.
- *Tobacco Control* online (http://tc.bmjjournals.com/), covering 16 years of research and the leading policy journal in the field.
- Tobacco.Org (http://www.tobacco.org/), Gene Borio's tobacco news archive from all over the world.
- Globalink news (http://news.globalink.org/), another depository for news stories on tobacco.
- Roswell Park Cancer Institute (http://roswell.tobaccodocuments.org/), includes Rick Pollay's massive collection of tobacco advertising.
- The Centers for Disease Control tobacco site (http://www.cdc.gov/tobacco/), providing a huge collection of all the Surgeon General Reports plus much more.
- Campaign for Tobacco-Free Kids (http://www.tobaccofreekids.org/), the USA's leading advocacy agency.
- ASH UK (http://www.ash.org.uk/), containing many of the hardest hitting reviews of tobacco industry conduct you will ever find.
- Legacy Tobacco Documents Library (http://legacy.library.ucsf.edu/), the motherload site for industry documents.
- PubMed (http://www.ncbi.nlm.nih.gov/entrez/query.fcgi?DB=pubmed), where you can find tobacco-related research from peer-reviewed journals.

Interview strategies[iii]

Many public health workers will have spent many hundreds of hours during their careers preparing presentations such as lectures and speeches for students, conferences and community meetings. The biggest of such occasions might be a national or international conference where perhaps several thousand people might listen to a plenary presentation in a huge auditorium. The far more common presentation will be to a room full of students, colleagues or consumers. Such occasions set up expectations that speakers will be suitably prepared and rehearsed, that they will have objectives, a planned beginning, middle and end to their speech or lecture, and that they will have suitable slides. Awareness of these expectations often drives speakers and lecturers to lengthy preparation.

The contrast here with the typical preparation made for a news interview is invariably stark. The best example from my own experience occurred in New Delhi, India, in 1985. I was giving a talk on tobacco control strategy to about 30 workers from the Voluntary Health Association of India. Immediately afterwards, I was approached by a young man with a tape recorder who asked if I had a few moments to give a short interview for his radio station. At the end of our impromptu chat I asked him what radio station he worked for. He worked for the central government broadcasting service and blithely informed me that the interview would be played the next day after the main news bulletins to an estimated listening audience of 200 million!

Such an example highlights the often casual and unprepared way that public health advocates approach opportunities to speak to unparalleled numbers of people, numbered among whom can be many hundreds of significant policymakers and politicians. This section outlines some of the more important strategies to be considered when being interviewed or when debating in the mass media.

There is an entire industry dedicated to training people (usually from industry and government and usually at great expense) to "perform" better on the media. If you expect to be interviewed a great deal by the media, consider investing in one of these courses. Ask other advocates if they can recommend a suitable agency or course.

There are three sorts of interviews that all advocates will encounter:

- The spur-of-the-moment phone call from a print or radio journalist who wants comment immediately. In the case of radio, this may mean that the interviewer will roll the tape, and within minutes what you say may be broadcast into perhaps millions of homes and cars.
- A prerecorded radio or TV interview. This will typically be edited to fit into the news format in which it will be broadcast.
- A live-to-air radio or TV interview, where everything you say, warts and all, will be broadcast.

When a journalist phones and you're unprepared

If a print or radio journalist phones and asks for a comment, it can often happen that you are caught unprepared: that you can't immediately think of anything sensible to say, or you don't have the relevant facts at your fingertips. In these situations, buy some time to think it over. Make an excuse (you're with someone; you need to look up a reference) and promise that you will call back within ten minutes. This will allow you time to consider your response, to frame it correctly and to work it into a sound bite or compelling quote (see below). Only in rare, red hot news situations will a journalist see such a request as unreasonable.

Objectives

With broadcast appearances you must pursue two objectives:

1   To be persuasive on the issues you have decided to pursue.
2   To make certain that your audience feels that you are a person they like and trust.

Here, it is important to cover certain key aspects.

Identify the ethical bottom line of your argument

Many viewers, listeners or readers will be only marginally aware of or interested in your issue. However, part of the way in which they assess whether they are on your side will be determined by the extent to which they are able to identify with your ethical "bottom line". Tobacco control is wringing wet with moral and ethical issues: cover-up, corruption and industry mendacity; protection of the innocent; thwarted rights to information, safety, redress and justice; community health versus company profits; and so on. It is important that you are aware of this dimension to your issue and use language that either explicitly or implicitly underscores your message with its ethical bottom line.

Mike Pertschuk[678] draws our attention to the advice of political scientist Ethel Klein, a leading strategist for public health advocacy campaigns on issues ranging from spousal abuse to handgun control. She laments that when issue advocates plan their "message" they invariably rush to hatching catchy slogans and clever soundbites. Or they concoct elaborate arguments to answer all the arguments put forward by their adversaries. Klein offers a different vision: "Good sound bites, and slogans – and speeches, policy solutions, meaningful statistics, arguments – all support and reinforce your message, but they are not what communications experts mean by 'message'. To communications professionals, your message is your organizing theme. And no media advocacy campaign can succeed without a powerful, coherent organizing theme, a theme that is at the same time logically persuasive, morally authoritative, and capable of evoking passion. A campaign message must speak at one and the same time to the brain and to the heart."

Authenticity

Audiences of media interviews will be particularly attuned to the extent to which you appear "real" or authentic when being interviewed. Public health advocates often argue for policy changes that are easily caricatured by their opponents as the dead hand of regulatory bureaucracy and government. A common tactic of those who are being opposed in tobacco control debates is to try to paint you and your group in some calculatingly pejorative way (meddlers, busybodies, warriors against pleasure, zealots, quasi-religious "crusaders", health Nazis, even people who would like to "adjust the temperature of your shower if they had the chance"[679]. Often these frames will succeed in capturing an audience's understanding of who they think you are and what you stand for. It is thus important for you to find ways of framing both the issues being debated and your opposition in equally powerful ways, and making what you are saying sound authentic – that you are personally committed to what you are saying – and not that you are merely mouthing the words of a dutiful employee or spokesperson for a committee's policy. Speaking in the first person and being anecdotal are two ways of doing this. Another is to personalise your arguments.

Personalising

Saul Alinsky advised that advocates should "Pick the target, freeze it, personalise it, and polarise it".[661] The community consumes many news stories as metaphorical battles between individuals representing particular values. When you appear on television speaking about your public health issue, only a fraction of the viewing audience will attend to what you are saying with anything remotely like the detail you might hope. Nearly everyone watching though, will form some opinion about you and your opposition's qualities as human beings. You will evoke a response from the range of very ordinary, everyday human reactions that we all have towards others.

Many tobacco control issues readily lend themselves to intensely personal framings with which audiences can identify: a child burnt and disfigured by a fire caused by a discarded cigarette could so easily be your own; it could be your 12-year-old to whom that shop is willing to sell cigarettes; the suburban bar worker who gets none of the same occupational health protections that you get in your workplace. Try to frame your concerns in these personally relevant sorts of ways rather than as statistical or clinical abstractions.

A study I conducted with Nicola Christofides on how the tobacco industry was portrayed in the Australian press showed eight subtexts that characterised press descriptions of the industry (callous merchants of death; conspiracy/cover-up; blood money; toxic Pied Pipers; corporate leviathans; beleaguered/legitimate industry; the tobacco industry as an index case of unethical or corrupt practice; and bumbling fools). Eighty-nine percent of references to the industry framed it negatively[220].

As well as addressing your opposition as (say) industry officials or politicians, in public debate address them in their roles as parents, citizens and human beings. This can dramatically reframe the platform from which they speak and create awkward appositions. Remember always that audiences often attend far more to the subtexts of news items and debates than to the overt content.

Advice for media performers

The Advocacy Institute offers the following advice about media performances.

- Find out all you can about the ground rules. What's the format? Who will moderate? Who else will appear on the programme? If this is a regular talk show or interview programme, try to watch or listen ahead of time or find colleagues who are familiar with the programme and can give you a feeling for its norms. Is the host interested in civil discourse or in provoking conflict and confrontation? What expectations do viewers have of the programme? Is it the equivalent of the Roman Colosseum or is it a serious-minded background briefing programme where slogans and adversarial talk will sound out of place? If you can't get the answers to these questions, or if you are uncomfortable with the answers you get, reconsider whether appearing will serve your goals. If the deck is stacked – the host obviously opposed, the questions likely to be ill-framed, the "culture" of the show too high-powered or trivial for your comfort – consider passing it up. Not all exposure is good exposure.

- Ask yourself, who is going to hear or see me? What do you want them to take away from the programme? How do you want to change their attitudes? What do you want them to be left with or to do?
- Plan in advance the main points you want to get across during the interview. Ask how long the segment or show is going to run. If you only have 3 minutes (not unusual on TV or radio interview programmes), concentrate on only one or two key points. If you have longer, you may want to add some key supporting arguments or data, but you probably can't effectively convey more than two main themes. Outline your points on a single piece of paper. Have it handy so you can glance at it during a break (or whenever necessary if on radio). After any breaks, emphasise points you haven't yet made. Repeat your key messages and bridge back to them as necessary.
- Make a list of foreseen questions and clear, concise answers to them.
- Check your facts and statistics. Be sure what you assert as fact is indeed fact. It is better to say nothing than to stretch the truth and be caught out. Don't be afraid to say you don't know the answer to a specific question, or that you're not certain of a specific fact.
- Don't try to win the wrong fight. Your opposition can be maddeningly provocative. Their claims and accusations may sting so sharply that an advocate is drawn into elaborate denials or quibbling over side issues. Ignore the provocations and return to your strong themes and moral high ground. Don't be passive or overly polite. Interrupt if your opponent is dominating the discussion, but try to do so in a manner that suggests an easy, conversational disagreement rather than hectoring, lecturing or a panicked feeling overcoming you.
- If your opponent is obviously rude and domineering, it is likely that many viewers or listeners will be preoccupied with this rather than with what he or she is saying. Quickly and calmly point this rudeness out. This will often trip up your opponent momentarily, allowing you to gain a debating advantage.
- Wordiness/mouthfuls. You're trying to persuade a general audience, not impress an audience of your scholarly peers. Don't ramble. Stay with one or two clear points at a time. Don't filibuster; come up for air. Let your opponent get a few words in edgeways, but not dominate the debate.
- Wasting opportunities/getting drawn off track. There's a danger in getting too comfortable with a charming, gracious interviewer and getting drawn off into an interesting side issue that does not advance your policy goals. You may think you've got all the time in the world, but even an hour-long talk show can pass by so quickly that you lose the opportunity to hammer home your main points.
- Being unprepared. This needs no explanation.
- Being over-prepared. If your words and mannerisms sound memorised or rehearsed, they lose much of their potency. Your arguments and main points should be thoroughly worked out ahead in comfortable, but not rigid formulas committed to memory.
- Relying on one's status or credentials. If you think that a sceptical host or a paid industry spokesperson will treat you respectfully because you have an impressive curriculum vitae or are a high-ranking executive of a prestigious organisation,

think again. On the other hand, if you are prepared to speak knowledgeably and with authority, then your credentials will help contrast and expose the hired–gun status of your opposition.

- Avoid "trading" scientific studies in a debate. This can go on indefinitely and the audience is never sure who has access to the most reliable and important studies.
- Wit and humour are wonderful weapons to disarm a sceptical host or hostile adversary, but not every would-be humorist is good at it. Don't reach for humour or sardonic slogans or labels unless unbiased friends or colleagues confirm that you're good at it. Otherwise, be serious and straight. It's safer.
- If you've been distracted and haven't heard a question, or if you simply need more time to think, don't be afraid to ask the questioner to repeat the question. But try not to let your mind wander! Time is precious in such settings.
- Dress appropriately.

Transitional phrases

Paul Eddington's masterful portrayal of fictitious British Prime Minister Jim Hacker in the television series *Yes, Prime Minister* contained the advice about being interviewed: "If you have nothing to say, say nothing. But better still, have something to say and say it, *no matter what they ask*. Pay no attention to the question, make your own statement. If they ask you the same question again, you just say 'that's not the question' or 'I think the more *important* question is this': Then you make another statement of your own, easy peasy." Transitional phrases can be used to move from what you have been asked to segue to the point you want to make. Some examples:

- But the point I'd like to make is . . .
- But the real point is . . .
- Another thing worth mentioning . . .
- Let me mention something else . . .
- There's something else I'd like to point out . . .
- Another point I'd like to make is . . .
- There's another aspect to that question that we should be focusing on . . .
- There's something else we should be looking at . . .
- If you don't mind, there's something more important we should be discussing . . .
- That's not really the issue. The issue is . . .
- That question raises an interesting point, but the more important point is . . .
- But the question I get asked most often is . . .
- I think the best way to answer that is to tell you what we're trying to do . . .
- The best way to answer that is to give you some background on . . .
- Let me answer that this way . . .
- If you're asking me [then phrase the question in your own terms] . . .
- Before I answer that, let me first point out . . .

Eight answers to the same question

An advocacy planning exercise I learned from American public health advocate Phil Wilbur, illustrates beautifully how a fully prepared interviewee can use a question to turn the definition of what is at issue in any number of planned directions. For example, if an interviewer asks "Why are smoking rates among young people going up?" at least eight different answers might be given, depending on your goal.

Goal 1: Demonstrate the effectiveness of your programme

Response: "The rates are going up, but only slightly. If we didn't have the policies and programmes we now have in place, they would probably be going up much faster" [and then go on to argue for the importance of more resources].

Goal 2: Demonstrate the ineffectiveness of your own programme

Response: "The increase is worrying us all. It's obvious that a lot more funding and effort needs to be put into preventing teenage smoking" [and then go on to argue for what is needed].

Goal 3: Support a specific piece of policy, legislation or programme

Response: "Rates are going up because we're not doing enough to keep them down. If the government would take the sales-to-minors law seriously and start removing tobacco licences from shopkeepers who sell, rather than just talking about it, we might get somewhere."

Goal 4: Turn attention onto the tobacco industry

Response: "Rates are going up because the industry wants them to go up – kids are their most important customers. Every open-air rock festival has a tobacco-sponsored 'chill out' tent. Tobacco companies are flavouring cigarettes with fruits and sugars to try to make them more palatable to kids. This has to be outlawed."

Goal 5: Show that the data aren't as bad as the questioner thinks

Response: "If you look at the figures closely, it is only occasional smoking that is rising only slightly. Heavier daily smoking continues to fall as it has for the last 10 years."

Goal 6: Give someone else media exposure

Response: "I'd be happy to answer that question for you, but today I'm with a young woman who until recently worked in tobacco promotions and has a few interesting things to say about her work."

Goal 7: Draw attention to another related issue

Response: "Smoking rates are going up because of the aggressive price discount-ing that's happening. Tobacco industry profits are such that they can still offer major discounts and keep profit margins. The government needs to increase tobacco tax to make cigarettes more expensive to children."

Goal 8: Reframe the issue to avoid blaming children

Response: "You know, when we see rates go up, people tend to think 'why are so many kids so stupid?' But society has a responsibility to protect children. If smoking rates are going up, we should be asking 'where are we falling down in not controlling the tobacco industry's efforts to get at them?'"

Practise being interviewed

There are commercial interview training companies in many countries that specialise in training people to be interviewed to their best advantage. These are often run by ex-journalists and tend to service political and corporate clients who usually have lots of money to pay for such training. Public health groups are seldom numbered among their clients.

Local community (non–commercial) radio stations typically have very small audiences, yet their radio journalists are often very eager to cover public health stories. It is tempting to think that the time it can take to provide interviews for such stations is hardly worth the effort. In terms of the small audience this may be true. However, the stations can provide you with invaluable practice at being interviewed: if you give a poor performance, few will have heard and you will be more the wiser for the next interview opportunity.

Rehearse with colleagues before you are to be interviewed. Get them to role-play hosts and opponents. However, don't memorise answers or points – they'll sound wooden. There's a paradox: we all seek the perfect soundbite (see below). But if it sounds more like a canned slogan than a spontaneous utterance, it loses its effect, especially if it is stale or an overused cliché.

Media bites or grabs

Knowing your issue in the detail that you do, it well may loom before you as complicated, complex and inextricably convoluted. Many public health issues *are* extremely complex. A critical ability that every public health advocate must possess is to be able to evaluate the essence of the problem that he or she is dealing with and to translate this essence into small, memorable elements that can fit into the time and space limitations of the news media and be consumed by its audiences. Such elements are known as media "bites" or "grabs". These are short, pithy quotes that serve as a central, characterising feature of a broadcast ("soundbites") or print news story. Essentially, they are attention-getting statements that have struck the news editor who cuts your interview down to usable length as being pivotal, emblematic or simply arresting in some way.

With rare exceptions, the clips used in radio and TV news bulletins are always prerecorded: only very occasionally, such as when the bulletin cuts to a reporter on the spot at a major news event, will live interviews be broadcast. This means that interviews you give for news bulletins will be edited to fit the format of the news bulletin. I selected and recorded at random a 30-minute evening TV news bulletin. Aside from advertising and "coming up" announcements, there were 19 stories in the news that night. These stories ran for an average of 66.8 seconds (range 2 minutes 19 seconds to a mere 13 seconds). "Talking heads" of "news actors" were shown 21 times in these stories, with the average talking time per interview being 7.8 seconds.

The obvious lesson here for any interview you give is that you have very little time – a few seconds and perhaps one or two sentences at most – to make the most important points that you hope will be broadcast. The situation with current affairs interview programmes or longer documentaries is considerably different, particularly if the interview is live-to-air.

At best, the media bite can serve to encapsulate both information and effective symbols for an audience that is increasingly used to quick bursts of information. A bite can compress your position in a quick, succinct or witty manner – capturing the attention of the media and the eventual consumer of the message. Like them or not, media bites are a central tool of media advocacy – ignore the "art" of producing good ones at your own peril.

It is not easy to define the qualities that make a successful media bite but here are some suggestions from the Advocacy Institute:

- Utilise concrete images that evoke a lively response, ones that are fresh, alive and surprising.
- Avoid sloganeering, shrillness and moralising.
- Stay brief, and divide longer ideas into short sentences.
- Humour is permissible, but avoid cuteness or frivolity that can downplay the seriousness of the problem. In competing for limited space or time, it is often the pithy or witty quote that gets included in the story. A well-conceived quip can deflate even your opposition's most carefully crafted attempt at legitimacy. Biting humour can also be effective in conveying an appropriate sense of outrage.
- Standard literary devices such as alliteration, rhyming, analogy, parallelism, puns and the like, can make a bite resonate with the journalist and the audience.
- Remember, the goal is not to earn yourself applause or laughs, but to advance your media advocacy goals.

Here are some memorable soundbites from Stan Glantz:

- "They've discovered a vaccine against lung cancer and have flushed it down the toilet" (commenting on the Californian Governor's decision to cut the State's anti-smoking media campaign).
- "The tobacco industry are like cockroaches: they spread disease and don't like the light. We need to turn on the lights and expose them."
- "If you want to control malaria, you have to control mosquitoes. If you want to control lung cancer, you have to control the tobacco industry."

Jargon and ghetto language

Many communications from public health activists suffer from being constipated by language that seems natural to them, but is confusing and alienating to many members of the public. Often this language is jargon – words and expressions that are the technical or specialised language of medicine and public health. Sometimes it is also "ghetto language" – a branch of jargon that is developed by groups or causes with a highly refined and politicised sense of their oppression. Ghetto language is often highly politically correct and wanders about in taken-for-granted notions of history and knowledge that can lose many potential listeners or readers.

Perhaps the main source of lapses into jargon is the classic mistake of confusing your public health objectives with your media objectives. For example, as someone working within a complicated area of public health, you may be constantly aware that greater attention to coordination of policies and programmes is required to effect improvements in your public health goal. "Coordination" may well be one of your public health objectives, but as a peg for media interest it is a kiss of death. The term "coordination" is hopelessly vague to members of the public, who generally will not share your insights into the problem. They will be attending to what you say, seeking to understand the problem you are expressing in terms of tangible issues with which they can relate. Improved coordination will mean something practical and concrete. It is this that you should talk about in media interviews, not the bureaucratic means of achieving it.

A few examples of public health jargon foisted too often on the public include:

- utilisation (use);
- proactive (active);
- intersectoral (people from different parts of government and the community);
- liaising (meeting with);
- cohort (group);
- substance use (drug use);
- policy (to many people, a "policy" is something they receive each year from their insurance company. They are not used to thinking of public health issues as reflecting "policies". Having a policy enacted may be your preoccupation, but the news-listening or newspaper-reading public will find discussion of the issue much more accessible if you address the reason for or the intended effects of the policy, rather than what sounds like some dull bureaucratic process).

Know your opposition

The more that you know about your opposition, the less likely it will be that you will be caught unprepared to deal with any tactic or strategy that they use. Knowing how your opposition thinks, its preoccupations, strengths, weaknesses and Achilles' heels, and relevant information about its principal members will also allow you to be more strategic in your approach to undermining its public and political support.

You should subscribe to or somehow join the mailing list for all magazines, journals, newsletters and bulletins published by your opposition (see "Mailing lists"). The tobacco industry is served by trade journals (*Tobacco Reporter*, *World Tobacco*, *Tobacco International*, *Tobacco Asia*, *Euro Tab*, *Smoke*, *Cigar Aficionado* and the Australian *Retail Tobacconist*), which regularly feature interviews, reports, information and candid gaffes that are indispensable to anyone wanting an inside view of the industry's preoccupations.

Make it a habit to buy examples of new products, especially when they first come onto the market. These will often be invaluable in demonstrating (e.g.) that a company can print small-run new packs in test markets, when it may be arguing to a national government that production of new packs with proposed new warnings would take years of preparation.

Open and maintain active files on your opposition. These should include details of their personnel and leadership, their annual reports, their leading shareholders, market share, market capitalisation value, and other products in their portfolio. Most importantly, maintain detailed "dirt" files on each policy issue so that you will always have damaging and embarrassing examples of what the industry has previously said about any issue. The tobacco industry's internal documents are a goldmine for such material on every conceivable issue. Thanks to what is now a huge amount of scholarship from researchers, who have sifted through over 60 million pages of internal documents and produced hundreds of reports and quote digests[iv], your work can be greatly reduced here.

Learning from other campaigners

There are very few public health causes that are not being addressed by others somewhere else in your country or internationally. Make contact with others who are engaging in the same advocacy efforts. You will avoid reinventing the wheel, and the flat tyre too! Making contact with such people will save you invaluable time, effort, expense and potential advocacy damage by learning from them. Read the papers and reports in your field. Ask others what these are. They will often be repositories of valuable information and perspectives. Globalink (see "Internet") is the best way I know of doing this. Questions are asked and answered daily from all over the world.

Letters to politicians

There is a widespread and naïve view that a penultimate step in getting a law changed or a policy implemented, is simply to write to the relevant politician. This view has it that if one's concerns reflect some sensible suggestion, perhaps drawing attention to some inconsistency in policy, and are expressed soundly, the politician will put the cogs into gear and the desired changes will be set in motion. The view is naïve in all sorts of ways, not the least being the assumption that your suggestion will be found in any way new or original. Most recommendations for change in major public health issues are verses from litanies that have been sung for many years.

Many politicians rarely read incoming letters, unless they are specially passed to them by staff as being particularly important. Neither do they write their own outgoing replies, especially when it concerns routine matters like points of view from members of the public on topical matters. Instead, advisers usually draft replies for the politician's signature. Often replies will be lifted out of a word-processing system, containing giveaway paragraphs like "I have received many letters from constituents on the subject of smoking in bars. The government's view on the changes you suggest is that . . . We thank you for your views which have been noted."

There are, however, ways that letter writing can help to make waves. Below are some suggestions that may enhance the chances of a politician reading, showing concern about, and perhaps even acting on the contents of letters.

How can you make the politician look good? Change frequently involves conflict and opposition. Every astute politician will be fully aware of the strength of the opposition to introducing any effective measures. The decision to implement any tough public health policy will not be taken lightly, and will be balanced against the likely political gains to be made by doing so. Letters to politicians can seed perspectives on the likely reception a stand against a public health problem will have ("an epoch-making decision for community health", "a principled decision in times of political spinelessness . . ." and so on). If you have members who represent large constituencies themselves, point this out to the politician. Always write and congratulate politicians when any worthwhile action is taken so they don't feel they have acted for nothing.

Volume is important. A trickle of letters can always be dismissed by a politician as unrepresentative, especially if over the months they seem to be coming from the same handful of people. A constant stream of letters, and great rushes in response to particular incidents, will be taken much more seriously. The tobacco industry knows the importance of keeping the letters pouring in: tobacco industry workers have been known to sign letters of complaint in response to smoking control announcements. However, the ones I've seen fell into the form-letter basket (see below) and so are readily dismissed.

Don't send form letters. Form letters are standard preprinted letters designed to be signed by your supporters and sent to politicians and other community influentials. They are meant to send a signal that there is widespread community concern about an issue. While form letters are commonly used by advocacy groups, there is almost universal consensus among politicians that, as with most petitions (see "Petitions"), they are a very ineffective means of communicating that those who send the letters actually care much about the issue. It takes little effort or commitment to sign your name on a letter you may not have even read. Politicians receive many examples of such letters and I have never heard a politician express anything but annoyance at the way they clutter up the office and require equally meaningless letters of acknowledgment to be sent to all who write.

The most inept example of this I have seen was a boxful of the same letter clearly written by the management of a local tobacco factory in Sydney, signed by corralled production-line workers, and sent into a health minister. His office staff simply put them all in one corner and had the most junior member of the office prepare single-sentence acknowledgement letters, which were then stamped with an office official's signature. The effect of the letters was to annoy the Minister, his staff and to add to the contempt he already held for those on the industry's side of the issue.

While there may be total agreement about the wording of the ideal letter on a public health subject, never distribute such letters as form letters for people to either sign or retype and send. A form letter will get a form reply and nothing will be accomplished other than to affirm to the politician that your group has no imagination or political acumen. It is even risky to distribute a form listing "essential points' to be made in letters. This may result in a flood of obvious paraphrases being sent, which will leave a similar poor impression.

It is best to produce a fact sheet for distribution to potential letter writers. The sheet should provide all factual material germane to the issue you hope to have people write about, as well as summaries of the various arguments and possible responses that writers can either raise or anticipate.

Who actually writes the politician's replies? Do some detective work and find out the name of the bureaucrat who deals with all correspondence relevant to your issue. There is a good chance that the person will be in this role because of his or her knowledge or background in public health, and therefore might be positively disposed to your concerns. Ask this person frankly what the politician's attitudes and positions are on the various aspects of public health policy – whether he or she is under instructions from the political party or cabinet to take a particular line, whether he or she has any personal convictions, positive or negative, about your issue, and most importantly, whether there are any issues that the bureaucrat feels are ripe for the politician to take action on.

Letters from powerful, important or well-known people. Letters from persons in positions of power and influence or from public celebrities almost by definition carry more weight than those from "ordinary" citizens. Professors, deans, heads of medical colleges, public interest groups with large memberships, trade unions, Nobel laureates, folk heroes and bodies representing children's interests all qualify here. It is even more impressive if several such people – say, the deans of all medical schools in the country – jointly sign a letter to a politician (see also "Open letters").

Send copies of your letters to influential people. It may be prudent to send copies of your letters to politicians to other influential groups such as journalists, key organisations or the opposition political party. You should indicate that you have done this at the foot of your letter. If the politician feels that your letter and his or her response is being read or anticipated not only by you, but by influential people in the community, they may consider your letter more urgently and seriously.

Consider publishing your correspondence. Even if you have no immediate plans to do so, it cannot hurt your efforts to explain in your letters to politicians that you are seeking information on his or her policies for a forthcoming article, report or book. This will help you obtain a serious and carefully worded reply, rather than some throwaway line that may later embarrass its signatory. Such a prompt may even cause some reconsideration of policy if the present policy looks archaic in the face of new information or compared with the policies of other states or nations. Care should be taken not to word such letters in belligerent terms or tones. Careful thought can produce letters that are uncompromising and to the point while not sounding hot-headed and "emotional". Think about how you react to angry letters you receive and ask yourself why a politician would feel any different. Always send copies of your correspondence and replies received to other groups in your network.

Letters to the editor

Although letters to the editor don't carry the implied weight of authority and expertise that editorials or op-ed pieces do (see "Editorials"; "Op-ed opinion page access"), they are one of the most read sections of newspapers, especially in quality newspapers, where the competition to get a letter published often results in a high standard of writing. Most large newspapers employ staff who do nothing else but read, select, edit and verify the identities of letter writers whose letters are short-listed. Apart from smaller, regional newspapers it is seldom that the actual editor of a major newspaper will read or select letters for publication.

Most letters page editors select one or two longer letters to publish as lead letters. Often these will be complemented with one or two smaller letters on the same subject. Letters editors with whom I have spoken shared common views about the nature of a letters page. Most were emphatic that the letters page was first and foremost a vehicle for "ordinary citizens" to express their views on topical matters. They took the view that advocacy groups, politicians, government departments and businesses were able to express their views in newspapers through the news pages or through paid advocacy advertising. Preference is therefore given to those who might express the same views as a lobby group, but who are writing as ordinary citizens.

This is not to say that letters pages will not publish letters from groups known to have a recognised position, but only that if they are to get published, such letters have to be outstandingly better than those sent in by ordinary citizens. The main exception to this is where a letter represents a reply or rejoinder to a previous letter that attacked or misrepresented your group or cause.

Major newspapers can receive several hundred letters each day. When there is an important or emotive news story, the number of letters can quadruple. Yet regardless of the number of letters received, it is rare for the letters page to be expanded. A fundamental first step when attempting to have a letter published is to find out the newspaper's policy on length.

Here are a few steps that will improve your chances of getting your letter printed and of making the impact you want to make:

- Be concise. Even if the paper you are writing to doesn't explicitly limit the length of letters it publishes, it will still be to your advantage to be as concise as possible. This rule applies to anyone who writes for a newspaper – editorialists, news reporters, columnists. With letters, brevity is critical.
- Stick to one angle or issue. This will help limit its length.
- Be timely. Newspapers will rarely print letters about subjects that are not in the news. Use a current news event or recently published article as a hook for making your letter timely. Decisions about the letters for the next day's edition are often made by mid-afternoon, so if the issue you are writing about is very topical, get your letter written and delivered quickly. Email the letter – a faxed letter needs retyping, which will lower its appeal in a busy office.
- Be familiar with the different styles and genres of letters that appear on a particular paper's letters page. Are they often whimsical? Literary? Ironic? Polemical? Colloquial or formal? Is there an apparent preference for wit or metaphorical language? These sorts of questions can be helpful in shaping your approach.
- Don't assume readers will know what you are writing about. If you are writing about pending legislation, explain (briefly) what that legislation is, what its effects will be, and when it will be decided. If you are writing in response to an article, editorial or previous letter, start your letter by saying which article you are responding to (refer to the headline or writer's name as the title) and when it appeared.
- Use your credentials. If you have personal experience or expertise in the subject area, mention it briefly ("As someone who has operated on over 500 cases of lung cancer . . .", "I work as a waiter in a busy city hotel . . ."). This will not only enhance your credibility but increase your chances of getting published.
- Be consistent, but original. If your organisation is planning a letter-writing campaign, make sure everyone knows the facts of the situation – two letters, ostensibly on the same side of the issue, that contradict each other will ring alarm bells for the editor. At the same time, don't send in "form letters" or letters that are clearly part of a write-in campaign. No newspaper will knowingly allow itself to be part of an organisation's propaganda efforts.
- Concentrate on the local angle. Newspapers are community-based organs and the letters page is where they interact with the community most explicitly. Any local angle on the subject you are writing about will increase the impact of your letter and increase its chances for publication.
- Be literate. Even with serious subjects, there is no need for letters to be totally dull and earnest. Obviously your spelling and grammar should be correct but try also to write with a little flourish. Metaphors, similes, satire, literary and

historical allusions, oxymorons and most importantly, wit, will make your letter more attractive to the letters editor and enhance its chances of being published. The letters editor of the *Sydney Morning Herald* counselled potential writers: "The elements I miss in the letters these days are wit and whimsy. A year ago they were still present but either hard times or a trend toward political correctness, or a combination of both, is killing those delightful qualities."

Two strategies are worth considering in trying to get letters published. First, attempt to get an authoritative letter published by an expert on the subject or by a well-known community member. Often such people will be glad to have a letter you write go out under their signature. Alternatively, try to flood the newspaper with letters from members of the community in an effort to represent widespread public opinion. If several different perspectives occur to you about how an issue might be treated in a letter, write separate letters using each approach and then quickly email them around your coalition members or supporters for them to sign and send in.

Local newspapers

Many advocates are dismissive of local suburban or small town newspapers because they feel that they are parochial, have comparatively small circulations and seldom if ever deal with issues likely to be compatible with significant public health advocacy. However, take the time to find out if your prejudices are justified. Often they will not be. Find out the circulation and whether anything is known about its readership. Find out whether the paper is at all interested in covering stories about public health and whether it has ever taken up the cudgels for a local cause such as banning smoking in an enclosed shopping mall. Think about how you might localise a state or national issue for a local area readership (see "Localisation" under "Creative epidemiology").

Young and ambitious editors and journalists working on local newspapers often nurture hopes that they can break a big story that will be picked up by a state or national news medium. If you sense that a local journalist has a sense of destiny and will "work" a local story into a state or national focus, give consideration to whether you might try to break the story locally first.

Mailing lists

Your opposition may be gathering names for databases of people it can enlist in support for its legislative proposals or in lobbying against yours. The tobacco industry has developed huge mailing lists from various giveaway or coupon marketing schemes. You should try to get on such mailing lists so that you know what they are up to and when. If you are well known to them they will not be willing to put you on mailing lists, so use a name not known to them. Another route onto mailing lists includes any petition you may be asked to sign. While the thought may be obnoxious, consider sending a small donation to your opposition (such as a smokers' rights group) – this will signal your support and may fast-track you onto their mailing list. You may need to consider safeguarding your privacy when handing out your address: tactics here include giving post office box numbers, or "safe house" addresses, where an arrangement can be made for you to collect mail. It can be interesting to use a range of different names. This will allow you to track which avenues led your "name" to be handed to which particular database.

If all this seems somewhat devious, be assured that your opposition is getting information about you in exactly the same sorts of ways (see "Infiltration"). The first rule of politics is to *be there*: if your opposition is cooking something up and you need to know about it, a certain degree of inventiveness and cunning is often required.

Your mailing list

If your group's newsletters say nothing important, then your opposition will not be bothered to get hold of them (and perhaps you should question the effort and expense of distributing such material! Far too many advocacy groups tie up much time and effort into producing newsletters that describe happenings that are old news to everyone who is in any way active in the issue). Assuming that your newsletters do contain important information about strategy or tactics, then the opposition will try to get on your mailing list too. This means that you should exercise some care in opening up your mailing list to just anyone. In soliciting membership or supporters, you may wish to think about ways of checking just who is joining. One way of doing this is to require all who join to go through some form of scrutiny. You can explain the need for this to people so that they do not see your questions or procedures as overly intrusive. Scrutiny could take the form of having joining members be nominated by existing, known and trusted members; and being unwilling to accept post box addresses from any member not well known to your group (this will allow you to check a "doubtful" name against the addresses given using a telephone directory – if there is no listing of the name given, you may have some cause to be suspicious).

Marginal seats

These are those electoral areas where a politician has only narrowly won or lost the previous political contest. In some situations, a political seat will hang on a dozen or so votes. Where governments are elected with only the narrowest of political margins, the importance of influencing a mere handful of voters in a marginal electorate to support your policies can take on national significance. Marginal seats are literally the political threads on which the life or death of whole governments and opposition parties can hang.

Marginal seats will be inordinately interesting to political leaders, particularly in the months and weeks preceding elections. If voters in these seats can be shown to be actively interested in your public health issue, it will be a foolish local politician who will ignore this interest. Reports sent by politicians in marginal seats to the central policy forums of their parties about local support for your issue, can transform a marginal issue into a high-profile concern. Accordingly, marginal seats are frequently the scenes of intense efforts to influence voters about both political parties and single issues. Your opposition will appreciate this too and it is likely that particular electorates within countries will be the focus of their efforts. If they succeed in gaining wide support for their cause in a marginal seat, irreparable damage can be done to your cause.

All public health advocates should know which political seats in their country are marginal. Efforts should then be made to foster supportive networks within each of these areas (see "Networks"). Email, mailing and contact lists of groups such as doctors, churches and community groups, should be compiled. Familiarity should be cultivated with the local media (reporters' names, copy deadlines and so on). This is the sort of activity that should be undertaken routinely, as part of the background preparation for advocacy work. Key opinion leaders in the area should be noted and efforts made to determine whether or not they are sympathetic to your issue. If they are, or look like they may be amenable to influence, they should be supplied with information, flattered by visits from any important campaign emissaries, and given supportive publicity via your own media access opportunities. The opposite course of action should apply to local politicians who oppose your cause.

If your organisation is bound by its constitution or rules to be non-party political, a traditional tactic here is for lobby groups to write letters to each politician in an electorate and invite them to state their views on particular questions. Their responses, including refusals or "no comments", can then be published in advertising or on leaflets and posters. Politicians advised about the public fate of their answers will think very carefully before replying.

Media cannibalism (or how media feed off each other)

In any news bulletin there will be some stories that are breaking for the first time, and others that are extensions of stories that have broken earlier in other media. So, in an important way, part of the definition of news is the circular statement that much news is what has already been determined to be news. (Some have even suggested that a lot of news in fact should be called "olds" because similar stories are retold repeatedly with new particulars, facts and news actors.) In practice this means that if one news agency decides that an issue is newsworthy, it will often be the case that its competitors will also conclude that the issue is newsworthy, even if they might have independently decided otherwise beforehand. For example, radio journalists seeking to fill breakfast and morning radio news programmes tend to use many of the stories that are printed in that morning's newspapers as their primary source, although naturally they will be keen to break stories that have come to light after the print media stories have gone to press. One radio in Sydney is jokingly referred to as "the Sydney Morning Herald for the visually impaired" because many journalists actually read out sections of stories live to air. Breakfast radio journalists obtain the newspapers in the early hours of the morning while the public is asleep. A story defined as major by that morning's print media will be very compelling to radio journalists.

Similarly, any major story that has been broken by radio or daytime television will be picked up by evening television and by print journalists writing their stories for the next morning's edition. Journalists who are covering a story that has already been broken in another medium will be seeking to extend the story in a way that makes it look like they are not simply repeating others' material. In these ways, the media are constantly cannibalising their fellow outlets.

For advocates, this means that they must think of news opportunities in two ways. Besides trying to interest the news media in original stories, they must place themselves in the position of journalists and be constantly anticipating ways in which to assist journalists in *extending* stories. Most successful public health advocates are avid news addicts: they get up early to read newspapers, they wake to radio news bulletins, have news programmes on in the car and watch news and current affairs programmes as much as they can.

Media conferences

Media conferences are a standard vehicle in any advocate's stable of strategies. Media conferences are essentially meetings where the media are invited *en masse* for a specific purpose. These purposes can include:

- releasing statements and providing detailed commentary;
- the launch of something new (books, reports, products, services, etc.);
- an opportunity to interview a celebrity or authority.

A media conference should be held whenever you anticipate that your story is likely to be of interest to a wide range of media. It is also important to put yourself in the media's shoes and ask whether there is any perceived advantage to them in covering your story face-to-face at a news conference, or whether it could just as adequately be covered by a journalist phoning you. If you conclude that the conference does not have obvious allure, then you will need to put thought into making it more tantalising.

Journalists regularly try to ascertain whether other media (and particularly their rivals) will be covering a story or attending a media conference. A missed story, particularly a big one, is considered very bad form in journalistic circles. So if you have the assurance from particular journalists that they will be attending your conference, it is a good idea to spread such information to other media in a passing mention.

The timing and place of media conferences are important. You should become familiar with the schedules and deadlines of the programmes or editions in which you want to have your story covered and hold the conference at a time that will allow the journalists to attend, write or edit their story, and allow for any other commitments that may be in their schedules. In planning the day for the conference, you should try to anticipate any competition from other stories (see "Slow news days") and consider that journalists will need to buy their lunch (so if you provide it, you may well tip the scales in favour of their attendance!).

When you hold media conferences, advantage should be taken of any venues that will be a poignant reminder of the more dramatic aspects of your public health issue. Rooms adjacent to cancer wards or general hospital locations are ideal. Someone active in your field will probably be connected with such a venue, and so holding a meeting there will not appear contrived or melodramatic.

In such locations, a major thrust of your opposition's position – that the health consequences of (e.g.) smoking or cigarette-caused burns are the exaggerated fabrications of fanatics – will be rendered an objection in the poorest possible taste.

Checklist for media conferences[v]

- Have the date, time and place been cleared with all speakers?
- Are the time and place suitable for the reporters from media you are most concerned to attract to the event or media conference?
- Are there any predictable media conflicts (i.e. other major events or media conferences you know about)?
- Is the room large enough?
- Are there plenty of electrical outlets for television lights?
- Will you need a public address system?
- Have people been assigned to clean up the room before and after the conference?
- Do you plan to serve refreshments? Has this been arranged?
- Who is sending out the media releases?
- Have you checked to see that the emails and recipients for the releases are still current?
- Who is making follow-up calls to editors and reporters? Are these people properly briefed about the event and the issue?
- Are visuals, charts, etc. required for the media conference?
- Does each speaker know what the other speakers are going to say?
- Is someone drafting a question-and-answer sheet for anticipated questions at the media conference?
- Has provision been made for each speaker to rehearse their presentations and answers to the anticipated questions?
- Are materials being prepared for a media kit?
  - media release
  - background information on speakers
  - fact sheet
  - organisational background
  - copies of speakers' statements

Media etiquette

Like any group of professionals, journalists have operating procedures that should be respected by anyone who chooses to interact with them.

- Respect deadlines. Whenever you talk with any journalist about a story, first ask them if they are on a deadline. If they are, respect it. One of the quickest ways to lose a journalist's respect is to call them with help on a story after their deadline has passed.
- Don't consider reporters to be your friends. After they've developed a friendly relationship with a journalist, many advocates are tempted to ask the journalist to "join the cause". Journalists sometimes make it plain to you, off the record, that they sympathise with your cause. However, there is a huge difference between them expressing this to you personally and their wishing to do anything more than report your story. Attempting to cross such a boundary may be embarrassing for the journalist, who may avoid subsequent contact with you. A journalist's job is to write about an issue, not to help you in your cause. This should be respected. Equally, journalists who write unfavourable stories are not necessarily your enemies. Agree to disagree with them. They may report your side differently next time. Do not tell a journalist anything that you do not wish to be reported.
- Follow up on promises. If journalists ask for information you don't have and you promise to provide it later, do so. Journalists depend on their sources. If you don't follow up on your promises you are not only making it difficult for them to do their job, but also you may seriously damage your credibility as a source.
- Don't be petty. If journalists fail to use your quote, or fail to give your organisation sufficiently prominent mention, don't act like they have failed to do their job. Their job is not to publicise you. This applies especially to the common practice of minor misquotation. Journalists will sometimes paraphrase what you have said, with the result that expressions or emphases are used that are not exactly what you would have preferred. It is wise to consider the impact on the journalist of any complaint you might make. It is preferable to be seen by journalists as a good and reliable source, than as a sensitive pedant to be treated with kid gloves or avoided.

Media logs

Most radio and TV stations keep a record or log of calls from the public who call up to praise, complain or otherwise comment on programmes. Sometimes callers are switched through to an answering machine; others summarise calls into a log book. Many lobbies arrange for their members and supporters to inundate such programmes with calls. In Australia, for example, the pro-gun and anti-abortion lobbies both swamp the switchboards of programmes that run items featuring spokespeople whom these lobbies oppose. Often the inundation is so obviously orchestrated that it is not taken seriously as sign of community feeling. However, the programme logs are set up because journalists and media management are keenly interested in taking the pulse of audiences in as many ways as possible. Encouraging your supporters to phone in their praise or criticism can thus be an important way of sending messages to key influentials in the media.

Some programmes do not seem to mind allowing you information about their programme logs, especially if you have been of assistance to them in making the programme or have appeared in it. Such access can provide some interesting insights into how the public reacted to you or your opposition.

Media releases (press releases)

A media release is simply a means of sending a statement to the media with the intention that it will make the issues contained in become news. If a media release achieves its purpose, it will almost invariably cause the media to contact the author or contact person listed on it. This means that you should be prepared to take matters further than they have been expressed in the release, which means that you should prepare some notes to prompt you when journalists begin to phone for interviews.

The checklist below gives some important points to cover in composing a media release. Some people baulk at the idea of putting their private phone numbers on a media release, fearing invasion of privacy or even security problems. Cellphone numbers are not listed with addresses. Use them. However, 24-hour contact is extremely important to the success of a media release. You must appreciate that the media do not work to a nine-to-five schedule, and that if they cannot reach you to check a story or conduct an interview, the story will often die and the whole point of putting out the release will be lost.

Checklist for media releases[v]

- Is the release on the organisation's letterhead?
- Is the release dated and marked for immediate release or embargoed until a specific day and time?
- Is the contact person's name and phone number (day and evening) listed at the top of the release?
- Is the headline short and pithy? Is it arresting, relevant and succinct?
- Is the copy doubled spaced?
- Does the first paragraph explain who, what, why, when and where?
- Have you quoted key individuals in the second and third paragraphs? Have you cleared the quotes with them first?
- Is each page marked with an abbreviated headline? (Try to keep the release to two pages – one is better – two can become separated on a journalist's desk and rendered useless.)
- Is a photo opportunity mentioned if there is one? If so, also send the release to the photo editor.

Meeting with the tobacco industry

Many of my colleagues receive approaches – some direct, but most through third parties – to meet with the tobacco industry. Many of these approaches are remarkably inept, gushing with the latest managerial phrases about "stakeholders" and "constructive engagement". The industry wants to use meetings as a means of advancing its various agendas. It will seek strategically to refer to such meetings as evidence that you both are "working together" when the reality is almost always that one or both of you are trying to gather intelligence to gut what the other side is doing. Under no circumstances should you ever meet with the industry in any situation where they are controlling the agenda, the invitees and the spin that will be put on the meeting.

I have met with tobacco industry people on a few occasions. I met with Swedish Match representatives a couple of times in my office out of open-mindedness to learn more about snus. I served for a short time on a Standards Australia committee examining reduced ignition propensity (RIP) cigarettes, on which three tobacco committees also sat. To have kept away would have risked two companies trying to eviscerate the process. If you learn that the tobacco industry is involved in any government or other official committees or forums, make sure that you get effective public health people onto the same committees.

If you do meet with them, use the occasion to ask all the difficult questions, and have their answers formally minuted and available for public scrutiny. When Philip Morris's David Davies addressed the National Press Club in Canberra on "The Politics of Harm Reduction", we prepared a set of questions that we distributed to the journalists, inviting them to select from them. These included:

- While we've been listening to you, about 40 of your best customers have died. How many will still die if they switch to "reduced harm" products? Has your industry ever produced a cigarette that caused lower death rates? What's different today?
- When people do wrong, civil society normally demands that they do four simple things: admit that they've done wrong; promise not to do it again; apologise to those they've harmed; and try to make good the damage that's been done. Mr Davies, has Philip Morris done any of these things? Will you commit to doing so here?
- Will you confirm that Philip Morris has taken out patent registrations on chemicals that are analogues of nicotine? Internal tobacco industry documents reveal that one of the reasons these have been developed is to "get around" potential regulation of nicotine by allowing your company to say that these are distinct products, not covered by regulations pertaining to nicotine. Is that true?
- [to be asked by guest with a respirator for her lung disease] Mr Davies, as you can see, I have to have oxygen to help me to breathe. Can I have your absolute guarantee that the new harm reduced products won't cause people to go through what I've been through?
- Your website says repeatedly that you do not want children to smoke. How much money does your company make each year from smoking by the young people you say you don't want to see smoking? If you are sincere about not wanting to see them smoke, why don't you hand back all the money you make each year to cancer charities and quit campaigns?

- Philip Morris now says that there is no such thing as a safe cigarette. But not long ago, Philip Morris said cigarettes had not been proven to be unsafe. Your former CEO, Geoff Bible, also said if your products were ever found to be unsafe that you would stop selling them. Are you here today to announce that Philip Morris will keep its promise not to sell unsafe cigarettes?
- Will Philip Morris agree to pay for stop-smoking medications to help your addicted customers who wish to quit smoking?

Similarly, if the industry tries to engage with you on your turf, do not allow them to use the occasion as a PR exercise. When the US Smokeless Tobacco Company (USSTC) submitted anodyne abstracts to the 13th World Conference on Smoking and Health in Washington DC in 2006, one of the scientific committee suggested that these be rejected, but that they be offered the following suggested topics:

- "The Use of Tobacco Sponsorship and Rodeo to Target Native American Youth: The USSTC Experience"
- "The Design of Oral Snuff Products and Nicotine Delivery: How to Graduate Novice Users into Tobacco Dependence: The USSTC Approach"
- "Reaching College Kids with your Message: How to Use Fraternity Sponsorship and other Events to Promote Tobacco Dependence among the Young: The USSTC Model"
- "Using Professional Athletes as Spokespeople and How to get your Message Free on Televised Sporting Events. USSTC and Major League Baseball"
- "Partnering with Your Friends: How to Promote Snuff Use as a Temporary Alternative to Smoking. The USSTC and Philip Morris Combined Use Program, a Win for All"
- "Toxins in Tobacco Products Why Should you Care? The USSTC Response"

A final word on the subject. In 2002 Philip Morris sought to bring European scientists together for a meeting. Professor Bertrand Dautzenberg, one of the authors of a call to boycott the meeting, put the effort in clear perspective in the French newspaper, *Le Monde*: "The makers of antipersonnel mines at least have the decency not to invite orthopedic surgeons to a symposium to talk about the risks associated with their products, or to get the surgeons' thoughts on the subject."

Networks and coalitions

In advocacy work, networks are generally informal webs of loosely affiliated groups and individuals who share common concerns. It is important to identify and make contact with other groups that might lend numbers, power, resources, prestige, inviolate credibility or some unique association to your tobacco control advocacy. There exist formidable networks such as medical associations and societies, the consumer movement, trade unions, parent groups, environmental groups, welfare agencies, churches, groups of people living with particular diseases, and international networks of issue-specific activists whose experience and contacts can prove invaluable to advocacy work.

Coalitions are more defined groupings of different interest groups that join forces around particular issues or specific tasks (e.g. to lobby for a particular piece of legislation or in protest against a particular policy). There are enormous advantages, and occasionally disadvantages, in forming a coalition. The principal one is all about strength in numbers and diversity. Individual agencies that might be hypersensitive to the *sequelae* of criticising government, may feel emboldened by joining with a large number of other agencies that are together prepared to do so. Similarly, if government is dismissive of advocacy for tobacco control as coming mostly from "the usual suspects" – the same small bunch of agencies – then the appearance of a coalition of groups containing names it normally respects can greatly change how governments see the tobacco control constituency. Individual groups within coalitions will often have their own publicity and information distribution networks through which your issue can be publicised, adding greatly to dissemination.

It is important to have all coalition members make specific personal, financial and institutional commitments to any advocacy initiative with which their name is associated. When you invite any group to join a coalition, you should take time to determine the degree of commitment that you might expect from the new group. Many coalitions have members that are merely passengers – dead weights to the efforts of others, who use up valuable resources by insisting on being kept informed and so on, but never really contributing. Early clarity about a group's involvement will benefit all concerned. Never let servicing the demands of the coalition subsume the reasons why the coalition was formed in the first place.

Online polls

Online polls about tobacco control issues are often run by newspapers and other media outlets on their websites. They can also be set up on your own organisation's website as a way of rapidly gathering data on community views on a particular proposal. Big news stories on "should this happen?" issues are often passed by news editors to their web editors, and polls set up. Sometimes hundreds of thousands of people vote on these national sites.

Online polls can attract criticism that they are unrepresentative of community opinion because people self-select to vote. However, this criticism can be levelled at any system of electoral voting in many of the world's democracies where voting is not compulsory. Those who self-select to vote in an online poll or in a non-compulsory voting election are those who care enough to express their opinion. If a huge number of people vote in support of a public health position, this can be useful ammunition in further advocacy.

Given the popularity of such polls, and their potential to be used by opponents of public health, advocates need to be vigilant about when the polls commence and conclude. Find out which media outlets run such polls, bookmark them, and then make it part of the start of your day quickly to check the daily online poll topic being run. You might also try proposing a particular poll – and the question – to a journalist who may have interviewed you on the subject, or directly to the staff at the media outlet in charge of the polls.

Once the poll is running, your task is to alert as many people as possible to the existence and timing of the poll. Email is essential here – the polls often change daily. Sometimes local area media outlets run such polls, and I have debated other advocates on the ethics of urging people who live outside an area to vote in the polls. Should I, living in Sydney, vote in an online poll in London about smoke-free pubs, for example? Those opposed to doing this argue that the only way that genuine local opinion on a topic like this can be gauged is for there to be a local vote confined to registered residents. But by allowing votes to be registered on the internet, those doing so are opening up the possibility of voting to anyone anywhere whose attention is brought to the website. We may all have noble thoughts about respecting the "intent" of local media to be only interested in views of genuine locals. But single-issue anti-public health lobby groups (anti-fluoride, anti-immunisation, pro-guns, pro-tobacco, etc.) very much make it their business to bring these polls to their own supporters' attentions. The result can sometimes be propaganda victories for these groups, which then trumpet the results. For the gullible and ill-educated, who can sometimes be in power, such "surveys" risk being used as evidence. And indeed, they *are* evidence of the ability of people to alert support to an opportunity to express their opinion.

If pro-tobacco interests triumph in one local area after another by flooding internet sites with votes, there are potentially domino effects whereby they can then refer to the "sensible" decisions taken by local government councils in different areas. Public health issues are rarely parochial issues, although they may be administered locally. Opposition to public health issues like smoking bans can "catch fire" very easily.

Op-ed opinion page access

Most papers publish an op-ed page opposite the editorial page. The op-ed page contains columns written by the paper's own columnists and syndicated columnists. In some cases, newspapers will publish guest columns or opinion pieces written by academics, experts and public authorities.

Although many newspapers consider it a high priority to maintain open access to their opinion pages, not all papers are receptive to publishing guest pieces from non-staffers, let alone special interest groups. If your paper is averse to running pieces by overt advocacy groups, you may be able to get your issue covered by having a sympathetic academic submit the piece under his or her name, which may lend the article extra authority in the eyes of the editors.

When you've decided what you want to write, email or phone the op-ed page editor to discuss the proposed contribution. Whenever someone in your group delivers an important speech, writes a column for a newsletter, or writes a summary of a report or study, consider whether or not that might be a good basis for a guest piece in the paper.

If your idea is accepted by the page editor, find out how long they would like the piece to be and when they need it. Observe the deadline. Be prepared for rejection and a wall of silence. All advocates know the frustrations and disappointment of being given the green light to submit a piece, only to never have it printed. I have had published over 120 opinion articles in newspapers, but have written probably twice that number. Opinion page editors receive many submissions on all manner of subjects. Some courteously let you know that they can't use a piece you send, while some leave you wondering. As an author, do not be cowed into thinking you cannot simultaneously send the same piece to other outlets, although the moment you hear it is accepted in one, you must immediately withdraw it from other newspapers.

Consider what the paper has already printed on the subject and decide how you could best contribute to the debate. Above all, be sensitive to the needs of newspapers to publish readable, engaging material. Ask yourself, and have others tell you before you send off your contribution, whether what you have written reads well. Would an ordinary reader who was inexpert or not close to the issue find it meaningful and interesting? Are you using bureaucratic or ghetto language (see "Jargon and ghetto language")? Do you make assumptions about the readers' knowledge that are unreasonable?

Open letters

Private letters to politicians run the risk of achieving nothing but a polite reply, with no one but staff knowing the extent and vehemence of community feeling towards your public health issue. Public or open letters are read by thousands, and millions in some countries. You should weigh up what effects you hope to achieve – gentle, polite persuasion or public confrontation – before deciding to write privately or publicly, as described below. An open letter is a letter published in a newspaper to a particular individual like a politician, the managing director of an industry that is affecting public health or a sporting hero who helps in tobacco promotions. Open letters should always ask direct questions that allow those to whom they are addressed no room for evasion. Open letters are the advocate's equivalent of politicians' parliamentary questions to their political opposition. Like parliamentary questions, open letters are on the public record, cannot easily be avoided, and allow the public to "eavesdrop" on a personal exchange about matters of public importance.

If your issue is one of public significance, the person "receiving" the open letter will hardly be able to avoid answering the questions asked, because any silence on their part is likely to be subject to inquiries from journalists. In other words, the open letter and its *sequelae* may well become news in itself.

The most direct way of publishing open letters is to run them as a paid advertisement. This may not be possible if your organisation has a small budget. However, fundraising or celebrity funding (see "Advertising in advocacy") may make this possible. Finally, open letters – and any responses – can be placed on your website, allowing a permanent record, sometimes read by thousands.

Opinion polls

Opinion polls on your issue, particularly those conducted in marginal seats (see "Marginal seats") or in the run-up to elections, are a time-honoured advocacy strategy. Favourable results from polls can be used to assure politicians that there is strong community support for your issue, and that any suggestion that your concerns are fringe or unrepresentative are unwarranted. Results from polls can also be useful as a focal point for media releases.

Commercial opinion poll organisations are polling the community for their clients all year round. They have infrastructures to deal with question design, sampling, interviewing (door-to-door or phone), analysis of results and reporting that are often highly efficient and frequently of a standard that will pass most tests of methodological acceptability. Many of these companies conduct "omnibus" surveys where they present a string of questions commissioned by different clients to samples of the population. The cost of having one or several questions added to these omnibus surveys can often be surprisingly affordable even to groups with modest budgets. If the cost is out of reach, consider pooling resources with some other members of your network to buy a few questions.

The public has a healthy disrespect for survey results. This can work both against your own use of polls, but also for you when you attack dubious poll results being promoted by your opponents. Your opponents' polls should be subject to scrutiny for practices such as leading or bias-inducing questions, series effects (the practice of asking a key question after several others, the answers to which virtually induce respondents into producing a desired answer), inadequate samples or lack of independence in those who conduct the poll. If you have a survey expert among your supporters, try routinely to submit your opposition's polls to this person for criticism.

Case study: call tampering

In the past, cricket in Australia long received huge sums from the *Benson & Hedges* tobacco company. When a politician tried to have a bill introduced to ban tobacco sponsorship of sport, an Australian cricketing association advertised that it had set up a public opinion voting phone line. The public were invited to phone and register their support or opposition to the proposed bill. However, callers to the line who wanted to register their support for the ban were told that only opposing calls were being recorded. Two days later, the Tobacco Institute of Australia published a large press advertisement where results of a "cricket poll" were stated as "90% opposed, 10% in favour" of the ban. The realities of the fabricated "poll" were then given high-profile exposure on primetime television[41] and made the subject of a formal complaint to the Advertising Standards Council, which upheld the complaint.

Opportunism

A media advocacy campaign is like a political campaign in which competing forces continually react to unexpected events, breaking news items, and opportunities, rather than conducting a static, preformed educational campaign. For this reason, opportunism is central to the nature of effective media advocacy. To describe someone as an opportunist is generally to cast a slur on their character. In advocacy, though, a nose for opportunism is an invaluable and indispensable trait. In fact, it is probably the single most important quality that an effective advocate can develop. There are innumerable examples in public health of quite unplanned media coups occurring through individuals having a nose for opportunities to exploit newsworthy events and issues by offering alternative angles that satisfy media appetites for "the other side". The most successful public health advocates have not taken a casual, serendipitous attitude to the search for opportunities, but actively cast about for new ways to raise public health issues onto the public agenda. There are few guidelines that can convert you into a good opportunist other than to advise that public health advocates should be constantly assessing opportunities that can provide a "peg" for a media comment. The Japan Tobacco case study (see Box) gives some examples.

Case study: Japan Tobacco

In 2001, Japan Tobacco announced it had bought rights to develop and market lung cancer vaccines. This opened up a huge opportunity for me to draw attention on a radio broadcast to a string of ironies in the tobacco industry's concern for health, all designed to increase public awareness of commercially driven ethical duplicity rampant throughout the industry:

> When Amatil owned WD & HO Wills in the 1980s, it also owned Lion Insurance. While Wills was busily denying that smoking causes cancer, their colleagues at Lion were busily whacking stiff premiums on smokers, presumably because they had a different view on whether smoking kills.
>
> In 1996 Philip Morris recalled its Kraft peanut butter from across Australia because of a salmonella scare[680], but down the corridor from Philip Morris's food division is its tobacco branch. There the official line – since at least 1954 – has been that they're concerned about customers' health. Back then, one official infamously remarked: "if any one of us believed that the product we were making and selling was in any way harmful to our customers' health – we'd voluntarily go out of business."
>
> Recently Philip Morris posted on its website the statement: "there's an overwhelming medical and scientific consensus that cigarette smoking causes lung cancer, heart disease, emphysema and other serious diseases in smokers. Smokers are far more likely to develop serious diseases, like lung cancer, than non-smokers. There is no 'safe' cigarette."
>
> So how is it that Philip Morris's tobacco products are still filling the shelves? What exactly is the ethical difference between a remote chance of dying from peanut butter poisoning and a very good chance of dying from lung cancer or heart

disease? And why didn't the cigarette boys walk up the corridor and tell their peanut butter pals to tough it out and simply post a note on their website explaining that "eating Kraft peanut butter might cause a serious dose of the squirts or even kill you"?

In the United States some of the largest health insurers and health maintenance organisation owners invest heavily in tobacco. What are we to make of this? It's simply a brilliant win–win financial strategy: the insurers collect premiums and pay few claims for non-smokers, while from smokers, they bank much higher premiums while profiting from the product that kills them. It's a bit like a combination vet/taxidermist who guarantees "regardless of the outcome, you'll have your pet back".

In acquiring rights to lung cancer vaccines and treatments, Japan Tobacco is playing the same game. One official talked of servicing "the cancer market". In the logic of the marketplace, the more cancer, the more desperate victims willing to open their wallets. This is vertical integration at its finest. Funeral parlour chains should expect takeover bids any day now.[681]

Case study: cyanide shocks!

Another example of creative opportunism involved the Food and Drug Administration's ban on all fruit imports from Chile because of some tainted grapes. At the Smoking Control Advocacy Resource Center in Washington DC, staff investigations found that the whole episode started because two grapes in Philadelphia were each found to contain three micrograms of cyanide. A quick check of information in recent US Surgeon General's reports showed that every single cigarette contains several hundred micrograms of cyanide. In fact, the sidestream smoke emitted from a single cigarette contains up to 110 micrograms of hydrogen cyanide, which is more potent than the sodium cyanide found in the grapes. All fruit imports from an entire country were banned because of two grapes containing a tiny fraction of only one of the poisons in cigarettes. That was news.

Parody

In 1987 the Australian Council on Smoking and Health in Perth published an "alternative" annual report for a fictitious tobacco company. Produced with a luscious glossy cover, the report featured a death yield table where brand shares of different cigarettes were apportioned into the total number of tobacco-caused deaths in Australia for that year. The report went on to explain that the directors of this fictitious tobacco company had now decided to accept the evidence on smoking and disease and quoted approvingly a resignation speech from a former chairman of Carreras Rothmans in Northern Ireland who said: "I could not quite get it [working for a tobacco company] squared with my conscience". The report was launched with all the pomp and ceremony of a real company report and attracted much media attention.

ASH UK and New Zealand have also recently published several "alternative" reports in response to BAT's drive into the corporate responsibility arena. With titles like "Trust us – we're socially responsible", "BAT's Big Wheeze – the Alternative Report",

"Behind the Mask – the Real Face of Corporate Responsibility" and "The Other Report to Society", these reports have provided vital counterweight material to BAT's greenwash exercise.

Petitions

Lists of names, addresses and signatures of people supporting your issue or demanding that a politician or authority take some action – are an age-old advocacy tactic. In the USA in approximately 20 states, they can be essential to the process of having referendums put to voters so that citizen-initiated laws can be enacted. Petitions can operate at the local neighbourhood level (e.g. having residents petition local government about the need for a smokefree shopping mall), in the workplace (e.g. to petition management to declare areas surrounding building entrances smoke-free) or on state and national issues.

Generally speaking, the effectiveness of petitions is directly proportional to the extent that they are perceived to represent a majority of citizens in a given area, coupled with the consideration of what sort of commitment is implied by someone troubling merely to sign their name. Small neighbourhood petitions that include the signatures of most residents are likely to make their point more forcibly to a local government body than comparatively large, community-wide petitions, which can be shown to be unrepresentative.

The principle that a chain is only as strong as its weakest link can apply to petitions. If a petition has names on it that can be shown to be fictitious ("Mr Elmer Fudd", or simply names that are shown not to exist at the address given), doubt can be cast on the whole petition. If you are aware or suspect that names on your opponents' petitions are fictitious, it can be devastating to alert the media to this. Equally, if you are in the business of collecting signatures yourself for a petition, it is wise to require all those who are signing to provide identification to the person collecting the signatures. The reason for this should be explained to those who are inconvenienced when signing.

It is also wise to put a lot of thought into how to collect lots of signatures most efficiently. The main way to do this is to avoid time-consuming methods such as door-to-door approaches, when opportunities exist to approach many people who gather together in places like workplaces, shopping centres, sporting events, queues, churches, meetings and so forth. "Snowballing" techniques (e.g. asking particularly keen signatories to take a copy of the petition sheet and collect signatures themselves) should also be considered. Online petitions can easily be organised at www.thepetitionsite.com.

Petitions of specialised, targeted groups can also be useful. Stan Shatenstein and I organised a petition of professional ethicists to condemn tobacco industry appropriation of the corporate responsibility movement, and were able to attract over 80 signatures including several of the world's leading ethicists. This list has been useful in subsequent advocacy in this issue. (see http://petition.globalink.org/view.php?code=extreme).

Pictures and graphics

Watch any news bulletin on TV and observe what is shown. Typically each item will commence with the newsreader in camera introducing the story. As he or she reads, it is common that a still shot or graphic illustrative of the story will be on screen behind the newsreader. Very early into the news piece, the film will cut to either file film or footage recorded that day about the story being dealt with. On big, dramatic on-the-spot items that are occurring while the news bulletin is going to air, the cut may be to a live shot involving a reporter.

Television is an essentially visual medium, and news producers are always keen to illustrate any story with an apposite and arresting scene. It is a very rare TV news story that does not feature film footage in some way. Advocates can take no interest in this aspect of their news stories, or they can take steps to try to influence what is shown as the story is being read. If you don't orchestrate how your story will be illustrated, the media will do it for you, and will sometimes get things horribly wrong, giving an emphasis to the story that may distract greatly from your ideal framing.

If you are going to be interviewed or photographed for a press story, think about the location where you will ask the media to meet you. Many television journalists and editors regard the "talking head" shot of a person being interviewed or making a speech as boring television, often more likely to end up on the cutting room floor than being broadcast. Anticipate this reaction, no matter how important you feel the news value of your story might be. If you can make your talking head points in a setting that is visually relevant to the issue at hand (e.g. in front of a tobacco factory, the company head office; a burns ward in a hospital if your issue is reduced ignition propensity (RIP) cigarettes). Such settings will generally appeal to media gatekeepers more than the usual talking head shot of an expert or spokesperson in front of a shelf of books or sitting at a desk.

The media are equally thirsty for good graphical depictions of the data you are dealing with. "Good" basically means simple and readily comprehensible to viewers or readers, expressing no more than one or two relationships between variables. Have colour versions of these ready for journalists who may be keen to include them in a story. I've more than once been asked by a journalist for a graphic that I used in a press conference.

Piggy-backing

Riding your story on the back of a stronger one that is running a good race in the media is a time-honoured media advocacy strategy. The idea is to latch onto the interest being shown by the media in a particular story and provide a new twist or angle that will enable the media to extend the life of the original story. The bigger the original story, the broader the shoulders on which your new-twist story can ride. If you see that there are apposite parallels or ironies with your issue in the reporting of a news story, the media will often find this worth reporting. Polished advocates will scour newspapers each day looking for piggy-backing opportunities.

Case study: Kerry Packer and the bigger picture

In October 1990, Australia's wealthiest man, publishing billionaire the late Kerry Packer, suffered a heart attack. For some minutes, Packer was clinically "dead", but was revived with a cardiac defibrillator carried by the ambulance that attended him. On his recovery, Packer donated $3.5 million to the NSW State Health Department to enable defibrillators to be installed in every ambulance in NSW. His magnanimity and concern to save lives was an instant headline story and the devices have since been referred to as "Packer whackers" by ambulance teams. At the time, Packer's Australian television network carried the rights to broadcast the summer-long tobacco-sponsored (*Benson & Hedges*) cricket. I wrote a letter to the *Sydney Morning Herald* praising Packer's generosity, but making the point that his concern to save people from deaths from heart disease would find fuller expression if he were publicly to refuse to continue accepting the tobacco-sponsored cricket on his television network. The letter generated considerable debate in the media.

Case study: privates and principles?

On the day that the eminent and high-profile Australian eye surgeon Professor Fred Hollows died with a last wish that instead of flowers donations be sent to his memorial Foundation to help support interocular lens factories and implant programmes in Eritrea, Nepal and Vietnam, a prominent Australian footballer was awarded $350 000 damages against a magazine that had run an unauthorised photograph that inadvertently showed his penis in an after-match shower. The footballer had argued that his reputation as a role model for children was endangered by the implication he had given permission for the photograph to be published. Supporters of the Hollows Foundation lost no time in making press comment that if the footballer was indeed sincere in his motivation, and that venal concerns were not paramount, then he would donate the awarded damages to the Foundation.

Precedents

These function like analogies. If this is like that, then this should be treated like that. In 2006, in an effort to counter an epidemic of graffiti, the New South Wales government proposed legislation to require spray cans to be hidden from public display in paint and hardware stores. Purchasers would need to be over 18 and have to ask a shop assistant to get the can from storage. Anne Jones of ASH quickly saw the precedent that this set for a concurrent debate about the public display of cigarettes in shops, and issued a press release making the strong point that if governments could act to hide spray cans from display to reduce their sales to young people, then they had the power to hide tobacco products from display too.

Press agencies

Press agencies like Reuters, United Press International and Australian Associated Press are journalistic agencies that cover stories and then distribute the stories to news outlets, often worldwide, which may have been unable to cover a story first hand. These agencies can be very important in obtaining maximum coverage. They have particular value in getting coverage for local issues that may have worldwide interest, but are not mammoth hard news stories that will have sold themselves worldwide. In public health, good examples of this are often research reports appearing in medical journals. These may not have been big enough news stories to make the front page of a national paper, but they may have been covered in some way by the national press. By giving a press agency an opportunity to cover such a story, it may well be picked up around the world, which in turn can sometimes give it an extra newsworthy boost at home (see "Media cannibalism").

Private sector alliances

A growing number of private sector companies are engaging in actions that are damaging to the tobacco industry. Their motives range from wishing to assist government policy, to projecting a non-smoking image to the public, to not wanting any public association with the industry. In 2005, the courier companies UPS, DHL and FedEx each announced that they would stop delivering cigarettes to US consumers[682–684] thus assisting in reducing internet sales that avoid tax and make access by minors easy. These policies followed an agreement in March 2005 by major credit card companies to refuse to allow their cards to be used in internet tobacco sales in the USA. Today, internet tobacco suppliers run credit card payments through a third party that receives the internet buyer's payments and then pays them to the internet tobacco seller.

Hotel chains like Westin have begun banning smoking completely on their premises. This is likely to grow as this feature becomes a routine part of first-class hospitality and guests begin revolting against those hotels to which smokers might begin to gravitate ("Let's not consider the X chain – last time we were there, do you remember how the rooms stank of tobacco smoke?"). Some supermarkets in Australia have been voluntarily experimenting with covering up tobacco displays, and several high-profile companies (McDonalds, Pfizer, ING) have refused to participate in corporate responsibility conferences where tobacco companies were due to appear[685].

Be vigilant for any business associations between the tobacco industry and other companies. Draw these associations to the attention of other agencies in your network, suggesting that they might like to approach those companies and urge them to reconsider their association, or that they themselves will not consider any commercial relationship with them as long as they have tobacco accounts. Public relations and advertising agencies with tobacco accounts will be particularly sensitive about this.

Publicising others' research

Scientific research published in medical and public health journals is regularly used as a source for news stories. Some medical journals employ public relations consultants or staff better to ensure that scientific articles in their journals are covered by the media. However, most do not, with the result that many potentially greatly newsworthy scientific articles are read only by a relative handful of specialists who subscribe to such specialist journals, who read them in libraries or by those who go searching for specialised stories on journal websites.

As described in Chapter 3, public health advocates can act as the absent public relations people for such journals by simply bringing the media's attention to potentially newsworthy articles. Serious public health advocates should be able to identify all of the main specialist journals favoured by researchers in their field. They should also routinely check new issues in their nearest public health library. It may be prudent to allocate an hour or so a week as time when someone with an eye for likely newsworthiness can scan through electronic databases like Current Contents for newly published papers. Those with newsworthy potential can then be obtained either by pay-per-view or from a friendly academic with access to electronic journals through their library. Contact the researchers and explain that you would like to see their work given a wider audience in the media. Ask if they would be amenable to talking with the media and suggest that you could prepare a press release, have them check it for accuracy, and then you would send it out to the media.

If the researchers have had no experience with the media, try to demystify the likely course of events that will follow for them if the media take an interest in the story. I followed this procedure in a pilot study to see whether we could increase news coverage of tobacco issues. Fifty-eight of 283 (20.5%) media reports in the study period were generated by our releases[686]. These would have almost certainly never seen the light of day without our efforts.

Radicalism

Many public health issues attract individuals who are impatient for change and unconstrained by conflicts of loyalty to an employing agency's policies. Their agenda for change may share much in common with yours, but go a great deal further in both goals and strategies. Often such individuals will alarm those who are working in or near "the system". The latter will complain that those with radical goals and strategies risk alienating those with power and influence to change things; they fear that radicalism will frighten moderates away from supporting an issue. Sometimes this will be true. As will have been obvious in Part I of this book, there are some "radical" ideas in tobacco control that are also thoroughly ignoble and deserved to be called that.

However, radical groups and ideas have often been of critical importance in the process of successful public health advocacy. Perhaps the most important historical function of radicalism is the way that it can redefine as moderation that which had formerly seemed radical. Before the emergence in the early 1980s of the Australian anti-tobacco billboard graffiti group BUGA UP, the calls by establishment health and medical organisations for total bans on tobacco advertising had seemed draconian to many sections of the Australian population. BUGA UP's wit and uncompromising spray-painted criticisms gradually transformed the mild-mannered positions of the establishment groups into commonplaces that were less confronting to governments not wanting to be seen to move ahead of public opinion. This resulted in a gradual drift by even conservative parties towards the centre ground, newly defined by BUGA UP's radicalism. The result was that within a decade, the tobacco advertising ban position drew all-party support.

Today's radical ideas that I believe will become part of tobacco control orthodoxy within a decade or two include regulation of the tobacco industry[419], the criminal prosecution of many of its executives[687], a drastic reduction in the number of retail outlets for tobacco, banning smoking in cars when children are on board[688], banning displays of tobacco products in shops[119], generic packaging, greatly increased tax on tobacco effectively to elevate it into the luxury price category (this already is the case for cigars, which are smoked far less frequently partly because of this), and smokers' licences[116].

Civil disobedience

There have been many instances of civil disobedience (law breaking) in the history of public health. The work of Greenpeace in the environmental health area is perhaps the most prominent contemporary example. Civil disobedience can carry with it a Robin Hood subtext (outlaws who work for the public good), which forces the public to confront which set of values it believes to be more important. BUGA UP members, for example, were constantly vilified by the tobacco and outdoor advertising industries as being "vandals" for altering the wording on outdoor advertising posters. BUGA UP was confident that the great majority of the public would perceive the vandalism of eyesore ephemera like advertising hoardings to be instantly understandable as being a lesser "wrong" than the flagrant courting of new recruits into smoking.

Reporters and journalists

Reporters and journalists are the media workers with whom public health advocates deal most. It is therefore important to understand how they work, how they see their jobs, what sort of things motivate and please them, and to generally try to see their work from their perspective. If you can do this, you will better be able to develop a mutually valued relationship with journalists (see also "Media etiquette").

The most important thing that should be said about your relationship with reporters and journalists is that they need you just as much as you need them. Understanding this can develop mutual respect, which can be rewarding for advocates and journalists alike: you will get your issues covered in the media and they will write stories that get published or broadcast, thereby helping their own career paths. If they do not know of your existence, or if they find your cause or the way you usually present it dull and lacking in newsworthiness, you will have no mutually beneficial relationship. However, if they know and respect you as a regular news source or commentator, they will seek you out as someone who helps them get their job done.

The second main point to be made about journalists is that they are journalists, not public health advocates. Their job is to produce copy that will pass upwards through the various editorial filters that operate in news organisations and into print or broadcast. To fulfil this goal, their stories have to satisfy the criteria of newsworthiness that were described in Chapter 3. Their job is *not* to be fifth-column public health educators. If their work *in fact* is effective public education or advocacy, then there will have been a happy coincidence of advocacy and the journalistic agenda. Often though, journalists will not give the same emphasis to a story that you would have wished. While you may be disappointed in this, it is thoroughly inappropriate to blame journalists for somehow falling short of a mark that you as an advocate have set for their work. To act in such a way would be to wholly misunderstand what journalists are there to do.

Advocates who work every day in a particular area are sometimes disappointed to discover that many in the media do not know about their expertise and dedication, or even their existence. This is true even for the advocates of well-established groups. Part of the reason for this is that staff changes in news organisations can be rapid: the reporters covering various rounds like health and medicine, politics or features tend to move on to other rounds quickly, so that the reporter you deal with next time may be new to the area and unaware of your group, the issues involved and the history of a particular debate.

Eventually, if you prove yourself to be an open, credible, dependable and trustworthy source, you won't have to worry about attracting the media's attention because they will come looking for you. However, becoming known as a good source can take time, so be patient.

The first step in establishing access to the media in your community is to let them know that you exist. Find out which reporters cover the issues on which you work. This may not be as obvious as it seems. Public health issues, for example, might at one time or another be covered by reporters on all of the following rounds: health; business; sport; cooking and leisure; legislation or politics. Stories about public health might also be assigned by editors of the national, state, local or business desks.

The best way to determine which reporters and editors are responsible for the issues that interest you is to read the paper and look at the bylines. If you're not a regular, careful reader, do some research. Most newspapers have back issues indexed by subject in their libraries, and will give you access to them. The major newspapers can also be found on file at libraries.

Once you have determined which reporters you need to know, initiate contact with them. You can do this by sending them a letter that advises them of your interests and areas of expertise. Tell them you would like to be put on their files of contacts and are willing to be consulted for future news stories, features, or opinion pieces.

Personal contact is even better, so don't hesitate to call a reporter. Remember, reporters make their living by talking to people. Tell the reporter who you are, what your background is and what your specialties are. Be succinct; never waste a reporter's time. Once you've introduced yourself and your areas of interest, you might try suggesting a future meeting. Some reporters like to make coffee dates to meet with new sources; others prefer to keep meetings shorter and less formal.

When you meet with the reporter, take advantage of the opportunity to discuss upcoming events, future story ideas or reactions you and your colleagues have had to stories written by that reporter in the past. (The best way to flatter reporters is to let them know you've read what they've written!) Again, let them know your areas of expertise and tell them you will be able to provide information about those areas in the future.

Some guidelines to keep in mind when you are talking to a journalist working on a story:

- Help to answer the question the journalist is pursuing, even if you're not comfortable with his or her framing of the story; but then suggest another angle for the story. Even if you fail to redirect it, help with the story. The reporter will be back, and you'll get another chance.
- Keep in mind how you would like to see the article framed. Articulate and return to the three or four key points you want to stress.
- Have in mind a key bite (see "Interview strategies"): the one phrase you would like to see in print, either as a quote or, even better, in the journalist's own words or as a headline.
- Rather than stretch your expertise, help reporters find the right expert. Be prepared to suggest other sources to help journalists prepare their stories: effective spokespeople who will help frame the issue well. A dilemma can arise here if the journalist asks your advice on who to interview for the "other side". Should you offer the names of those in your opposition whom you regard as being their most capable spokespeople? Or should you refer the journalist to your opposition's most inept representatives? One view is that you should avoid the temptation to steer reporters to ineffective opposition spokespeople whose poor performances will make your side look stronger. Those who hold to this view argue that when journalists realise that you may have set them up with a weaker other side to the story they are preparing, they will not thank you for having manipulated them and may well not come back to you on later occasions. However, if you sense (as often occurs) that the journalist is sympathetic to your cause, they may be only too willing to allow your opposition to portray their case in a deleterious way.
- Be willing *not* to be quoted. For example, if you are advocating for smoke-free bars, and you have a supportive bar worker who is willing to speak, push such people forwards. If you direct the journalist to good sources, journalists will remember this and come back to you next time.

Journalists and editors can have short memories. While you will probably have a special interest in the media coverage that has been given to your public health issue over recent years, it is likely that you will encounter many journalists who have only a superficial acquaintance with your issue. While you may live and breathe the memory of particular legislative battles, legal cases or lobbying campaigns, a journalist may never have heard of such incidents. Many journalists in my experience are relatively young (early 20s) and so would have been still at school or even not born when you may have been at the frontline on some aspect of your issue.

This observation applies also to research findings. In the early 1980s I issued a press release that challenged the tobacco industry to name the chemical additives that were being used to flavour, preserve and regulate the burning temperature of cigarettes. The subtexts of the issue were "cover-up and secretiveness by industry" and the related issue of the public's right to product information. The release attracted significant media coverage. In subsequent years, I have resurrected the same issue several times in deliberate releases and on several other occasions in response to slow news day "fishing expeditions" (when journalists phone regular news sources to see if they have any potential news stories simmering).

On each of these subsequent occasions, I have used virtually the same source material, the same framing of the issues involved, and the same soundbites. Journalists seldom say "that's an old story", but have run the stories as if they were original. If you are contemplating resurrecting old stories, be aware that newspapers have electronic files on each issue that will generally be searched for background material. If you are being overly repetitive or have not been straightforward with the journalist about the story being an old one, you may risk losing your credibility. Nonetheless, all public health advocates have similar tales to tell about stories that seem to be irresistible to the press.

Create your own press list. Even if your press list contains only a handful of entries at its inception, each should include the following information: name; title; publication; issue areas covered; address; phone and fax numbers; and any idiosyncrasies that may be relevant to your issue (e.g. the reporter may have had a relative killed by a drunk driver; have mentioned that they have a relative affected by a disease you are working to prevent or care for; may have a reputation for preferring press meetings where there is plenty of food and drink; and so on).

As new stories develop, make use of your press list and maintain your press relationships by contacting them with new information, story ideas and good leads. If you have close contacts with one or a few key journalists, you may want to offer them "exclusive" stories.

Finally, keep a copy of every story that you help to generate. This will also help to determine whom you should contact for follow-up and related future stories. In addition, sharing your successes with others can make it easier for them to generate publicity in their own communities. After all, once a story is reported, it is old news only to the paper that reported it. To all other media outlets, it may still be an opportunity.

Scream test

The first principle in effective tobacco control is that if the tobacco industry "screams", you know you're doing the right thing. If there is a deafening silence, you need hardly bother. If they want to work with you, it's time to have a serious review of what you are advocating and whether you are being blind-sided by a wider industry agenda you haven't fully appreciated.

Very early in my career I attended a lunchtime postgraduate seminar in the Economics Department at my university to listen, incognito, to a *Rothmans'* marketing analyst who, as part of his masters degree, was describing how his company gathered intelligence on the effect of virtually any variable on sales. Each stock delivery to every retail outlet in the country was entered in a hand-held computer and the data relayed for analysis. In this way, the company had data on sales movements for their brands, separately and in aggregate, day-by-day, shop-by-shop, suburb-by-suburb. They could relate these changes to any macroeconomic variable such as changes in disposable income, unemployment levels, or consumer confidence, but also to tobacco control variables such as tax rises, health education campaigns, a powerful television documentary, or the launch of a new quit smoking pharmaceutical. The industry knows almost instantly whether something is affecting sales, and by looking back over longer periods, it can discern the synergies of different interventions and policies, and those of its own marketing initiatives. If something is negatively affecting sales, it is elementary that the industry will seek to oppose it, arguing wherever it can, that its concerns are about far more noble matters.

There are some today who argue that the iron-clad validity of the scream test has waned, with the industry's supposed capitulation on its policy of denying the health risks of tobacco said to have ushered it into a more responsible era. Whatever changes the industry has made, none of these give it a moment's pause ruthlessly to pursue its bottom line. Chapter 7 described some of the very worst recent marketing and public relations ploys that the leading companies have used in their post "we've changed" rebirthing period. The tobacco industry's recent investment and publicity for its various ostensible anti-smoking initiatives, as discussed in Chapter 7, is the apotheosis of this duplicity. As discussed at length in Chapter 4, much of the industry's rejuvenated interest in harm reduction is little more than an effort to arrest cessation and to tide smokers over times when smoking bans reduce use.

Shareholders

Public declarations by reputable companies and individuals that they will not invest in a tobacco company for ethical reasons can be newsworthy and may cause other groups to reflect on their position. The ethical investment movement in your country will be a useful ally in suggesting ways of promoting divestment of tobacco shares, often complicated when pension and superannuation funds invest many employees' contributions in portfolio investments that include tobacco stocks. Nonetheless, there remain many companies and individuals who retain total discretion in which stocks they invest in. If these can be convinced to dispose of tobacco stocks, someone else of course will buy them, including the companies themselves.

However, divestment is important for its shaming potential (see "Shaming"), providing yet another vehicle for the community to learn about the industry and why it should be spurned by civil society.

Keep an updated list of the directors and major shareholders of all tobacco companies operating in your country. This can serve as a useful ready-reference for understanding the web of vested interests that is likely to support the tobacco industry. Make special note of any significant joint directorships (e.g. newspapers, broadcasting and hospital boards) that might raise public concern. In 2001, it came to the attention of ASH UK's Clive Bates that Derek Bonham, chairman of Imperial Tobacco, had for some time been a director of GlaxoSmithKline, manufacturers of Zyban and nicotine replacement products. A rapid global protest followed, organised through the internet, where key tobacco control individuals threatened to cut all ties with the pharmaceutical company if Bonham was not axed. He rapidly "voluntarily stood down" with the incident being reported in the press[689].

Case study: named and shamed

In 1985, David Player, then Director General of the British Health Education Council, funded the public interest group, Social Audit, to compile a list of tobacco shareholders in Britain whose investment in tobacco was ethically questionable. Player believed that if news got out to the public that groups concerned with health were having a bet on tobacco both ways, that many of the public would see this as hypocritical and the overall effort against tobacco would suffer. Shareholdings of public companies can be searched by computer. Key words like "Doctor", "Royal", "Medical", "Hospital", "Children", etc. were submitted to the computer and a massive list emerged. These were listed in a special report published by the British Medical Association (BMA) under the following headings:

- Institutions in health and related areas
- Organisations concerned with children's welfare
- Educational establishments
- Church and related organisations
- Agencies involved in welfare and relief work
- Official and national agencies
- Local government authorities
- Pension funds

Initially, a suggestion was made to write to all the shareholders listed in the report prior to its publication, suggesting that they may wish to review their policy in light of the health effects of tobacco. But in the heat of the revelations, this suggestion was not taken up and the report was published and covered widely by the press. Predictably, this led to a mixed reaction. Some groups named declared publicly that they would be selling all their tobacco shares while others were drawn into justifying their retention. But the worst result was undoubtedly the public scrap that ensued between a cancer charity with shares and the BMA, the former accusing the latter of not consulting them and implying a motive of humiliation. Anyone contemplating a similar exercise should definitely keep their findings private until shareholding groups have at least been given a chance to reconsider. Otherwise it is likely to be a case of "divide and rule" in your opposition's favour.

Some tobacco control advocates buy a small number of shares in tobacco companies. The chief advantages of this are that it will place you on their mailing list for annual reports and news of the company. It will also allow you to attend shareholder meetings and functions such as annual general meetings. Such attendances can be used to great advocacy advantage if strategic questions are asked from the floor. Reporters often attend these meetings and your presence may provide good copy[690]. Protesting shareholders have disrupted meetings and caused them to move to other locations[691]. If different members of your coalition each buy shares and attend the shareholders meetings, your protest questions will appear to be coming not merely from individuals but from a seemingly larger number of shareholders seated throughout the meeting.

Slow news days

News should be understood as a product manufactured by the news gathering process. This means that when there are fewer people actually gathering news, there will be correspondingly fewer news stories being gathered and competing for the limited space in print, radio or television news outlets. At such times, the chances of any given story being picked up by a reporter and published are much higher than normal. The chances are made even greater by the correspondence of slow news gathering periods with lower activity periods in the community generally. Weekends, particularly Sundays, public holidays and summer holiday periods, are the most obvious slow news days that can be exploited. Remember also that these times can be disastrous times to stage press conferences: skeleton staff operate in many media and if a bigger story than yours breaks, these staff will probably be drawn away from yours and it is unlikely that substitute journalists will be available to take over. At the end of the day there is no way of knowing when a bigger story than yours will break: it's just that the probability of this happening is less on slow news days.

Strategic research

It is important to anticipate how research might enhance your advocacy objectives. Is your opposition constantly alluding to community support for its position? Do you suspect that this support is not all it seems? Is there a critical piece of missing information or perspective that, were it available, might dramatically alter the terms in which an issue is being debated? Most areas of public health advocacy have several such gaps and the strategic use of research to plug them is a very common tactic used by advocates.

It should be emphasised that the risks of losing credibility both within your own professional or community constituency and with the media by conducting or promoting shoddy research are great indeed. Strategic research should *never* be understood as a synonym for poor quality research. However, nearly every piece of research has the potential to snake down a myriad of inconsequential and confusing pathways determined by over-cautiousness or an overly zealous respect for comprehensiveness. Strategic research can often be simple, conducted quickly and of high quality within the objectives set for it.

Call a meeting of your most strategically imaginative colleagues once a year and brainstorm all the questions that "if only" you had information on. This can produce a long wish list, which in turn may throw up suggestions of how different questions might be quickly researched and what advocacy initiatives these might feed into.

Case study: damned by statistics

Philip Morris in Australia argued persistently that its small, inexpensive packs of 15 cigarettes ("kiddie packs") were not marketed with children in mind, despite an overtly teenage-oriented advertising campaign. A quick survey comparing school children and adults from the same area showed otherwise: 57% of smoking children had bought a pack of 15s in the past month compared with only 8% of adult smokers.[692] As a result, Philip Morris's argument was quickly diffused and the small packs banned in South Australia, causing a domino effect around all the other Australian states in the following few years.

Talent (spokespeople)

The media refer to news actors (those who appear in the news) as "talent", a reference that reflects the essentially dramaturgic nature of the way media workers conceive of news. News should be considered as a daily social drama, populated by casts of heroes, villains, victims and ordinary people. It is vital that advocates consider how to populate these often vitally relevant social dramas with the most influential people possible.

Many public health causes feature spokespeople who are so distractingly bad in some aspect of their presentation that they all but destroy any advantage their issue may have in media representations. Broadcast journalists who judge you as poor talent will be very reluctant to call on you again. The result can be an avoidable neglect of your issue, simply because of its identification with such people as being difficult to work with or boring to audiences and the journalists themselves. On the other hand, an engaging, articulate, credible and skilled media advocate can attract inordinate positive attention to an issue, way beyond that achieved by someone with less "talent".

Many organisations assume that the importance of a media appearance warrants the most senior person in the organisation being the obvious spokesperson to deal with the media. The Advocacy Institute comments:

> Your best spokesperson may or may not be you – or the boss. The head of your organisation may be the right name on a press release, or the named

author of an op-ed article, but not an experienced or effective broadcast presence. Your organisational culture may encourage volunteers to speak for the organisation while professional staff members are expected to remain in the background. That may be a fine practice for many occasions – but not for handling a professionally trained adversary. Of course, choosing the right spokesperson sometimes requires exquisite tact and considerable courage.

(http://www.alcoholpolicymd.com/take_action/checklist_2.htm)

If your issue or organisation is labouring under the burden of an inappropriate spokesperson, especially one who is in a managerial or executive role, it may be possible to address this issue through the services of outside media consultants whose independence may allow them to make the point that underlings within the organisation cannot. Equally, instituting some form of evaluation of media performances, through focus groups of either members of the public or relevant experts, may produce information and feedback that will be useful. Finally, the acid test of how well your organisation's "talent" is viewed by the media will be the extent to which the media return for comment on other occasions, especially in relation to news stories where they have some discretion on who to interview.

The tobacco control lobby occasionally labours under the unfortunate public image legacy of some of its activists, many of whom were the last word in puritanism and everything that represents dullness. To such people, smoking was a self-indulgent evil and tobacco the devil's weed. Smoking was a symptom of some more fundamental moral turpitude and so it was smokers more than smoking that was at the heart of what they reviled. Think about the characteristic vaudeville representation of the non-smoker and imagine most people's response to a word-association exercise using "anti-smoker" and it is easy to see some of the difficulties that still beset the field today. Many probably still believe that, given some rein, people taking a stance against smoking would like to stop everyone drinking, lace everyone up, turn the music down at your party, take all sweets out of children's mouths, and ban sex and probably laughing too. How many who might otherwise stop and think about smoking, dismiss or relegate the message because of this pious and totally unnecessary wrapper?

Talkback (access) radio

Radio programmes that are open for listeners to phone in and talk on air can provide a host of opportunities for you to place a message in front of mass audiences at no cost. The Australian Prime Minister John Howard has said of the medium: "I think that people on talkback radio have more influence now than many print journalists . . . Now your comments . . . and the way in which your listeners hear what I say . . . I believe has a very significant influence in conditioning public attitudes. Now that's just a fact of media life and I think it's got to be recognized." [Radio 3AW, Melbourne, 14 May 1997.] Talkback radio is perhaps the least scientific of polls, but political parties "are nonetheless convinced of the power of callers to swing opinion: that's why they have armies of volunteers constantly calling up the big radio shows to have their say"[693].

The talkback genre is meant to create the illusion of a form of random sampling of public views on issues. It is radio's equivalent of the way newspapers sometimes run a series of vox pop one-line responses to a news item by people intercepted in shopping malls. Talkback is seen by radio programmers as something different to the soliciting of expert or lobby group views on an issue. Talkback occasionally features people with authority or expertise phoning in, but generally, it is seen by stations as an access medium for the person-in-the-street. This means that you should probably treat it in the way it is intended to function and identify yourself as simply a person with a view on the issue being discussed. Alternatively, you can describe yourself as someone with some special interest or expertise in the issue (e.g. "Hello, I'm a doctor, and I've been listening to some of your callers arguing that these gruesome pack warnings are over the top. I'd like to tell you about a patient of mine I saw this morning with throat cancer . . ."). However, it is best to avoid being seen as a member of a lobby group trying to exploit the medium. The station is likely to want to control access for such groups through an invitation to be interviewed.

While many callers to talkback radio are genuine, unaffiliated "ordinary" people, a surprising number would probably turn out to be rather more calculating. Many political parties and lobby groups deliberately try to "stack" talkback programmes in attempts to convey to listeners that there is widespread support for their issue or position. It is common practice, for example, for staffers in politicians' offices to use up any spare moments trying to phone through calls to talkback programmes. This occurs especially when the politician they work for is in the studio taking calls (here, they feed preferred questions and ladle out praise) or when the political opposition is there (here, they go on the attack).

The important thing to remember is that neither the radio host nor the audience has any way of knowing that a caller is anything more than just that: an ordinary person with an opinion. If these opinions can be articulated with reference to the key principles discussed throughout this book, and if they appear to be coming in from the public one after the other, valuable advocacy reaching thousands or sometimes millions of people can occur.

Getting on air

As anyone who has tried to get through to a talkback programme knows, it can be difficult – all lines are often full. Knowing this, many callers phone up the programme in advance and have been waiting on the line unbeknown to listeners for many minutes. You must be prepared to do this too. This means that you must know when the talkback segment of different radio programmes usually commence or when the host announces what the subject of that day's talkback will be (some stations have "open-line" talkback, where any subject can be raised by listeners). Assuming the former, you can then decide whether on that day it will be worth your while phoning through. If there is a big news story breaking around your issue, the chances that it will be covered on talkback are greater than normal. It may be wise to activate the first few limbs of your telephone tree if a talkback session looks promising.

When you phone through, your call will be answered by a programme researcher or producer. Generally, this person will ask you your first name and what you want to talk about. Keywords from this information will often be relayed to a monitor visible to the radio host in the studio. Sometimes, the host will not go to air with the calls in the order they come in, but rather choose calls that balance one another. Others use the monitor to screen out callers with views they don't want to broadcast. If this is working against your issue, you can only know about this from experience. If it happens, you may decide that the only way to get on air is to appear to have changed your mind about what you want to say when you are actually talking to the host on air.

It is a good idea to draw up a week's calendar of all radio stations, marking each day with the stations that broadcast talkback programmes during particular hours. Code or somehow note against each programme anything that might be important to your issue (e.g. host known to be on/offside with your cause). To save time looking up station phone numbers and fumbling with the dial, pre-set radio station access lines into your office phones better to ensure that your call can get through.

Targeting or narrowcasting

Sending a message through the airwaves to reach as many people as possible is called "broadcasting"; targeting the audiences you need to reach through the right medium is called "narrowcasting". When you are seeking to persuade active citizens or community leaders to support your policies, it is important to target your media initiatives to those media that your target audience reads or views, and respects, and to frame and express your position in ways that will elicit the best response from the target group with whom you are most concerned. Effective media advocacy starts with an understanding of how an issue relates to the prevailing public opinions and values of your target group; only then can media messages be designed that will broaden an advocate's base of public support.

Research can help advocates determine how the public views various issues. Even fairly simple, low-cost research can help monitor public attitudes and perceptions within your community. National polls can also help reveal which of your policy initiatives is misconceived or distorted by segments of the public and, therefore, needs reframing. Qualitative research, such as focus groups, is another useful tool for indicating how the public feels about issues and the ways that these are being discussed. Armed with an understanding of the public's dominant concerns, advocates can successfully begin to frame an issue or actively work to reframe it if it is being typically discussed in unproductive ways.

When developing your messages, keep your target audience firmly in mind. Constantly ask yourself if the message being formulated is likely to be appropriate for the chosen group. An anti-tobacco message designed for policymakers will probably not be effective for reaching adolescents.

In using any particular media outlet, you need to understand what kind of language and tone that particular audience responds to. The audience for a local public radio channel may be far more interested in scientific discourse than those who enjoy the combative give and take of a local call-in talk show. As a result, it is your responsibility to make sure that your media advocacy message is suited for your audience.

Just as your message must be tailored to the specific audience you have in mind, you must also adjust your material to the medium that you use. A wordy magazine advertisement would not be as effective on a billboard. In short, each medium has varying strengths and weaknesses that you should keep in mind as you formulate your media advocacy.

Editorial pages are usually far less well read than sport or front page sections of newspapers, but they are read intensely by the community leaders who help shape public policy. In many countries, public broadcasting stations have smaller audiences than commercial stations, but reach large segments of those active citizens whom political scientists call the "attentive public".

By using the appropriate medium, you can reach your target audience. For example, if you want to reach people in the medical profession, there are a variety of periodicals that cater only to medical professionals, and a number that target members of specific medical specialties. Spreading your message in these periodicals would help you to reach your specific audience and therefore to accomplish your media advocacy goals.

It is important to be aware of who you believe to be your most important media audience. Messages can sound like they are aimed at all viewers, but in fact can be directly aimed at a few key politicians in the listening or viewing audience. As you develop your media advocacy projects, identify your target audience. Ask yourself to whom your media advocacy strategy should be targeted. Do you want to reach the general public? How about policymakers? Do you only want your message to be tailored to activists already on your side? Or do you want to target people who are "on the fence" and could easily be persuaded to take action for your cause?

Whistle-blowers

Whistle-blowers, people who break ranks from their expected duty of confidentiality and give the "inside story" – usually about corruption, duplicity or dirty dealings, hold immense fascination for the media. Jeff Wigand – "The Insider" – is probably the most famous tobacco industry whistle-blower[694], but there have been several others, such as Bill Farone[695], Fred Gulson[696], Paul Mele and Gary Huber[697]. Whistle blowers carry with them subtexts of bravery, uncommonness and truth-telling, which give them intrinsic newsworthiness. Whistle-blowers can be anyone from very senior people in organisations right down to humble workers who have witnessed things that they feel the public should know about. Disgruntled or disaffected relatives or lovers of people in organisations also sometimes blow the whistle.

Rather than waiting for whistle-blowers to take the initiative, it can be an interesting exercise to advertise that you are interested in having confidential discussions with people who may be sympathetic with your objectives (see "Infiltration"). You should, however, be clear about the legal implications of inducing whistle-blowing, and ensure that you do not break the law.

Two organisations with a wealth of information about whistleblowing are the Government Accountability Project (www.whistleblower.org) and the National Whistleblower Center (www.whistleblowers.org).

Wolves in sheep's clothing

If your opposition has been having a credibility crisis with the media, it may have resorted to the common strategy of "third party strategy": funding and supporting seemingly "independent" community and business groups to do its bidding, untainted by having any direct connection with them. These groups typically have names that incorporate sound, respectable values, the idea being to render attacks on their particular positions as attacks on the invincible values behind which they shelter. The tobacco industry has an impressive record of funding or otherwise supporting such groups, particularly around the passive smoking issue. Some of these groups include the Freedom Organisation for the Right to Enjoy Smoking Tobacco (FOREST), the California Business and Restaurant Alliance, Californians for Fair Business Policy, Restaurants for a Sensible Voluntary Policy, and Healthy Buildings International[177], the latter a regular front for the industry and subject of a searing piece of investigative journalism in *The Nation*[698].

As discussed above under "Talent", the credibility of those delivering a message can be critical to how believable and persuasive they are seen to be. Your opposition will often seek to frame or label you in some pejorative way. The objective here is to distract audiences from considering your message, by making them become preoccupied by the values that you supposedly represent. Front groups, cloaked in the respectability of a label like "freedom" or "fairness", can step into a debate with you with a head start in the eyes of an unsuspecting audience.

If you suspect that a group is being funded by your opposition, investigate the connection and if it is confirmed, use this information ruthlessly. If you are successful, you may quickly shift the frame around their respectable presence to the probably more powerful one of deception and the "wolf in sheep's clothing".

Notes

i   This section is an edited version of Chapman S. Advocacy for public health: a primer. *J Epidemiol Community Health* 2004;**58**:361–65.

ii   http://www.siu.edu/~cesl/students/support/eap/eap2_speedread2.html

iii Entire books and training programmes have been devoted to this area. One of the best books I have read in this area is Dickinson S. *How to Take on the Media*. London: Weidenfeld & Nicolson, 1990.

iv   For a complete list see www.library.ucsf.edu/tobacco/docsbiblio.html

v   Adapted from Bobo K, Kendall J, Max S. *Organize! Organizing for Social Change. A Manual for Activists in the 1990s*. Washington: Seven Locks Press, 1991.

References

1   Chapman S, Lupton D. *The Fight for Public Health: Principles and Practice of Media Advocacy.* London: BMJ Publishing, 1994.

2   Chapman S. Great expectorations!: the decline of public spitting: lessons for passive smoking? *BMJ* 1995;**311**:1685–6.

3   World Bank. *Curbing the Epidemic: Governments and the Economics of Tobacco Control.* Development in practice. Washington DC: World Bank, 1999.

4   Woodward SD. Trends in cigarette consumption in Australia. *Aust NZ J Med* 1984;**14**:405–7.

5   Australian Institute of Health and Welfare. *2004 National Drug Strategy Household Survey: Detailed Findings.* Drug statistics series, no. 16. Canberra: AIHW, 2005.

6   New South Wales Central Cancer Registry. *Lung Cancer Age Standardised Incidence Rates NSW.* Sydney: Cancer Institute NSW, 2005 (http://www.statistics.cancerinstitute.org.au).

7   Australian Institute of Health and Welfare. *Epidemic of Coronary Heart Disease and its Treatment in Australia.* Cardiovascular disease series, no. 20. Canberra: AIHW, 2002.

8   Smith M. Mopping up the advertising world. *Sydney Morning Herald* 5 Jul 1979:10.

9   Chapman S. A David and Goliath story: tobacco advertising and self-regulation in Australia. *BMJ* 1980;**281**:1187–90.

10 Chapman S. Civil disobedience and tobacco control: the case of BUGA UP. *Tob Control* 1996;**5**:179–85.

11 Wakefield M, Miller C, Woodward S. Community perceptions about the tobacco industry and tobacco control funding. *Aust NZ J Public Health* 1999;**23**:240–4.

12 Chapman S. Advertising and psychotropic drugs: place of myth in ideological reproduction. *Soc Sci Med-Med Soc* 1979;**13**:751.

13 Chapman S. *Over Our Dead Bodies: Port Arthur and Australia's Fight for Gun Control.* Sydney: Pluto Press, 1998.

14 World Health Organization Tobacco Free Initiative. *Facts and Figures about Tobacco.* Geneva: WHO, 2006 (http://www.who.int/tobacco/fctc/tobacco%20factsheet%20for%20COP4.pdf).

15 McKie J, Richardson J. The rule of rescue. *Soc Sci Med* 2003;**56**:2407–19.

16 Godfrey C, Parrott S, Coleman T et al. The cost-effectiveness of the English smoking treatment services: evidence from practice. *Addiction* 2005;**100**(Suppl. 2):70–83.

17 Parrott S, Godfrey C. Economics of smoking cessation. *BMJ* 2004;**328**:947–9.

18 World Health Organization. *An International Treaty for Tobacco Control.* Geneva: WHO, 2003 (http://www.who.int/features/2003/08/en).

19 Joint United Nations Programme on HIV/AIDS (UNAIDS), World Health Organization. *AIDS Epidemic Update: Special Report on HIV Prevention.* Geneva: UNAIDS, WHO, 2005 (http://www.unaids.org/epi/2005/doc/report_pdf.asp).

20 Peden M, McGee K, Krug EG (eds). *Injury: a Leading Cause of the Global Burden of Disease 2000.* Geneva: WHO, Dept of Injuries and Violence Prevention, 2002 (http://whqlibdoc.who.int/publications/2002/9241562323.pdf).

21 Krug EG, Dahlberg LL, Mercy JA et al. (eds). *World Report on Violence and Health.* Geneva: WHO, 2002 (http://www.who.int/violence_injury_prevention/violence/world_report/en/full_en.pdf).

22 Zumla A, Mullan Z. Turning the tide against tuberculosis. *Lancet* 2006;**367**:877–8.

23 Peden M, Scurfield R, Sleet D et al. (eds). *World Report on Road Traffic Injury Prevention.* Geneva: WHO, 2004 (http://www.who.int/world-health-day/2004/infomaterials/world_report/en/index.html).

24 World Health Organization. *Guidelines for the Treatment of Malaria.* Geneva: WHO, 2006 (http://www.who.int/malaria/docs/TreatmentGuidelines2006.pdf).

25 Lopez AD, Mathers CD, Ezzati M et al. Global and regional burden of disease and risk factors, 2001: systematic analysis of population health data. *Lancet* 2006;**367**:1747–57.

26 Centers for Disease Control and Prevention. Annual smoking-attributable mortality, years of potential life lost, and productivity losses: United States, 1997–2001. *MMWR Morb Mortal Wkly Rep* 2005;**54**:625–8.

27 Murray CJL, Lopez AD (eds). *The Global Burden of Disease: a Comprehensive Assessment of Mortality and Disability from Diseases, Injuries, and Risk Factors in 1990 and Projected to 2020.* Global burden of disease and injury series, Vol. 1. Cambridge, MA: Harvard School of Public Health on behalf of the World Health Organization and the World Bank, 1996.

28 Simpson D. Turkey: upping up the anti. *Tob Control* 2003;**12**:245–6.

29 Cardis E, Krewski D, Boniol M et al. Estimates of the cancer burden in Europe from radioactive fallout from the Chernobyl accident. *Int J Cancer* 2006;**119**:1224–35.

30 International Agency for Research on Cancer. The cancer burden from Chernobyl in Europe: press release no. 168. Lyon: IARC, 2006 (http://www.iarc.fr/ENG/Press_Releases/pr168a.html).

31 Arendt H. *Eichmann in Jerusalem: a Report on the Banality of Evil.* London: Faber and Faber, 1963.

32 Wakefield M, McLeod K, Smith KC. Individual versus corporate responsibility for smoking-related illness: Australian press coverage of the Rolah McCabe trial. *Health Promot Int* 2003;**18**:297–305.

33 Arthur D. Little, Philip Morris CR. Public finance balance of smoking in the Czech Republic. 28 Nov 2000. Philip Morris (http://legacy.library.ucsf.edu/tid/jxn10c00).

34 Campbell Johnson Limited. A public relations strategy. 20 Nov 1978. Philip Morris (http://legacy.library.ucsf.edu/tid/uus39e00).

35 Royal College of Physicians of London. *Smoking and Health: a Report on Smoking in Relation to Cancer of the Lung and other Diseases.* London: Pitman Medical, 1962.

36 American Academy of Anti-Aging Medicine. *Accomplishments* (http://www.worldhealth.net/p/89.html).

37 American Academy of Anti-Aging Medicine. Official position statement on the truth about human aging, 2002 (http://www.worldhealth.net/p/96,333.html).

38 von Eschenbach AC. Message from the director July 2004. US National Cancer Institute. 2004 (http://nano.cancer.gov/about_alliance/message_director.asp).

39 Elvik R. Can injury prevention efforts go too far?: reflections on some possible implications of Vision Zero for road accident fatalities. *Accid Anal Prev* 1999;**31**:265–86.

40 Lowy DR, Frazer IH. Chapter 16: Prophylactic human papillomavirus vaccines. *J Natl Cancer Inst Monogr* 2003:111–6.

41   Doll R, Peto R, Boreham J et al. Mortality from cancer in relation to smoking: 50 years' observations on British doctors. *Br J Cancer* 2005;**92**:426–9.

42   Peto R, Lopez AD, Boreham J et al. *Mortality from Smoking in Developed Countries 1950–2000: All Developed Countries.* Geneva: UICC, 2006 (http://www.ctsu.ox.ac.uk/%7Etobacco/C0003.pdf).

43   Ezzati M, Lopez AD. Estimates of global mortality attributable to smoking in 2000. *Lancet* 2003;**362**:847–52.

44   Shatenstein S, Chapman S. The banality of tobacco deaths. *Tob Control* 2002;**11**:1–2.

45   Chapman S, Haddad S, Sindhusake D. Do work-place smoking bans cause smokers to smoke "harder"?: results from a naturalistic observational study. *Addiction* 1997;**92**:607–10.

46   Chapman S. Tobacco Control Supersite (http://tobacco.health.usyd.edu.au).

47   Doll R, Peto R, Boreham J et al. Mortality in relation to smoking: 50 years' observations on male British doctors. *BMJ* 2004;**328**:1519.

48   Oakes W, Chapman S, Borland R et al. "Bulletproof skeptics in life's jungle": which self-exempting beliefs about smoking most predict lack of progression towards quitting? *Prev Med* 2004;**39**:776–82.

49   Diehm C, Kareem S, Lawall H. Epidemiology of peripheral arterial disease. *Vasa* 2004;**33**:183–9.

50   Thornton J, Edwards R, Mitchell P et al. Smoking and age-related macular degeneration: a review of association. *Eye* 2005;**19**:935–44.

51   Nomura K, Nakao M, Morimoto T. Effect of smoking on hearing loss: quality assessment and meta-analysis. *Prev Med* 2005;**40**:138–44.

52   Pihlstrom BL, Michalowicz BS, Johnson NW. Periodontal diseases. *Lancet* 2005;**366**:1809–20.

53   Cooper C, Westlake S, Harvey N et al. Review: developmental origins of osteoporotic fracture. *Osteoporos Int* 2006;**17**:337–47.

54   Millett C, Wen LM, Rissel C et al. Smoking and erectile dysfunction: findings from a representative sample of Australian men. *Tob Control* 2006;**15**:136–9.

55   Centers for Disease Control and Prevention. Cigarette smoking-attributable morbidity: United States, 2000. *MMWR Morb Mortal Wkly Rep* 2003;**52**:842–44.

56   Halbert RJ, Natoli JL, Gano A et al. Global burden of COPD: systematic review and meta-analysis. *Eur Respir J* 2006;**28**:523–32.

57   Fries JF. Aging, natural death, and the compression of morbidity. *N Engl J Med* 1980;**303**:130–5.

58   Goodin RE. The ethics of smoking. *Ethics* 1989;**99**:574–624.

59   Goodin RE. *No Smoking: the Ethical Issues.* Chicago: University of Chicago Press, 1989.

60   Mill JS. On Liberty (1859). In: RW (ed.) *Three Essays.* Oxford: Oxford University Press, 1975:1–141.

61   Chapman S, Carter M. "Avoid health warnings on all tobacco products just as long as we can": a history of Australian tobacco industry efforts to avoid, delay and dilute health warnings on cigarettes. *Tob Control* 2003;**12**(Suppl. 3):iii13–22.

62   Tobacco Institute of Australia. Submission to Senate Community Affairs Reference Committee Inquiry into Tobacco Industry and the Costs of Tobacco-Related Illness, 1994.

63   Murray W. [Letter to Hon. N. Greiner, Premier of NSW]. 26 Jun 1992. Philip Morris (http://legacy.library.ucsf.edu/tid/ifj19e00).

64   Carter SM, Chapman S. Smoking, disease, and obdurate denial: the Australian tobacco industry in the 1980s. *Tob Control* 2003;**12**(Suppl. 3):iii23–30.

65   Wakefield M, Morley C, Horan JK et al. The cigarette pack as image: new evidence from tobacco industry documents. *Tob Control* 2002;**11**(Suppl. 1):i73–80.

66   Webb WH. Status of the Marlboro Development Programme. 7 Dec 1984. Philip Morris (http://legacy.library.ucsf.edu/tid/gmr98e00).

67   Viscusi WK. *Smoking: Making the Risky Decision.* New York: Oxford University Press, 1992.

68   Wakefield M, Freeman J, Donovan R. Recall and response of smokers and recent quitters to the Australian National Tobacco Campaign. *Tob Control* 2003;**12**(Suppl. 2):ii15–22.

69   Yang G, Fan L, Tan J et al. Smoking in China: findings of the 1996 National Prevalence Survey. *JAMA* 1999;**282**:1247–53.

70   Mullins R, Borland R, Hill D. *Smoking Knowledge, Attitudes and Behaviour in Victoria: Results from the 1990 and 1991 Household Surveys.* Victorian Smoking and Health Program Quit Evaluation Studies, Vol. 6. Melbourne: Victorian Smoking and Health Program, 1995:1–30 (http://www.quit.org.au/downloads/QE/QE6/QE6Home.html).

71   Commonwealth Department of Health and Aged Care. Review of health warnings on tobacco products in Australia: discussion paper. Canberra: DHAC, 2001 (http://www.health.gov.au/internet/wcms/publishing.nsf/Content/health-pubhlth-strateg-drugs-tobacco-warnings.htm/$FILE/tobacco.pdf).

72   Scollo M, Lal A. *The Causal Links and Associations with Active and Passive Smoking and Specific Diseases and Medical Conditions.* Carlton, Vic.: VicHealth Centre for Tobacco Control, 2002 (http://www.vctc.org.au/health/causes_&_associations.pdf).

73   Mitchell P, Chapman S, Smith W. "Smoking is a major cause of blindness". *Med J Aust* 1999;**171**:173–4.

74   Watson P, Ashwathnarayan R, Lynch HT et al. Tobacco use and increased colorectal cancer risk in patients with hereditary nonpolyposis colorectal cancer (Lynch syndrome). *Arch Intern Med* 2004;**164**:2429–31.

75   Borland R. What do people's estimates of smoking related risk mean? *Psychol Health* 1997;**12**:513–21.

76   Weinstein ND, Marcus SE, Moser RP. Smokers' unrealistic optimism about their risk. *Tob Control* 2005;**14**:55–9.

77   Canadian Cancer Society. *Controlling the Tobacco Epidemic: Selected Evidence in Support of Banning all Tobacco Advertising and Promotion, and Requiring Large, Picture-based Health Warnings on Tobacco Packages.* Ottawa: Canadian Cancer Society, International Union Against Cancer, 2001.

78   Weinstein ND. Smokers' recognition of their vulnerability to harm. In: Slovic P (ed.) *Smoking: Risk, Perception & Policy.* Thousand Oaks, CA: Sage Publications, 2001:81–96.

79   Lipkus IM, Hollands JG. The visual communication of risk. *J Natl Cancer Inst Monogr* 1999:149–63.

80   Elliott & Shanahan (E&S) Research. Developmental research for new Australian health warnings on Tobacco Products Stage 2: prepared for Population Health Division, Department of Health and Ageing. Canberra: Dept of Health and Ageing, 2003 (http://www.health.gov.au/internet/wcms/Publishing.nsf/Content/health-pubhlth-strateg-drugs-tobacco-warnings.htm/$FILE/warnings_stage2.pdf).

81   Australia Department of Health and Ageing. Australian cigarette ingredient information (http://www.health.gov.au/internet/wcms/publishing.nsf/content/health-pubhlth-strateg-drugs-tobacco-ingredients.htm).

82   Chapman S. "Keep a low profile": pesticide residue, additives, and freon use in Australian tobacco manufacturing. *Tob Control* 2003;**12**(Suppl. 3):iii45–53.

83   Vagg R, Chapman S. Nicotine analogues: a review of tobacco industry research interests. *Addiction* 2005;**100**:701–12.

84   DiFranza JR, Rigotti NA, McNeill AD et al. Initial symptoms of nicotine dependence in adolescents. *Tob Control* 2000;**9**:313–19.

85   Knopick P. [Memorandum to W. Kloepfer]. 9 Sep 1980. Tobacco Institute (http://legacy.library.ucsf.edu/tid/yol92f00).

86   Robins LN. The sixth Thomas James Okey Memorial Lecture – Vietnam veterans' rapid recovery from heroin addiction: a fluke or normal expectation? *Addiction* 1993;**88**:1041–54.

87   Robins LN, Helzer JE, Davis DH. Narcotic use in southeast Asia and afterward: an interview study of 898 Vietnam returnees. *Arch Gen Psychiatry* 1975;**32**:955–61.

88   Robins LN, Davis DH, Nurco DN. How permanent was Vietnam drug addiction? *Am J Public Health* 1974;**64**(Suppl.):38–43.

89   United States Office of the Assistant Secretary for Health and Surgeon General. *The Health Consequences of Smoking: Nicotine Addiction: a Report of the Surgeon General.* DHHS publication no. (CDC) 88–8406. Rockville, MD: U.S. Dept. of Health and Human Services, Office on Smoking and Health, 1988 (http://www.cdc.gov/tobacco/sgr/sgr_1988/index.htm).

90   Becker G, Murphy K. A theory of rational addiction. *J Political Economy* 1988;**96**:675–700.

91   Ranieri v. Ranieri (1973) 7 South Australian State Reports 418, 429 (Sangster J), 1973.

92   Bowater v. Rowley Regis Corporation [1944] 1 King's Bench Reports 476, 479.

93   The Roper Organization. A study of public attitudes towards cigarette smoking and the tobacco industry in 1978. Vol 1. May 1978. Tobacco Institute (http://legacy.library.ucsf.edu/tid/qje03f00).

94   Chapman S, Borland R, Hill D et al. Why the tobacco industry fears the passive smoking issue. *Int J Health Serv* 1990;**20**:417–27.

95   Chapman S, Borland R, Scollo M et al. The impact of smoke-free workplaces on declining cigarette consumption in Australia and the United States. *Am J Public Health* 1999;**89**:1018–23.

96   Champion D, Chapman S. Framing pub smoking bans: an analysis of Australian print news media coverage, March 1996–March 2003. *J Epidemiol Community Health* 2005;**59**:679–84.

97   Collins DJ, Lapsley HM. *Counting the Cost: Estimates of the Social Costs of Drug Abuse in Australia in 1998–9.* Canberra: Commonwealth Dept of Health and Ageing, 2002 (http://www.health.gov.au/internet/wcms/publishing.nsf/content/health-pubhlth-publicat-mono.htm/$file/mono49.pdf).

98   Warner KE, Fulton GA, Nicolas P et al. Employment implications of declining tobacco product sales for the regional economies of the United States. *JAMA* 1996;**275**:1241–6.

99   Buck D, Godfrey C, Raw M et al. *Tobacco and Jobs: the Impact of Reducing Consumption on Employment in the UK.* York: Society for the Study of Addiction and Centre for Health Economics, University of York, 1995.

100 Francey N, Chapman S. "Operation Berkshire": the international tobacco companies' conspiracy. *BMJ* 2000;**321**:371–4.

101 Hurt RD, Robertson CR. Prying open the door to the tobacco industry's secrets about nicotine: the Minnesota Tobacco Trial. *JAMA* 1998;**280**:1173–81.

102 Slade J, Bero LA, Hanauer P et al. Nicotine and addiction: the Brown and Williamson documents. *JAMA* 1995;**274**:225–33.

103 Lupton D, Chapman S. Death of a heart surgeon: reflections on press accounts of the murder of Victor Chang. *BMJ* 1991;**303**:1583–6.

104 National Heart Foundation of Australia. *Heart Transplants and Organ Donation.* NHFA, 2004 (http://www.heartfoundation.com.au/downloads/Heart_Transplants_ Organ_Don_2004.pdf).

105 Bailar JC, 3rd, Gornik HL. Cancer undefeated. *N Engl J Med* 1997;**336**:1569–74.

106 Critchley JA, Capewell S, Unal B. Life-years gained from coronary heart disease mortality reduction in Scotland: prevention or treatment? *J Clin Epidemiol* 2003;**56**:583–90.

107 Thun MJ, Jemal A. How much of the decrease in cancer death rates in the United States is attributable to reductions in tobacco smoking? *Tob Control* 2006;**15**:345–7.

108 Chapman S. Tough on drugs – weak on tobacco. *Med J Aust* 2000;**172**:612–14.

109 Chapman S. The paradox of prevention. *BMJ* 1996;**313**:1104.

110 World Health Organization. *Smoking and its Effects on Health.* Geneva: WHO, 1975.

111 Gray N (ed.). *Lung Cancer Prevention: Guidelines for Smoking Control.* UICC technical report series no. 28. Geneva: International Union Against Cancer, 1977.

112 Roemer R, Taylor A, Lariviere J. Origins of the WHO Framework Convention on Tobacco Control. *Am J Public Health* 2005;**95**:936–8.

113 Assunta M, Chapman S. Health treaty dilution: a case study of Japan's influence on the language of the WHO Framework Convention on Tobacco Control. *J Epidemiol Community Health* 2006;**60**:751–6.

114 Kozlowski LT, O'Connor RJ, Giovino GA et al. Maximum yields might improve public health – if filter vents were banned: a lesson from the history of vented filters. *Tob Control* 2006;**15**:262–6.

115 Connolly GN, Alpert HR, Rees V et al. Effect of the New York State cigarette fire safety standard on ignition propensity, smoke constituents, and the consumer market. *Tob Control* 2005;**14**:321–7.

116 Chapman S, Liberman J. Ensuring smokers are adequately informed: reflections on consumer rights, manufacturer responsibilities, and policy implications. *Tob Control* 2005;**14**(Suppl. 2):ii8–13.

117 Carr-Gregg MR, Gray AJ. "Generic" packaging: a possible solution to the marketing of tobacco to young people. *Med J Aust* 1990;**153**:685–6.

118 Hammond D, Fong GT, McDonald PW et al. Graphic Canadian cigarette warning labels and adverse outcomes: evidence from Canadian smokers. *Am J Public Health* 2004;**94**:1442–5.

119 Dewhirst T. POP goes the power wall?: taking aim at tobacco promotional strategies utilised at retail. *Tob Control* 2004;**13**:209–10.

120 Connolly GN. Smokes and cyberspace: a public health disaster in the making. *Tob Control* 2001;**10**:299.

121 Wilkes MS, Kravitz RL. Medical researchers and the media: attitudes toward public dissemination of research. *JAMA* 1992;**268**:999–1003.

122 Otten AL. The influence of the mass media on health policy. *Health Aff (Millwood)* 1992;**11**:111–18.

123 Blecic DD. Monograph use at an academic health sciences library: the first three years of shelf life. *Bull Med Libr Assoc* 2000;**88**:145–51.

124 Wallack LM, Dorfman L, Jernigan D et al. *Media Advocacy and Public Health: Power for Prevention.* Newbury Park, CA: Sage, 1993.

125 Wallack LM, Woodruff K, Dorfman L et al. *News for a Change: an Advocate's Guide to Working with the Media.* Thousand Oaks, CA: Sage, 1999.

126 Siegel M, Doner L. *Marketing Public Health: Strategies to Promote Social Change.* Gaithersburg, MD: Aspen, 1998.

127 Ryan C. *Prime Time Activism: Media Strategies for Grassroots Organising.* Boston: South End Press, 1991.

128 Parisi P. Toward a philosophy of framing: news narratives for public journalism. *Journalism Mass Comm* 1997;**74**:673–86.

129 Dwyer T, Ponsonby AL. The decline of SIDS: a success story for epidemiology. *Epidemiology* 1996;**7**:323–5.

130 Ma T, Guo J, Wang F. The epidemiology of iodine-deficiency diseases in China. *Am J Clin Nutr* 1993;**57**:264S–66S.

131 Bower C, Miller M, Payne J et al. Folate promotion in Western Australia and the prevention of neural tube defects. *Aust NZ J Public Health* 2004;**28**:458–64.

132 Rein M. *Social Science and Public Policy.* New York: Penguin, 1976.

133 Lawrence G, Bammer G, Chapman S. 'Sending the wrong signal': analysis of print media reportage of the ACT heroin prescription trial proposal, August 1997. *Aust NZ J Public Health* 2000;**24**:254–64.

134 Blows S, Ivers RQ, Chapman S. "Banned from the streets I have paid to use": an analysis of Australian print media coverage of proposals for passenger and night driving restrictions for young drivers. *Inj Prev* 2005;**11**:304–8.

135 Durkin SJ, Germain D, Wakefield M. Adults' perceptions about whether tobacco companies tell the truth in relation to issues about smoking. *Tob Control* 2005; **14**:429–30.

136 Assunta M, Fields N, Knight J et al. "Care and feeding": the Asian environmental tobacco smoke consultants programme. *Tob Control* 2004;**13**(Suppl. 2):ii4–12.

137 Chapman S. "We are anxious to remain anonymous": the use of third party scientific and medical consultants by the Australian tobacco industry, 1969 to 1979. *Tob Control* 2003;**12**(Suppl. 3):iii31–37.

138 Drope J, Chapman S. Tobacco industry efforts at discrediting scientific knowledge of environmental tobacco smoke: a review of internal industry documents. *J Epidemiol Community Health* 2001;**55**:588–94.

139 Rupp JP, Billings DM, Covington & Burling. Asia ETS consultant status report. 14 Feb 1990. Philip Morris (http://legacy.library.ucsf.edu/tid/zzd58d00).

140 Witte K. The manipulative nature of health communication research: ethical issues and guidelines. *Am Behav Sci* 1994;**38**:285–93.

141 Chapman S. Unraveling gossamer with boxing gloves: problems in explaining the decline in smoking. *BMJ* 1993;**307**:429–32.

142 Chapman S. The news on smoking: newspaper coverage of smoking and health in Australia, 1987–88. *Am J Public Health* 1989;**79**:1419–21.

143 Borland R, Mullins R, Trotter L et al. Trends in environmental tobacco smoke restrictions in the home in Victoria, Australia. *Tob Control* 1999;**8**:266–71.

144 Chapman S, Borland R, Lal A. Has the ban on smoking in New South Wales restaurants worked?: a comparison of restaurants in Sydney and Melbourne. *Med J Aust* 2001;**174**:512–15.

145 Brackenridge RDC. *Medical Selection of Life Risks: a Comprehensive Guide to Life Expectancy for Underwriters and Clinicians.* London: The Nature Press, 1985.

146 Chapman S. Shared accommodation – non-smokers wanted! *Tob Control* 1992;**1**:248.

147 Chapman S, Wakefield MA, Durkin SJ. Smoking status of 132,176 people advertising on a dating website: are smokers more "desperate and dateless"? *Med J Aust* 2004;**181**:672–4.

148 Fichtenberg CM, Glantz SA. Effect of smoke-free workplaces on smoking behaviour: systematic review. *BMJ* 2002;**325**:188.

149 Chang JS, Selvin S, Metayer C et al. Parental smoking and the risk of childhood leukemia. *Am J Epidemiol* 2006;**163**:1091–100.

150 Hughes JR, Keely J, Naud S. Shape of the relapse curve and long-term abstinence among untreated smokers. *Addiction* 2004;**99**:29–38.

151 Hyland A, Li Q, Bauer JE et al. Predictors of cessation in a cohort of current and former smokers followed over 13 years. *Nicotine Tob Res* 2004;**6**(Suppl. 3):S363–9.

152 Chapman S. The limitations of econometric-analysis in cigarette advertising studies. *Br J Addict* 1989;**84**:1267–74.

153 Durrant R, Wakefield M, McLeod K et al. Tobacco in the news: an analysis of newspaper coverage of tobacco issues in Australia, 2001. *Tob Control* 2003;**12**(Suppl. 2):ii75–81.

154 Walsh RA, Tzelepis F, Paul CL et al. Environmental tobacco smoke in homes, motor vehicles and licensed premises: community attitudes and practices. *Aust NZ J Public Health* 2002;**26**:536–42.

155 Heironimus J. Impact of workplace restrictions on consumption and incidence. 21 Jan 1992. Philip Morris (http://legacy.library.ucsf.edu/tid/uue06e00).

156 National Cancer Institute. *Population Based Smoking Cessation: Proceedings of a Conference on What Works to Influence Cessation in the General Population.* Smoking and tobacco control monograph no. 12. Bethesda, MD: U.S. Dept of Health and Human Services Public Health Service, National Institutes of Health National Cancer Institute, 2000.

157 Samet JM, Burke TA. Turning science into junk: the tobacco industry and passive smoking. *Am J Public Health* 2001;**91**:1742–4.

158 Ong EK, Glantz SA. Tobacco industry efforts subverting International Agency for Research on Cancer's second-hand smoke study. *Lancet* 2000;**355**:1253–9.

159 Colley JR, Holland WW, Corkhill RT. Influence of passive smoking and parental phlegm on pneumonia and bronchitis in early childhood. *Lancet* 1974;**2**:1031–4.

160 Hirayama T. Non-smoking wives of heavy smokers have a higher risk of lung cancer: a study from Japan. *Br Med J (Clin Res Ed)* 1981;**282**:183–5.

161 Connolly GN, Wayne GD, Lymperis D et al. How cigarette additives are used to mask environmental tobacco smoke. *Tob Control* 2000;**9**:283–91.

162 National Health and Medical Research Council. *The Health Effects of Passive Smoking.* Canberra: NHMRC, 1986.

163 National Health and Medical Research Council. *The Health Effects of Passive Smoking: a Scientific Information Paper.* Canberra: NHMRC, 1997.

164 Woodward SD, Winstanley MH. Lung cancer and passive smoking at work: the Carroll case. *Med J Aust* 1990;**153**:682–4.

165 Francey N, Soulos G. *When Smoke Gets in Your Eyes – Nose, Throat, Lungs and Bloodstream.* Woolloomooloo, NSW: NSW Cancer Council, 2001.

166 Chapman S, Woodward S. Australian court decision on passive smoking upheld on appeal. *BMJ* 1993;**306**:120–2.

167 Chapman S, Woodward S. Australian court rules that passive smoking causes lung cancer, asthma attacks, and respiratory disease. *BMJ* 1991;**302**:943–5.

168 Walsh RA, Tzelepis F. Support for smoking restrictions in bars and gaming areas: review of Australian studies. *Aust NZ J Public Health* 2003;**27**:310–22.

169 Wainwright R. Club and pub staff want smoking banned at work. *Sydney Morning Herald* (Sydney, NSW) 7 May 2001:5.

170   Harper T, Martin J. Trojan horses: how the tobacco industry infiltrates the smoke-free debate in Australia. *Aust NZ J Public Health* 2002;**26**:572–3.

171   Cains T, Cannata S, Poulos R et al. Designated "no smoking" areas provide from partial to no protection from environmental tobacco smoke. *Tob Control* 2004; **13**:17–22.

172   Al-Delaimy W, Fraser T, Woodward A. Nicotine in hair of bar and restaurant workers. *NZ Med J* 2001;**114**:80–3.

173   Siegel M, Skeer M. Exposure to secondhand smoke and excess lung cancer mortality risk among workers in the "5 B's": bars, bowling alleys, billiard halls, betting establishments, and bingo parlours. *Tob Control* 2003;**12**:333–8.

174   Eisner MD, Smith AK, Blanc PD. Bartenders' respiratory health after establishment of smoke-free bars and taverns. *JAMA* 1998;**280**:1909–14.

175   Scollo M, Lal A, Hyland A et al. Review of the quality of studies on the economic effects of smoke-free policies on the hospitality industry. *Tob Control* 2003;**12**: 13–20.

176   Trotter L, Chapman S. "Conclusions about exposure to ETS and health that will be unhelpful to us": How the tobacco industry attempted to delay and discredit the 1997 Australian National Health and Medical Research Council report on passive smoking. *Tob Control* 2003;**12**(Suppl. 3):iii102–6.

177   Chapman S, Penman A. "Can't stop the boy": Philip Morris' use of Healthy Buildings International to prevent workplace smoking bans in Australia. *Tob Control* 2003;**12**(Suppl. 3):iii107–12.

178   Bero LA, Montini T, Bryan-Jones K et al. Science in regulatory policy making: case studies in the development of workplace smoking restrictions. *Tob Control* 2001;**10**:329–36.

179   Stewart BW, Semmler PC. Sharp v. Port Kembla RSL Club: establishing causation of laryngeal cancer by environmental tobacco smoke. *Med J Aust* 2002;**176**:113–16.

180   Eggleton G, Clayton Utz. Notes for presentation. 17 Jan 1994. Philip Morris (http://legacy.library.ucsf.edu/tid/chh29e00).

181   Dearlove JV, Bialous SA, Glantz SA. Tobacco industry manipulation of the hospitality industry to maintain smoking in public places. *Tob Control* 2002;**11**:94–104.

182   Magzamen S, Charlesworth A, Glantz SA. Print media coverage of California's smoke-free bar law. *Tob Control* 2001;**10**:154–60.

183   Bryan-Jones K, Chapman S. Political dynamics promoting the incremental regulation of secondhand smoke: a case study of New South Wales, Australia. *BMC Public Health* 2006;**6**:192.

184   Repace J. *An Air Quality Survey of Respirable Particles and Particulate Carcinogens in Delaware Hospitality Venues Before and After a Smoking Ban.* Bowie, MD: Repace Associates, 2003.

185   Jacobson P, Zapawa LM. Clean indoor air restrictions: progress and promise. In: Rabin RL, Sugarman SD (eds) *Regulating Tobacco.* Melbourne: Oxford University Press, 2001:207–44.

186   Balbach ED, Traynor MP, Glantz SA. The implementation of California's tobacco tax initiative: the critical role of outsider strategies in protecting Proposition 99. *J Health Polit Policy Law* 2000;**25**:689–715.

187   Givel M, Glantz S. Failure to defend a successful state tobacco control program: policy lessons from Florida. *Am J Public Health* 2000;**90**:762–67.

188   Jacobson PD, Wasserman J, Raube K. *The Political Evolution of Anti-smoking Legislation.* Santa Monica, CA: RAND, 1992.

189 Nielsen LB. American tobacco policy in the 20th century: the importance of attention, mobilization, and causal stories. Paper presented at The Annual Meeting of The Midwest Political Science Association, Palmer House Hilton, Chicago, IL, April 3–6, 2003.

190 Australian Hotels Association. Urgent alert to hoteliers and their patrons. 9 Sep 2004 (http://tobacco.health.usyd.edu.au/site/supersite/resources/pdfs/AHAletter.pdf).

191 Lund M. *Smoke-free Bars and Restaurants in Norway.* Oslo: National Institute for Drug and Alcohol Research (SIRUS), 2005 (http://www.globalink.org/documents/2005smokefreebarsandrestaurantsinNorway.pdf).

192 New Zealand Ministry of Health. The smoke is clearing: anniversary report 2005: initial data on the impact of the smoke-free environments law change since 10 December 2004. Wellington: Ministry of Health, 2005 (http://tobacco.health.usyd.edu.au/site/supersite/resources/pdfs/NZ_SmokeClearing.pdf).

193 New York City Department of Finance, New York City Department of Health & Mental Hygiene, New York City Department of Small Business Services, et al. *The State of Smoke-free New York City: a one year review.* Mar 2004 (http://tobacco.health.usyd.edu.au/site/supersite/resources/pdfs/SmokeFreeCityReportFinal328.pdf).

194 Kingdon JW. *Agendas, Alternatives, and Public Policies.* Boston: Little, Brown, & Co, 1984.

195 Stone DA. *Policy Paradox: the Art of Political Decision Making.* New York: Norton, 1997.

196 Studlar DT. *Tobacco Control: Comparative Politics in the United States and Canada.* Ontario: Broadview Press, 2002.

197 Arnold RD. *The Logic of Congressional Action.* New Haven, CT: Yale University Press, 1990.

198 Oliver R, Paul-Shaheen P. Translating ideas into actions: entrepreneurial leadership in state health care reforms. *J Health Polit Policy Law* 1997;**22**:721–88.

199 Chapman S. Pub smoking in Australia: 20 years of fiddling and burning. Part 1. *Online Opinion* 21 Feb 2005 (http://www.onlineopinion.com.au/view.asp?article=3062).

200 Chapman S. Pub smoking in Australia: 20 years of fiddling and burning. Part 2. *Online Opinion* 22 Feb 2005 (http://www.onlineopinion.com.au/view.asp?article=3064).

201 Glantz SA, Balbach ED. *Tobacco War: Inside the California Battles.* Berkeley: University of California Press, 2000.

202 Muggli ME, Hurt RD, Blanke DD. Science for hire: a tobacco industry strategy to influence public opinion on secondhand smoke. *Nicotine Tob Res* 2003;**5**:303–14.

203 Philip Morris Asia Region. Corporate Affairs review. 1997. Philip Morris (http://legacy.library.ucsf.edu/tid/ojk45c00).

204 Ebrahim S, Smith GD. Systematic review of randomised controlled trials of multiple risk factor interventions for preventing coronary heart disease. *BMJ* 1997;**314**:1666–74.

205 Lando HA, Pechacek TF, Pirie PL et al. Changes in adult cigarette smoking in the Minnesota Heart Health Program. *Am J Public Health* 1995;**85**:201–8.

206 Community intervention trial for smoking cessation (COMMIT): II. Changes in adult cigarette smoking prevalence. *Am J Public Health* 1995;**85**:193–200.

207 Community Intervention Trial for Smoking Cessation (COMMIT): I. Cohort results from a four-year community intervention. *Am J Public Health* 1995;**85**:183–92.

208 Ebrahim S, Smith GD. Effects of government policies on health behaviour must be studied. *BMJ* 1998;**317**:886.

209   Wakefield MA, Chaloupka FJ. Improving the measurement and use of tobacco control "inputs". *Tob Control* 1998;**7**:333–5.

210   Brodie M, Hamel EC, Altman DE et al. Health news and the American public, 1996–2002. *J Health Polit Policy Law* 2003;**28**:927–50.

211   Box Office Guru (http://www.boxofficeguru.com).

212   Davis R. Doling out soundbites in the presidential campaign. *Tob Control* 1996; **5**:317–19.

213   Menashe CL, Siegel M. The power of a frame: an analysis of newspaper coverage of tobacco issues – United States, 1985–1996. *J Health Commun* 1998;**3**:307–25.

214   Lupton D. Medical and health stories on the Sydney Morning Herald's front page. *Aust J Public Health* 1995;**19**:501–8.

215   Shiffman S, Sweeney CT, Ertischek MD et al. Tobacco cessation and weight loss: trends in media coverage. *Am J Health Behav* 2006;**30**:363–74.

216   Potter J, Wetherell M, Chitty A. Quantification rhetoric: cancer on television. *Discourse Soc* 1991;**2**:333–65.

217   Chapman S, Leask JA. Paid celebrity endorsement in health promotion: a case study from Australia. *Health Promot Int* 2001;**16**:333–38.

218   Chapman S. Lots of huff over Russell's puff. *The Australian* 25 Jul 2002:12.

219   Chapman S. Do as I say, not as I do: how famous faces muddle the message on cancer [opinion]. *Sydney Morning Herald* 3 Nov 2003:13.

220   Christofides N, Chapman S, Dominello A. The new pariahs: discourse on the tobacco industry in the Sydney press, 1993–97. *Aust NZ J Public Health* 1999;**23**:233–9.

221   Wallace C. Free drugs trade: say no. *The Australian* 31 Oct 2003:11.

222   Pryer W, Amalfi C. Gas heater firms 'like tobacco companies'. *West Australian* 25 Jun 2004.

223   Warner KE. The effects of the anti-smoking campaign on cigarette consumption. *Am J Public Health* 1977;**67**:645–50.

224   Reid DJ, Killoran AJ, McNeill AD et al. Choosing the most effective health promotion options for reducing a nation's smoking prevalence. *Tob Control* 1992;**1**: 185–97.

225   Pierce JP, Gilpin EA. News media coverage of smoking and health is associated with changes in population rates of smoking cessation but not initiation. *Tob Control* 2001;**10**:145–53.

226   Laugesen M, Meads C. Advertising, price, income and publicity effects on weekly cigarette sales in New Zealand supermarkets. *Br J Addict* 1991;**86**:83–9.

227   Cummings KM, Sciandra R, Markello S. Impact of a newspaper mediated quit smoking program. *Am J Public Health* 1987;**77**:1452–3.

228   McCombs M, Ghanem S. The convergence of agenda setting and framing. In: Reese SD, Gandy OH, Grant AE (eds) *Framing Public Life: Perspectives on Media and our Understanding of the Social World*. Mahwah, NJ: Lawrence Erlbaum Associates, 2003.

229   Tuchman G. *Making News: a Study in the Construction of Reality*. New York: Free Press, 1978.

230   Malone R, Boyd E, Bero L. Science in the news: journalists' construction of passive smoking as a social problem. *Soc Stud Sci* 2000;**30**:1–23.

231   Iyengar S. *Is Anyone Responsible?: How Television Frames Political Issues*. Chicago: University of Chicago Press, 1991.

232   Morley D. *Television, Audiences, and Cultural Studies*. London: Routledge, 1992.

233   Bell A. *The Language of News in the Media*. London: Basil Blackwell, 1991.

234 Sandefur T, Brown & Williamson. Hearing of the Health and Environment Subcommittee of the House Energy and Commerce Committee Tobacco Products. 23 Jun 1994. Lorillard (http://legacy.library.ucsf.edu/tid/tum60e00).

235 Entman RM. Framing: toward clarification of a fractured paradigm. *J Commun* 1993;**43**:51–8.

236 Kennedy GE, Bero LA. Print media coverage of research on passive smoking. *Tob Control* 1999;**8**:254–60.

237 Lima JC, Siegel M. The tobacco settlement: an analysis of newspaper coverage of a national policy debate, 1997–98. *Tob Control* 1999;**8**:247–53.

238 Ott W, Switzer P, Robinson J. Particle concentrations inside a tavern before and after prohibition of smoking: evaluating the performance of an indoor air quality model. *J Air Waste Manage* 1996;**46**:1120–34.

239 Ji BT, Shu XO, Linet MS et al. Paternal cigarette smoking and the risk of childhood cancer among offspring of nonsmoking mothers. *J Natl Cancer Inst* 1997;**89**:238–44.

240 Rodriguez C, Tatham LM, Thun MJ et al. Smoking and fatal prostate cancer in a large cohort of adult men. *Am J Epidemiol* 1997;**145**:466–75.

241 Brewer MS, Sprouls GK, Russon C. Consumer attitudes toward food safety issues. *J Food Safety* 1994;**14**:63–76.

242 Resurreccion AVA, Galvez FCF, Fletcher SM et al. Consumer attitudes toward irradiated food: results of a new study. *J Food Prot* 1995;**58**:193–6.

243 Sandman PM. Hazard versus outrage in the public perception of risk. In: Covello VT, McCallum DB, Pavlova MT (eds) *Effective Risk Communication*. New York: Plenum Press, 1989:45–9.

244 California Environmental Protection Agency Office of Environmental Health Hazard Assessment. *Environmental Tobacco Smoke: Health Effects of Exposure to Environmental Smoke: Final Draft for Scientific, Public and SRP Review: Feb 1997.* Sacramento, CA: California EPA, 1997.

245 Jamrozik K, Chapman S, Woodward A. How the NHMRC got its fingers burnt. *Med J Aust* 1997;**167**:372–4.

246 Mindell J. An assessment of the feasibility of health authorities generating unpaid mass media publicity in the long term. *Health Educ J* 1997;**56**:125–33.

247 Gascoigne T, Metcalfe J. Incentives and impediments to scientists communicating through the media. *Sci Commun* 1997;**18**:265–82.

248 Entwistle V. Reporting research in medical journals and newspapers. *BMJ* 1995;**310**:920–3.

249 Cornwall J. *Just for the Record: the Political Recollections of John Cornwall.* Kent Town, S. Aust: Wakefield Press, 1989.

250 Chapman S, Reynolds C. Regulating tobacco – the South Australian Tobacco Products Control Act, 1986: its development and passage through Parliament. *Community Health Stud* 1987;**11**:9s–15s.

251 Connolly GN, Winn DM, Hecht SS et al. The reemergence of smokeless tobacco. *N Engl J Med* 1986;**314**:1020–7.

252 Sachdev P, Chapman S. Availability of smokeless tobacco products in South Asian grocery shops in Sydney, 2004. *Med J Aust* 2005;**183**:334.

253 Winstanley M, Woodward S, Walker N. Smokeless tobacco: Legislative controls. In: *Tobacco in Australia: Facts and Issues 1995*, 2nd edn. Carlton South, Vic: Victorian Smoking and Health Program (Quit Victoria), 1995:chap. 9.4 (http://www.quit.org.au/quit/FandI/fandi/c09s4.htm).

254 Fagerstrom KO, Schildt EB. Should the European Union lift the ban on snus?: evidence from the Swedish experience. *Addiction* 2003;**98**:1191–5.

255 European Parliament and Council. Directive 2001/37/EC of the European Parliament and of the Council of 5 June 2001 on the approximation of the laws, regulations and administrative provisions of the Member States concerning the manufacture, presentation and sale of tobacco products. *Official Journal of the European Union: Legislation* 2001;**L194** (Vol. 44):26–35.

256 Wodak A. Harm reduction: Australia as a case study. *Bull NY Acad Med* 1995;**72**: 339–47.

257 Elliott AJ, Chapman S. 'Heroin hell their own making': construction of heroin users in the Australian press 1992–97. *Drug Alcohol Rev* 2000;**19**:191–201.

258 Stratton K, Shetty P, Wallace R et al. *Clearing the Smoke: Assessing the Science Base for Tobacco Harm Reduction*. Washington, DC: National Academy Press, 2001.

259 Levy DT, Mumford EA, Cummings KM et al. The relative risks of a low-nitrosamine smokeless tobacco product compared with smoking cigarettes: estimates of a panel of experts. *Cancer Epidemiol Biomarkers Prev* 2004;**13**:2035–42.

260 Henningfield JE, Fagerstrom KO. Swedish Match Company, Swedish snus and public health: a harm reduction experiment in progress? *Tob Control* 2001;**10**:253–7.

261 McDaniel PA, Smith EA, Malone RE. Philip Morris's Project Sunrise: weakening tobacco control by working with it. *Tob Control* 2006;**15**:215–23.

262 Henningfield JE, Rose CA, Giovino GA. Brave new world of tobacco disease prevention: promoting dual tobacco-product use? *Am J Prev Med* 2002;**23**:226–8.

263 Martin EG, Warner KE, Lantz PM. Tobacco harm reduction: what do the experts think? *Tob Control* 2004;**13**:123–8.

264 Nordgren P, Ramstrom L. Moist snuff in Sweden: tradition and evolution. *Br J Addict* 1990;**85**:1107–12.

265 Foulds J, Ramstrom L, Burke M et al. Effect of smokeless tobacco (snus) on smoking and public health in Sweden. *Tob Control* 2003;**12**:349–59.

266 Ramstrom LM, Foulds J. Role of snus in initiation and cessation of tobacco smoking in Sweden. *Tob Control* 2006;**15**:210–14.

267 Food and Drug Administration et al. v. Brown and Williamson Tobacco Corporation et al., no. 98-1152, 529 U.S. 120 (March 21, 2000).

268 Philip Morris International Management SA. Our business environment: supporting effective legislation. 2006 (http://www.philipmorrisinternational.com/PMINTL/pages/eng/busenv/Bus_environment.asp).

269 Kessler D. The control and manipulation of nicotine in cigarettes. *Tob Control* 1994;**3**:362–9.

270 DiFranza JR, Savageau JA, Rigotti NA et al. Development of symptoms of tobacco dependence in youths: 30 month follow up data from the DANDY study. *Tob Control* 2002;**11**:228–35.

271 Wayne GF, Connolly GN. How cigarette design can affect youth initiation into smoking: Camel cigarettes 1983–93. *Tob Control* 2002;**11**(Suppl. 1):i32–9.

272 Sutton CD, Robinson RG. The marketing of menthol cigarettes in the United States: populations, messages, and channels. *Nicotine Tob Res* 2004;**6**(Suppl. 1):S83–91.

273 Collins CC, Moolchan ET. Shorter time to first cigarette of the day in menthol adolescent cigarette smokers. *Addict Behav* 2005;**8**:1460–4.

274 Garten S, Falkner RV. Role of mentholated cigarettes in increased nicotine dependence and greater risk of tobacco-attributable disease. *Prev Med* 2004;**38**: 793–8.

275   Henningfield JE, Benowitz NL, Ahijevych K et al. Does menthol enhance the addictiveness of cigarettes?: an agenda for research. *Nicotine Tob Res* 2003;**5**:9–11.

276   Bates C, Jarvis MJ, Connolly G. *Tobacco Additives: Cigarette Engineering and Nicotine Addiction.* London: Action on Smoking and Health, UK, 1999 (http://www.ash.org.uk/html/regulation/html/additives.html#_Toc5014).

277   IARC Working Group on the Evaluation of Carcinogenic Risk to Humans. *Tobacco Smoke and Involuntary Smoking.* IARC monographs on the evaluation of carcinogenic risks to humans, no. 83. Lyon, France: International Agency for Research on Cancer, 2004:84.

278   Henningfield J, Pankow J, Garrett B. Ammonia and other chemical base tobacco additives and cigarette nicotine delivery: issues and research needs. *Nicotine Tob Res* 2004;**6**:199–205.

279   Laugesen M, Duncanson M, Fraser T et al. Hand rolling cigarette papers as the reference point for regulating cigarette fire safety. *Tob Control* 2003;**12**:406–10.

280   Bialous SA, Yach D. Whose standard is it, anyway?: how the tobacco industry determines the International Organization for Standardization (ISO) standards for tobacco and tobacco products. *Tob Control* 2001;**10**:96–104.

281   Kozlowski LT, O'Connor RJ, Sweeney CT. Cigarette design. In: *Risks Associated with Smoking Cigarettes with Low Machine-measured Yields of Tar and Nicotine.* Smoking and Tobacco Control Monograph, no. 13. Bethesda, MD: US Department of Health and Human Services, National Institutes of Health, National Cancer Institute, 2001:13–37.

282   Dunn WL, Johnstone ME. Market potential of a health cigarette. Jun 1966. Philip Morris (http://legacy.library.ucsf.edu/tid/bdw67e00).

283   Fields N, Chapman S. Chasing Ernst L Wynder: 40 years of Philip Morris' efforts to influence a leading scientist. *J Epidemiol Community Health* 2003;**57**:571–8.

284   Wynder EL, American Association of Cancer Research. Text taken from IBM recorder and preprint studies in tobacco carcinogenesis. 11 Apr 1964. Philip Morris (http://legacy.library.ucsf.edu/tid/ejg12a00).

285   Wynder EL, Hoffmann D. Reduction of tumorigenicity of cigarette smoke: an experimental approach. *JAMA* 1965;**192**:88–94.

286   Parascandola M. Lessons from the history of tobacco harm reduction: the National Cancer Institute's Smoking and Health Program and the "less hazardous cigarette". *Nicotine Tob Res* 2005;**7**:779–89.

287   Russell MA. The nicotine addiction trap: a 40-year sentence for four cigarettes. *Br J Addict* 1990;**85**:293–300.

288   Sheehy P. [Note to Mr Crawford regarding cigarette improvement]. 18 Dec 1986. British American Tobacco (http://bat.library.ucsf.edu/tid/pxb01a99).

289   Pollay RW, Dewhirst T. The dark side of marketing seemingly "Light" cigarettes: successful images and failed fact. *Tob Control* 2002;**11**(Suppl. 1):i18–31.

290   Tcheng J. Merit advertising brief. 27 Jul 1987. Philip Morris (http://legacy.library.ucsf.edu/tid/ikx32e00).

291   British American Tobacco Company Limited. Conference on Marketing Low Delivery Products January 1982: Marketing news supplement. Apr 1982. Brown & Williamson (http://legacy.library.ucsf.edu/tid/urf14f00).

292   King B, Borland R. What was "light" and "mild" is now "smooth" and "fine": new labelling of Australian cigarettes. *Tob Control* 2005;**14**:214–15.

293   Peeler CE. Cigarette testing and the Federal Trade Commission: a historical overview. In: *The FTC Cigarette Test Method for Determining Tar, Nicotine, and Carbon*

Monoxide Yields of US Cigarettes. Smoking and Tobacco Control Monograph 7; NIH Publication No. 96-4028. Bethesda, MD: US Department of Health and Human Services, Public Health Service, National Institutes of Health, 1996:1–8.

294 Kozlowski LT, O'Connor RJ. Cigarette filter ventilation is a defective design because of misleading taste, bigger puffs, and blocked vents. *Tob Control* 2002; **11**(Suppl. 1):i40–50.

295 Isaac PF, Rand MJ. Cigarette smoking and plasma levels of nicotine. *Nature* 1972;**236**:308–10.

296 Shemer I. Cigarette smoking and plasma levels of nicotine: Nature, April 7, 1972. 14 Apr 1972. Philip Morris (http://legacy.library.ucsf.edu/tid/wma48e00).

297 Goodman BL, Meyer LF. Summary of human smoker simulator program. 19 Aug 1977. Philip Morris (http://legacy.library.ucsf.edu/tid/boq08e00).

298 Wickham JE. Saratoga 120 and Plus 120 cigarettes – Australia. 30 Oct 1975. Philip Morris (http://legacy.library.ucsf.edu/tid/ssx54e00).

299 Balint LE. Philip Morris Limited (Australia) C.I. report no. 38. May 1980. Philip Morris (http://legacy.library.ucsf.edu/tid/kgo06e00).

300 Ruff R. Philip Morris Limited (Australia) C.I. report no. 84. Jun 1994. Philip Morris (http://legacy.library.ucsf.edu/tid/vcp96e00).

301 Evans G, Johnson G, Frizzell M. A study of the smoke yield of vented filter cigarettes. Australian Government Analytical Laboratories (unpublished MS), 1993.

302 Foster AA. Synopsis of A.A. Foster's trip report: U.S.A., U.K., Switzerland, Nov. 1st–30th, 1974. 13 Feb 1975. Philip Morris (http://legacy.library.ucsf.edu/tid/gpl98e00).

303 *Final Report on the Work of ISO/TC 126/WG 9 Smoking Methods for Cigarettes*. 14 March 2006.

304 Chapman S, Heidemann A, Woodward S. Were asbestos-filtered Kent cigarettes sold in Australia? *Aust NZ J Public Health* 1996;**20**:218–19.

305 Longo WE, Rigler MW, Slade J. Crocidolite asbestos fibers in smoke from original Kent cigarettes. *Cancer Res* 1995;**55**:2232–5.

306 Celanese Corporation. Cytrel smoking products: [press release]. 28 Mar 1974. British American Tobacco (http://www.healthservices.gov.bc.ca/guildford/pdf/112/00011362.pdf).

307 Thun MJ, Burns DM. Health impact of "reduced yield" cigarettes: a critical assessment of the epidemiological evidence. *Tob Control* 2001;**10**(Suppl. 1):i4–11.

308 Slade J. The tobacco epidemic: lessons from history. *J Psychoactive Drugs* 1989; **21**:281–91.

309 Slade J, Connolly GN, Lymperis D. Eclipse: does it live up to its health claims? *Tob Control* 2002;**11**(Suppl. 2):ii64–70.

310 Foy JW, Bombick BR, Bombick DW et al. A comparison of in vitro toxicities of cigarette smoke condensate from Eclipse cigarettes and four commercially available ultra low-"tar" cigarettes. *Food Chem Toxicol* 2004;**42**:237–43.

311 Pauly JL, Lee HJ, Hurley EL et al. Glass fiber contamination of cigarette filters: an additional health risk to the smoker? *Cancer Epidemiol Biomarkers Prev* 1998;**7**:967–79.

312 Fagerstrom KO, Hughes JR, Rasmussen T et al. Randomised trial investigating effect of a novel nicotine delivery device (Eclipse) and a nicotine oral inhaler on smoking behaviour, nicotine and carbon monoxide exposure, and motivation to quit. *Tob Control* 2000;**9**:327–33.

313 Fagerstrom KO, Hughes JR, Callas PW. Long-term effects of the Eclipse cigarette substitute and the nicotine inhaler in smokers not interested in quitting. *Nicotine Tob Res* 2002;**4**(Suppl. 2):S141–5.

314   Lee EM, Malson JL, Moolchan ET et al. Quantitative comparisons between a nicotine delivery device (Eclipse) and conventional cigarette smoking. *Nicotine Tob Res* 2004;**6**:95–102.

315   Breland AB, Acosta MC, Eissenberg T. Tobacco specific nitrosamines and potential reduced exposure products for smokers: a preliminary evaluation of Advance. *Tob Control* 2003;**12**:317–21.

316   Shiffman S, Pillitteri JL, Burton SL et al. Smoker and ex-smoker reactions to cigarettes claiming reduced risk. *Tob Control* 2004;**13**:78–84.

317   O'Connor RJ, Hyland A, Giovino GA et al. Smoker awareness of and beliefs about supposedly less-harmful tobacco products. *Am J Prev Med* 2005;**29**:85–90.

318   United Kingdom Parliament. *Select Committee on Health Minutes of Evidence: Memorandum by Gallaher Group Plc: the tobacco industry and the health risks of smoking (TB 8)*. 2000 (http://www.publications.parliament.uk/pa/cm199900/cmselect/cmhealth/27/0011319.htm).

319   Caraballo RS, Pederson LL, Gupta N. New tobacco products: do smokers like them? *Tob Control* 2006;**15**:39–44.

320   Associated Press. Reynolds American Completes Conwood deal: Reynolds American acquires Conwood for $3.5 billion in notes, loans and cash. 2006 (http://biz.yahoo.com/ap/060531/reynolds_american_acquisition.html?.v).

321   Gray N. Reflections on the saga of tar content: why did we measure the wrong thing? *Tob Control* 2000;**9**:90–4.

322   Swedish Match North Europe AB. *Swedish Gothiatek Snus* (http://www.gothiatek.com/templates/index.aspx?page_id=24).

323   Commonwealth of Massachusetts Executive Office of Health and Human Services Department of Public Health. MDPH issues challenge to U.S. snuff makers and warns consumers of high cancer risk tied to smokeless tobacco, 21 August. 2001 (http://www.mass.gov/dph/media/2001/pr0821a.htm).

324   Norwegian Directorate for Health and Social Affairs. Bruk av snus i 2005. 2006 (http://www.shdir.no/tobakk/statistikk/bruk_av_snus_/bruk_av_snus_i_2005_38008).

325   Rosen M, Alfredsson L, Hammar N et al. Attack rate, mortality and case fatality for acute myocardial infarction in Sweden during 1987–95: results from the national AMI register in Sweden. *J Intern Med* 2000;**248**:159–64.

326   Critchley JA, Unal B. Health effects associated with smokeless tobacco: a systematic review. *Thorax* 2003;**58**:435–43.

327   Royal College of Physicians of London. *Protecting Smokers, Saving Lives: the Case for a Tobacco and Nicotine Regulatory Agency*. Salisbury: Sarum Colorview Group, 2002.

328   Bates C, Fagerstrom K, Jarvis MJ et al. European Union policy on smokeless tobacco: a statement in favour of evidence based regulation for public health. *Tob Control* 2003;**12**:360–7.

329   Boffetta P, Aagnes B, Weiderpass E et al. Response to comments by Drs. Rutqvist, Lewin, Nilsson, Ramstrom, Rodu and Cole further to the publication of the manuscript "smokeless tobacco use and risk of cancer of the pancreas and other organs". *Int J Cancer* 2006;**118**:1586–7.

330   Boffetta P, Aagnes B, Weiderpass E et al. Smokeless tobacco use and risk of cancer of the pancreas and other organs. *Int J Cancer* 2005;**114**:992–5.

331   Machado F, Rodriguez JR, Leon JP et al. Tamoxifen and endometrial cancer. Is screening necessary?: a review of the literature. *Eur J Gynaecol Oncol* 2005; **26**:257–65.

332   Benowitz NL, Gourlay SG. Cardiovascular toxicity of nicotine: implications for nicotine replacement therapy. *J Am Coll Cardiol* 1997;**29**:1422–31.

333   Cummings KM, Hyland A, Giovino GA et al. Are smokers adequately informed about the health risks of smoking and medicinal nicotine? *Nicotine Tob Res* 2004;**6**(Suppl. 3):S333–40.

334   Dasgupta P, Rastogi S, Pillai S et al. Nicotine induces cell proliferation by beta-arrestin-mediated activation of Src and Rb-Raf-1 pathways. *J Clin Invest* 2006;**116**:2208–17.

335   Heeschen C, Jang JJ, Weis M et al. Nicotine stimulates angiogenesis and promotes tumor growth and atherosclerosis. *Nat Med* 2001;**7**:833–9.

336   Heeschen C, Weis M, Cooke JP. Nicotine promotes arteriogenesis. *J Am Coll Cardiol* 2003;**41**:489–96.

337   West KA, Brognard J, Clark AS et al. Rapid Akt activation by nicotine and a tobacco carcinogen modulates the phenotype of normal human airway epithelial cells. *J Clin Invest* 2003;**111**:81–90.

338   Hatsukami DK, Giovino GA, Eissenberg T et al. Methods to assess potential reduced exposure products. *Nicotine Tob Res* 2005;**7**:827–44.

339   WHO Study Group on Tobacco Product Regulation. *Report on Threshold Limits for Toxic Constituents in Cigarette Smoke*. Geneva: World Health Organization, 2006.

340   O'Connor RJ, Kozlowski LT, Flaherty BP et al. Most smokeless tobacco use does not cause cigarette smoking: results from the 2000 National Household Survey on Drug Abuse. *Addict Behav* 2005;**30**:325–36.

341   O'Connor RJ, Flaherty BP, Quinio Edwards B et al. Regular smokeless tobacco use is not a reliable predictor of smoking onset when psychosocial predictors are included in the model. *Nicotine Tob Res* 2003;**5**:535–43.

342   Kozlowski LT, O'Connor RJ, Edwards BQ et al. Most smokeless tobacco use is not a causal gateway to cigarettes: using order of product use to evaluate causation in a national US sample. *Addiction* 2003;**98**:1077–85.

343   Hall WD, Lynskey M. Is cannabis a gateway drug?: testing hypotheses about the relationship between cannabis use and the use of other illicit drugs. *Drug Alcohol Rev* 2005;**24**:39–48.

344   Kozlowski LT, O'Connor RJ, Edwards BQ. Some practical points on harm reduction: what to tell your lawmaker and what to tell your brother about Swedish snus. *Tob Control* 2003;**12**:372–3.

345   Kozlowski LT, O'Connor RJ. Apply federal research rules on deception to misleading health information: an example on smokeless tobacco and cigarettes. *Public Health Rep* 2003;**118**:187–92.

346   Bayer R, Gostin LO, Javitt GH et al. Tobacco advertising in the United States: a proposal for a constitutionally acceptable form of regulation. *JAMA* 2002;**287**:2990–5.

347   World Health Organization. *WHO Framework Convention on Tobacco Control*. Geneva: WHO, 2005 (http://www.who.int/tobacco/framework/WHO_FCTC_english.pdf).

348   Bryan Cave [Attorneys to United States Tobacco]. Response to Advisory Opinion regarding the acceptability of communicating in advertising that smokeless tobacco are considered to be a significantly reduced risk alternative as compared to cigarette smoking. Submission to Hon DS Clark, Secretary Federal Trade Commission, Washington DC, 2002 Feb 2.

349   Davies D. The politics of harm reduction: a perspective on public policy approaches to a controversial industry and product. Philip Morris International.

2005 (http://www.philipmorrisinternational.com/PMINTL/pages/eng/press/speeches/DDavies_20050323.asp).

350   Doran CM, Shakeshaft AP, Gates JA et al. Current prescribing patterns of bupropion in Australia. *Med J Aust* 2002;**177**:162.

351   Gertner J. Incendiary device. *New York Times Magazine* 12 Jun 2005.

352   Tindle HA, Rigotti NA, Davis RB et al. Cessation among smokers who used "light" cigarettes: results from the 2000 National Health Interview Survey. *Am J Public Health* 2006;**96**:1498–504.

353   British American Tobacco. About smokeless snus. 2006 (http://www.bat.com/oneweb/sites/uk__3mnfen.nsf/vwPagesWebLive/DO6CKJNP?opendocument&SID=&DTC=&TMP=1).

354   Morgan Stanley Research. UST: further from the precipice, but still significant L-T issues. 19 Sep 2006.

355   US Federal Trade Commission. Smokeless tobacco report for the years 2000 and 2001. Washington, DC: FTC, 2003 (http://www.ftc.gov/os/2003/08/2k2k1smokeless.pdf).

356   Mumford EA, Levy DT, Gitchell JG et al. Smokeless tobacco use 1992–2002: trends and measurement in the Current Population Survey–Tobacco Use Supplements. *Tob Control* 2006;**15**:166–71.

357   Alcabes P. Blowing smoke about tobacco. *Washington Post* 30 May 2006 (http://www.washingtonpost.com/wp–dyn/content/article/2006/05/29/AR2006052900734.html?referrer=emailarticle).

358   Dagens Industri (Sweden). 2004, May 19.

359   Gupta PC, Ray CS. Smokeless tobacco and health in India and South Asia. *Respirology* 2003;**8**:419–31.

360   Idris AM, Ahmed HM, Mukhtar BI et al. Descriptive epidemiology of oral neoplasms in Sudan 1970–1985 and the role of toombak. *Int J Cancer* 1995;**61**:155–8.

361   Ayo-Yusuf OA, Swart TJ, Pickworth WB. Nicotine delivery capabilities of smokeless tobacco products and implications for control of tobacco dependence in South Africa. *Tob Control* 2004;**13**:186–9.

362   Gray N, Henningfield JE, Benowitz NL et al. Toward a comprehensive long term nicotine policy. *Tob Control* 2005;**14**:161–5.

363   Silagy C, Lancaster T, Stead L et al. Nicotine replacement therapy for smoking cessation. *The Cochrane Database of Systematic Reviews* 2006, issue 2 (http://www.cochrane.org/reviews/en/ab000146.html).

364   Baillie AJ, Mattick RP, Hall W. Quitting smoking: estimation by meta-analysis of the rate of unaided smoking cessation. *Aust J Public Health* 1995;**19**:129–31.

365   Miller FG, Rosenstein DL. The nature and power of the placebo effect. *J Clin Epidemiol* 2006;**59**:331–5.

366   Shiffman S, Ferguson SG, Gwaltney CJ et al. Reduction of abstinence-induced withdrawal and craving using high-dose nicotine replacement therapy. *Psychopharmacology (Berl)* 2006;**184**:637–44.

367   Niaura R, Sayette M, Shiffman S et al. Comparative efficacy of rapid-release nicotine gum versus nicotine polacrilex gum in relieving smoking cue-provoked craving. *Addiction* 2005;**100**:1720–30.

368   Dale LC, Hurt RD, Offord KP et al. High-dose nicotine patch therapy: percentage of replacement and smoking cessation. *JAMA* 1995;**274**:1353–8.

369   Shamasunder B, Bero L. Financial ties and conflicts of interest between pharmaceutical and tobacco companies. *JAMA* 2002;**288**:738–44.

370 SmokeFree New Zealand (http://www.smokefree.co.nz).

371 Science and Environmental Health Network. Wingspread Conference on the Precautionary Principle, 26 January 1998 (http://www.sehn.org/wing.html).

372 Gee D, Krayer von Krauss MP. Late lessons from early warnings: towards precaution and realism in research and policy. *Water Sci Technol* 2005;**52**:25–34.

373 National Health and Medical Research Council. *Report of the 92nd Session.* Canberra: NHMRC, 1981:18.

374 Fink W, Moser F, Speck M. Agricultural chemicals, 25 January to 20 February 1978. Feb 1978. Philip Morris (http://legacy.library.ucsf.edu/tid/fvm23e00).

375 Counts ME, Hsu FS, Laffoon SW et al. Mainstream smoke constituent yields and predicting relationships from a worldwide market sample of cigarette brands: ISO smoking conditions. *Regul Toxicol Pharmacol* 2004;**39**:111–34.

376 Gray N, Zaridze D, Robertson C et al. Variation within global cigarette brands in tar, nicotine, and certain nitrosamines: analytic study. *Tob Control* 2000;**9**:351.

377 Fischer S, Spiegelhalder B, Preussmann R. Tobacco-specific nitrosamines in commercial cigarettes: possibilities for reducing exposure. *IARC Sci Publ* 1991;**105**: 489–92.

378 Fischer S, Spiegelhalder B, Preussmann R. Tobacco-specific nitrosamines in European and USA cigarettes. *Arch Geschwulstforsch* 1990;**60**:169–77.

379 Fischer S, Castonguay A, Kaiserman M et al. Tobacco-specific nitrosamines in Canadian cigarettes. *J Cancer Res Clin Oncol* 1990;**116**:563–8.

380 Fischer S, Spiegelhalder B, Preussmann R. Tobacco-specific nitrosamines in mainstream smoke of West German cigarettes: tar alone is not a sufficient index for the carcinogenic potential of cigarette smoke. *Carcinogenesis* 1989;**10**:169–73.

381 Hoffmann D, Hoffmann I. The changing cigarette: chemical studies and bioassays. In: *Risks Associated with Smoking Cigarettes with Low Machine-measured Yields of Tar and Nicotine.* Smoking and Tobacco Control Monograph 13. Bethesda, MD: US Department of Health and Human Services, National Institutes of Health, National Cancer Institute, 2001:159–91.

382 Kaiserman MJ. *The Canadian Benchmark: Myths and Realities.* Ottawa: Health Canada, 2003.

383 Hecht SS. Biochemistry, biology, and carcinogenicity of tobacco-specific N-nitrosamines. *Chem Res Toxicol* 1998;**11**:559–603.

384 World Health Organization TobReg Committee. *Report on Threshold Limits for Toxic Constituents in Cigarette Smoke.* Geneva: WHO, 2006.

385 King B, Borland R, Fowles J. Mainstream smoke emissions of Australian and Canadian cigarettes. *Nicotine Tob Res* (in press).

386 Collishaw N. *Tales of Toxic Tobacco: BAT Research on the Harmful Properties of Smoke.* Physicians for a Smoke-Free Canada, 2000 (http://www.smoke-free.ca/pdf_1/documentresearchpdf/toxictobacco.pdf).

387 Teo KK, Ounpuu S, Hawken S et al. Tobacco use and risk of myocardial infarction in 52 countries in the INTERHEART study: a case-control study. *Lancet* 2006;**368**:647–58.

388 Henley SJ, Thun MJ, Connell C et al. Two large prospective studies of mortality among men who use snuff or chewing tobacco (United States). *Cancer Causes Control* 2005;**16**:347–58.

389 Norberg M, Stenlund H, Lindahl B et al. Contribution of Swedish moist snuff to the metabolic syndrome: a wolf in sheep's clothing? *Scand J Public Health* 2006; **34**:576–83 (http://www.journalsonline.tandf.co.uk/link.asp?id=jqh56824k1667256).

390   Peto R, Doll R, Buckley JD et al. Can dietary beta-carotene materially reduce human cancer rates? *Nature* 1981;**290**:201–8.

391   Ziegler RG, Mayne ST, Swanson CA. Nutrition and lung cancer. *Cancer Causes Control* 1996;**7**:157–77.

392   Speizer FE, Colditz GA, Hunter DJ et al. Prospective study of smoking, antioxidant intake, and lung cancer in middle-aged women (USA). *Cancer Causes Control* 1999;**10**:475–82.

393   Hennekens CH, Buring JE, Manson JE et al. Lack of effect of long-term supplementation with beta carotene on the incidence of malignant neoplasms and cardiovascular disease. *N Engl J Med* 1996;**334**:1145–9.

394   Omenn GS, Goodman GE, Thornquist MD et al. Effects of a combination of beta carotene and vitamin A on lung cancer and cardiovascular disease. *N Engl J Med* 1996;**334**:1150–5.

395   Albanes D, Heinonen OP, Huttunen JK et al. Effects of alpha-tocopherol and beta-carotene supplements on cancer incidence in the Alpha-Tocopherol Beta-Carotene Cancer Prevention Study. *Am J Clin Nutr* 1995;**62**:1427S–30S.

396   Goodman GE, Thornquist MD, Balmes J et al. The Beta-Carotene and Retinol Efficacy Trial: incidence of lung cancer and cardiovascular disease mortality during 6-year follow-up after stopping beta-carotene and retinol supplements. *J Natl Cancer Inst* 2004;**96**:1743–50.

397   Ziegler RG. *The Olestra Project: Carotenoids and Human Cancer* (http://www.hsph.harvard.edu/Academics/nutr/olestra/o4.html).

398   Irwin D. Nitrosamines. 26 May 1999. British American Tobacco (http://bat.library.ucsf.edu/tid/evj34a99).

399   Irwin D, British American Tobacco. SRG mini symposium: [emails]. 20 Jan 2000. Brown & Williamson (http://legacy.library.ucsf.edu/tid/ekp71d00).

400   Irwin D. Costing the Earth: BBC TV programme, 2 May 2000. British American Tobacco (http://tobacco.health.usyd.edu.au/site/gateway/docs/pdf2/pdf/BAT325153707.PDF).

401   Chapman S. New disclosures in additives from New Zealand. *Tob Control* 1994;**3**:206–7.

402   Philip Morris Limited (Australia). Letter to Australian Department of Health: draft. 29 Mar 2000. Philip Morris (http://legacy.library.ucsf.edu/tid/gxi95c00).

403   Commonwealth Department of Health. Voluntary agreement for the disclosure of the ingredients of cigarettes. 2000 (http://www.health.gov.au/pubhlth/strateg/drugs/tobacco/agreement.pdf).

404   Proctor C. Smoking issues. Sep 1994. British American Tobacco (http://tobacco.health.usyd.edu.au/site/gateway/docs/pdf2/pdf/BAT502581860_1870.PDF).

405   Francis P. [Telex to F. Resnik]. 10 Feb 1981. Philip Morris (http://legacy.library.ucsf.edu/tid/mbn68e00).

406   Hutchens R. Australian cigarette specifications. 2 Dec 1993. R.J. Reynolds (http://legacy.library.ucsf.edu/tid/oyc73d00).

407   Brindle J, WD & HO Wills (Australia) Ltd. Ingredient MGE-7 [Letter to J. Webb]. 6 Jul 1984. Brown & Williamson (http://legacy.library.ucsf.edu/tid/pgz21f00).

408   Hackney P, Rothmans of Pall Mall (Australia) Limited. ITC-14 [Material Safety Data Sheet] and ITC 14 Flavour [Fax to W. Allen, RJ Reynolds]. 2 Nov 1993. R.J. Reynolds (http://legacy.library.ucsf.edu/tid/qyc73d00).

409   King W, Borland R, Christie M. Way-out developments at BATCO. *Tob Control* 2003;**12**:107–8.

410 Green S. C.A.C. II – Salamander: developments in scientific field 1976/77. 18 Apr 1977. British American Tobacco (http://tobacco.health.usyd.edu.au/site/gateway/docs/pdf2/pdf/BAT110069827_9829.PDF).

411 Lewis MJ, Wackowski O. Dealing with an innovative industry: a look at flavored cigarettes promoted by mainstream brands. *Am J Public Health* 2006;**96**:244–51.

412 Carpenter CM, Wayne GF, Pauly JL et al. New cigarette brands with flavors that appeal to youth: tobacco marketing strategies. *Health Aff (Millwood)* 2005;**24**: 1601–10.

413 Connolly GN. Sweet and spicy flavours: new brands for minorities and youth. *Tob Control* 2004;**13**:211–12.

414 British American Tobacco Australia. Submission No. 46 to the Inquiry into Tobacco Smoking in New South Wales. 2006 (http://www.parliament.nsw.gov.au/prod/parlment/committee.nsf/0/2B14B998DDA58536CA2571620017ECD2).

415 British American Tobacco Australia Limited. Australia ingredients report, 1 March 2004–1 March 2005. 2005 (http://www.health.gov.au/internet/wcms/publishing.nsf/Content/health-pubhlth-strateg-drugs-tobacco-ingredients.htm/$FILE/bata.pdf).

416 Baker RR, Pereira da Silva JR, Smith G. The effect of tobacco ingredients on smoke chemistry. Part I: Flavourings and additives. *Food Chem Toxicol* 2004; **42**(Suppl.):S3–37.

417 Gray N. The need for tobacco regulation. *Tob Control* 2006;**15**:145.

418 Henningfield JE, Benowitz NL, Connolly GN et al. Reducing tobacco addiction through tobacco product regulation. *Tob Control* 2004;**13**:132–5.

419 Borland R. A strategy for controlling the marketing of tobacco products: a regulated market model. *Tob Control* 2003;**12**:374–82.

420 Callard C, Thompson D, Collishaw N. Transforming the tobacco market: why the supply of cigarettes should be transferred from for-profit corporations to non-profit enterprises with a public health mandate. *Tob Control* 2005;**14**:278–83.

421 Liberman J. The future of tobacco regulation: a response to a proposal for fundamental institutional change. *Tob Control* 2006;**15**:333–8.

422 Warner KE, Burns DM. Hardening and the hard-core smoker: concepts, evidence, and implications. *Nicotine Tob Res* 2003;**5**:37–48.

423 Peto R. Global tobacco mortality: monitoring the growing epidemic. In: *Proceedings of the Tenth World Conference on Tobacco or Health, 24–28 August, Beijing, China*, 1997.

424 Centers for Disease Control and Prevention. State-specific prevalence of cigarette smoking and quitting among adults – United States, 2004. *MMWR Morb Mortal Wkly Rep* 2005;**54**:1124–7.

425 Health Canada. *Tobacco Control Programme, Health Canada Supplementary Tables, CTUMS Annual 2004 (February–December 2004)* (http://www.hc-sc.gc.ca/hl-vs/alt_formats/hecs-sesc/pdf/tobac-tabac/research-recherche/stat/ctums-esutc/2004/table-2004_e.pdf).

426 United Kingdom Office for National Statistics. *2004/05 General Household Survey* (http://www.statistics.gov.uk/ghs/).

427 Walsh RA, Paul CL, Tzelepis F et al. Quit smoking behaviours and intentions and hard-core smoking in New South Wales. *Health Promot J Austr* 2006;**17**:54–60.

428 Biener L, Reimer RL, Wakefield M et al. Impact of smoking cessation aids and mass media among recent quitters. *Am J Prev Med* 2006;**30**:217–24.

429 Chapman S. Stop-smoking clinics: a case for their abandonment. *Lancet* 1985;**i**:918–20.

430 Illich I. *Disabling Professions*. London: Marion Boyars, 1977.

431 Foulds J, Steinberg MB, Williams JM et al. Developments in pharmacotherapy for tobacco dependence: past, present and future. *Drug Alcohol Rev* 2006;**25**:59–71.

432   Klesges RC, Johnson KC, Somes G. Varenicline for smoking cessation: definite promise, but no panacea. *JAMA* 2006;**296**:94–5.

433   Janis IL, Feshbach S. Effect of fear-arousing communications. *J Abnorm Psychol* 1953;**48**:78–92.

434   Curry SJ, Grothaus L, McBride C. Reasons for quitting: intrinsic and extrinsic motivation for smoking cessation in a population-based sample of smokers. *Addict Behav* 1997;**22**:727–39.

435   Chapman S. For debate: the means/ends problem in health promotion. *Med J Aust* 1988;**149**:256,258–60.

436   Pierce JP, Macaskill P, Hill D. Long-term effectiveness of mass media led antismoking campaigns in Australia. *Am J Public Health* 1990;**80**:565–9.

437   Fischhoff B, Slovic P, Lichtenstein S. Lay foibles and expert fables in judgments about risk. *Am Stat* 1992;**36**:240–55.

438   Denissenko MF, Pao A, Tang M et al. Preferential formation of benzo[a]pyrene adducts at lung cancer mutational hotspots in P53. *Science* 1996;**274**:430–2.

439   Witte K. Putting the fear back into fear appeals: the extended parallel process model. *Communication Monogr* 1992;**59**:329–49.

440   Donovan RJ, Henley N. Negative outcomes, threats and threat appeals: towards a conceptual framework for the study of fear and other emotions in social marketing. *Soc Market Q* 1997;**4**:56–67.

441   Sutton S. Shock tactics and the myth of the inverted U. *Br J Addict* 1992;**87**:517–19.

442   Carroll T, Rock B. Generating Quitline calls during Australia's National Tobacco Campaign: effects of television advertisement execution and programme placement. *Tob Control* 2003;**12**(Suppl. 2):ii40–4.

443   Miller CL, Wakefield M, Roberts L. Uptake and effectiveness of the Australian telephone Quitline service in the context of a mass media campaign. *Tob Control* 2003;**12**(Suppl. 2):ii53–8.

444   Holman CD, Donovan RJ, Corti B et al. Banning tobacco sponsorship: replacing tobacco with health messages and creating health-promoting environments. *Tob Control* 1997;**6**:115–21.

445   Bal DG, Kizer KW, Felten PG et al. Reducing tobacco consumption in California: development of a statewide anti-tobacco use campaign. *JAMA* 1990;**264**:1570–4.

446   Biener L, Harris JE, Hamilton W. Impact of the Massachusetts tobacco control programme: population based trend analysis. *BMJ* 2000;**321**:351–4.

447   Fiore MC, Novotny TE, Pierce JP et al. Methods used to quit smoking in the United States: do cessation programs help? *JAMA* 1990;**263**:2760–5.

448   Zhu S, Melcer T, Sun J et al. Smoking cessation with and without assistance: a population-based analysis. *Am J Prev Med* 2000;**18**:305–11.

449   Cokkinides VE, Ward E, Jemal A et al. Under-use of smoking-cessation treatments: results from the National Health Interview Survey, 2000. *Am J Prev Med* 2005;**28**:119–22.

450   Lindstrom M, Isacsson SO. Smoking cessation among daily smokers, aged 45–69 years: a longitudinal study in Malmo, Sweden. *Addiction* 2002;**97**:205–15.

451   Cohen S, Lichtenstein E, Prochaska JO et al. Debunking myths about self-quitting: evidence from 10 prospective studies of persons who attempt to quit smoking by themselves. *Am Psychol* 1989;**44**:1355–65.

452   Jarvis M. Patterns and predictors of smoking cessation in the general population. In: Bolliger C, Fagerström KO (eds) *The Tobacco Epidemic*. Basel: Karger, 1997: 151–64.

453   Tocque K, Barker A, Fullard B. Are stop smoking services helping to reduce smoking prevalence?: new analysis based on estimated number of smokers. *Tobacco Control Research Bulletin (SmokeFree North West)* 2005 (3)Mar:1–13 (http://www.cph.org.uk/cph_pubs/reports/SM/SFNW3_mar05.pdf).

454   Action on Smoking and Health UK. *UK Tobacco Control Policy and Expenditure: an Overview.* 2006 (http://www.ash.org.uk/html/policy/uktobpolicy.html).

455   Ferguson J, Bauld L, Chesterman J et al. The English smoking treatment services: one-year outcomes. *Addiction* 2005;**100**(Suppl. 2):59–69.

456   Milne E. NHS smoking cessation services and smoking prevalence: observational study. *BMJ* 2005;**330**:760.

457   Stapleton JA, Sutherland G. Effective NHS smoking cessation services. *BMJ* 2005; e-letter 19 Mar 2005 (http://bmj.bmjjournals.com/cgi/eletters/330/7494/760).

458   Parrott S, Godfrey C, Raw M et al. Guidance for commissioners on the cost effectiveness of smoking cessation interventions: Health Educational Authority. *Thorax* 1998;**53**(Suppl. 5, pt 2):S1–38.

459   Tengs TO, Adams ME, Pliskin JS et al. Five-hundred life-saving interventions and their cost-effectiveness. *Risk Anal* 1995;**15**:369–90.

460   Altria. *For Smokers Who Want to Quit, a Nationwide Program – QuitAssist™, June 24, 2005* (http://www.altria.com/media/press_release/03_02_pr_2005_06_24_01.asp).

461   Zhu S-H. Increasing cessation in the population: quit attempts vs. successful quit attempts. Paper presented at 13th World Conference on Tobacco or Health, July 12–15 2006, Washington DC, USA.

462   Wakefield M, Szczypka G, Terry-McElrath Y et al. Mixed messages on tobacco: comparative exposure to public health, tobacco company- and pharmaceutical company-sponsored tobacco-related television campaigns in the United States, 1999–2003. *Addiction* 2005;**100**:1875–83.

463   West R, Sohal T. "Catastrophic" pathways to smoking cessation: findings from national survey. *BMJ* 2006;**332**:458–60.

464   Larabie LC. To what extent do smokers plan quit attempts? *Tob Control* 2005;**14**:425–8.

465   Cummings KM, Hyland A. Impact of nicotine replacement therapy on smoking behavior. *Annu Rev Public Health* 2005;**26**:583–99.

466   Shiffman S, Gitchell J, Pinney JM et al. Public health benefit of over-the-counter nicotine medications. *Tob Control* 1997;**6**:306–10.

467   Hughes JR, Shiffman S, Callas P et al. A meta-analysis of the efficacy of over-the-counter nicotine replacement. *Tob Control* 2003;**12**:21–7.

468   Hu T, Sung HY, Keeler TE et al. Cigarette consumption and sales of nicotine replacement products. *Tob Control* 2000;**9**(Suppl. 2):ii60–3.

469   Centers for Disease Control and Prevention. Cigarette smoking among adults: United States, 1999. *MMWR Morb Mortal Wkly Rep* 2001;**50**:869–73.

470   Thorndike AN, Biener L, Rigotti NA. Effect on smoking cessation of switching nicotine replacement therapy to over-the-counter status. *Am J Public Health* 2002; **92**:437–42.

471   Pierce JP, Gilpin EA. Impact of over-the-counter sales on effectiveness of pharmaceutical aids for smoking cessation. *JAMA* 2002;**288**:1260–4.

472   Bansal MA, Cummings KM, Hyland A et al. Stop-smoking medications: who uses them, who misuses them, and who is misinformed about them? *Nicotine Tob Res* 2004;**6**(Suppl. 3):S303–10.

473   Bolton LE, Cohen JB, Bloom PN. Does marketing products as remedies create "get out of jail free cards"? *J Consumer Research* 2006;**33**:71–81.

474 Novotny TE, Cohen JC, Yurekli A et al. Smoking cessation and nicotine replacement therapies. In: Chaloupka FJ, Jha P (eds) *Tobacco Control in Developing Countries*. Oxford: Oxford Medical Publications, 2000:287–307.

475 Grigg M, Glasgow H. Subsidised nicotine replacement therapy. *Tob Control* 2003;**12**:238–9.

476 O'Dea D. *An Economic Evaluation of the Quitline Nicotine Replacement Therapy (NRT) Service. Prepared for the New Zealand Ministry of Health, June 28*. 2004 (http://www.ndp.govt.nz/publications/economicevaluation-quitlinenrtservice.pdf).

477 Cummings KM, Fix B, Celestino P et al. Reach, efficacy, and cost-effectiveness of free nicotine medication giveaway programs. *J Public Health Manag Pract* 2006;**12**:37–43.

478 Cummings KM, Hyland A, Fix B et al. Free nicotine patch giveaway program 12-month follow-up of participants. *Am J Prev Med* 2006;**31**:181–4.

479 Jha P, Chaloupka FJ. The economics of global tobacco control. *BMJ* 2000;**321**: 358–61.

480 Van Kinh H, Ross H, Levy DT et al. The effect of imposing a higher, uniform tobacco tax in Vietnam. *Health Res Policy Syst* 2006;**4**:6.

481 Liang L, Chaloupka FJ. Differential effects of cigarette price on youth smoking intensity. *Nicotine Tob Res* 2002;**4**:109–14.

482 Ranson MK, Jha P, Chaloupka FJ et al. Global and regional estimates of the effectiveness and cost-effectiveness of price increases and other tobacco control policies. *Nicotine Tob Res* 2002;**4**:311–19.

483 Chaloupka FJ, Cummings KM, Morley CP et al. Tax, price and cigarette smoking: evidence from the tobacco documents and implications for tobacco company marketing strategies. *Tob Control* 2002;**11**(Suppl. 1):i62–72.

484 Philip Morris (Australia) Limited. Status report on anti-industry activities in Australia. 15 Apr 1983. Philip Morris (http://legacy.library.ucsf.edu/tid/ujl85e00).

485 Philip Morris International. The perspective of PM International on smoking and health issues. 27 Mar 1985. Philip Morris (http://legacy.library.ucsf.edu/tid/tus98e00).

486 Schwab C. Quitting share vs MSA share, by cigarette attribute: [attachments to memo re: Cigarette attributes and quitting]. 4 Mar 1993. Philip Morris (http://legacy.library.ucsf.edu/tid/wue06e00).

487 Farrelly MC, Bray JW, Office on Smoking and Health. Response to increases in cigarette prices by race/ethnicity, income, and age groups – United States, 1976–1993. *MMWR Morb Mortal Wkly Rep* 1998;**47**:605–9.

488 Marsh A, McKay S. *Poor Smokers*. London: Policy Studies Institute, 1994.

489 United Kingdom Office for National Statistics. *Smoking Habits in Great Britain*. 2006 (http://www.statistics.gov.uk/cci/nugget.asp?id=313).

490 Action on Smoking and Health UK. *Tobacco Smuggling – Introduction* (http://www.ash.org.uk/?smuggling).

491 Joossens L, Raw M. How can cigarette smuggling be reduced? *BMJ* 2000;**321**: 947–50.

492 Warner KE. Clearing the airwaves: the cigarette ad ban revisited. *Policy Anal* 1979;**5**:435–50.

493 Lewitt EM, Coate D, Grossman M. The effect of government regulation teenage smoking. *J Law Econ* 1981;**24**:545–69.

494 Balbach ED, Glantz SA. Tobacco control advocates must demand high-quality media campaigns: the California experience. *Tob Control* 1998;**7**:397–408.

495 Campaign for Tobacco-Free Kids. *Tobacco Industry Interference with State Efforts to Prevent and Reduce Tobacco Use*. 1999 (http://www.tobaccofreekids.org/research/factsheets/pdf/0078.pdf).

496 Association of Schools of Public Health. Legacy press release 22 Aug 2005 – American Legacy Foundation v. Lorillard – truth® ads will continue to save lives! 2005 (http://www.asph.org/document.cfm?page=772).

497 Various. Insights from Australia's National Tobacco Campaign. *Tob Control* 2003;**12**(Suppl. 2).

498 Siegel M. The effectiveness of state-level tobacco control interventions: a review of program implementation and behavioral outcomes. *Annu Rev Public Health* 2002;**23**:45–71.

499 Pierce JP, Gilpin EA, Emery SL et al. Has the California tobacco control program reduced smoking? *JAMA* 1998;**280**:893–9.

500 Hu TW, Sung HY, Keeler TE. Reducing cigarette consumption in California: tobacco taxes vs an anti-smoking media campaign. *Am J Public Health* 1995;**85**:1218–22.

501 Russell MA, Wilson C, Taylor C et al. Effect of general practitioners' advice against smoking. *Br Med J* 1979;**2**:231–5.

502 Dickinson JA, Wiggers J, Leeder SR et al. General practitioners' detection of patients' smoking status. *Med J Aust* 1989;**150**:420–2, 425–6.

503 Young JM, Ward JE. Implementing guidelines for smoking cessation advice in Australian general practice: opinions, current practices, readiness to change and perceived barriers. *Fam Pract* 2001;**18**:14–20.

504 Copeman RC, Swannell RJ, Pincus DF et al. Utilization of the "Smokescreen" smoking-cessation programme by general practitioners and their patients. *Med J Aust* 1989;**151**:83–7.

505 Silagy C, Muir J, Coulter A et al. Lifestyle advice in general practice: rates recalled by patients. *BMJ* 1992;**305**:871–4.

506 Britton J, Lewis S. Trends in the uptake and delivery of smoking cessation services to smokers in Great Britain. *J Epidemiol Community Health* 2004;**58**:569–70.

507 Borland R, Segan CJ. The potential of quitlines to increase smoking cessation. *Drug Alcohol Rev* 2006;**25**:73–8.

508 Tomson T, Helgason AR, Gilljam H. Quitline in smoking cessation: a cost-effectiveness analysis. *Int J Technol Assess Health Care* 2004;**20**:469–74.

509 An LC, Schillo BA, Kavanaugh AM et al. Increased reach and effectiveness of a statewide tobacco quitline after the addition of access to free nicotine replacement therapy. *Tob Control* 2006;**15**:286–93.

510 Etter JF. The internet and the industrial revolution in smoking cessation counselling. *Drug Alcohol Rev* 2006;**25**:79–84.

511 Bock B, Graham A, Sciamanna C et al. Smoking cessation treatment on the Internet: content, quality, and usability. *Nicotine Tob Res* 2004;**6**:207–19.

512 Walters ST, Wright JA, Shegog R. A review of computer and Internet-based interventions for smoking behavior. *Addict Behav* 2006;**31**:264–77.

513 Chapman S, Smith W. Deception among quit smoking lottery entrants. *Am J Health Promot* 1994;**8**:328–30.

514 Chapman S, Smith W, Mowbray G et al. Quit and win smoking cessation contests: how should effectiveness be evaluated? *Prev Med* 1993;**22**:423–32.

515 Thomas R, Perera R. School-based programmes for preventing smoking. *Cochrane Database Syst Rev* 2006;**3**:CD001293.

516   Peterson AV Jr, Kealey KA, Mann SL et al. Hutchinson Smoking Prevention Project: long-term randomized trial in school-based tobacco use prevention – results on smoking. *J Natl Cancer Inst* 2000;**92**:1979–91.

517   Wiehe SE, Garrison MM, Christakis DA et al. A systematic review of school-based smoking prevention trials with long-term follow-up. *J Adolesc Health* 2005;**36**: 162–9.

518   White V, Hayman J, Wakefield M et al. *Trends in Smoking Among Victorian Secondary School Students 1984–2002.* CBRC research paper series, no. 4. Melbourne, Vic: Centre for Behavioural Research in Cancer, The Cancer Council Victoria, 2003 (http://www.cancervic.org.au/cbrc-papers/rps4-2003.pdf).

519   Farkas AJ, Distefan JM, Choi WS et al. Does parental smoking cessation discourage adolescent smoking? *Prev Med* 1999;**28**:213–18.

520   Bricker JB, Peterson AV Jr, Leroux BG et al. Prospective prediction of children's smoking transitions: role of parents' and older siblings' smoking. *Addiction* 2006;**101**: 128–36.

521   Bricker JB, Rajan KB, Andersen MR et al. Does parental smoking cessation encourage their young adult children to quit smoking?: a prospective study. *Addiction* 2005;**100**:379–86.

522   White V, Tan N, Wakefield M et al. Do adult focused anti-smoking campaigns have an impact on adolescents?: the case of the Australian National Tobacco Campaign. *Tob Control* 2003;**12**(Suppl. 2):ii23–9.

523   Wakefield M, Chaloupka F. Effectiveness of comprehensive tobacco control programmes in reducing teenage smoking in the USA. *Tob Control* 2000;**9**:177–86.

524   Hill D. Why we should tackle adult smoking first. *Tob Control* 1999;**8**:333–5.

525   Landman A, Ling PM, Glantz SA. Tobacco industry youth smoking prevention programs: protecting the industry and hurting tobacco control. *Am J Public Health* 2002;**92**:917–30.

526   Teague CE. Research planning memorandum on some thoughts about new brands of cigarettes for the youth market: draft confidential report. 1973. R.J. Reynolds (http://legacy.library.ucsf.edu/tid/act68d00).

527   Chapman S. Tobacco giant's anti-smoking course flops. *BMJ* 2001;**323**:1206.

528   Hung S. Smoking & health meeting. 14 Feb 1973. Philip Morris (http://legacy.library.ucsf.edu/tid/owq24e00).

529   Slavitt JJ. Re: Sting operations. 9 May 1994. Philip Morris (http://legacy.library.ucsf.edu/tid/brz16e00).

530   Tilson M, Canadian Cancer Society. *A Critical Analysis of Youth Access Laws.* Ontario: Canadian Cancer Society, 2002 (http://www.cancer.ca/vgn/images/portal/cit_776/48/38/69664397cw_criticalanalysisyouthaccesslaws_en.pdf).

531   Fichtenberg CM, Glantz SA. Youth access interventions do not affect youth smoking. *Pediatrics* 2002;**109**:1088–92.

532   Ling PM, Landman A, Glantz SA. It is time to abandon youth access tobacco programmes. *Tob Control* 2002;**11**:3–6.

533   White V, Scollo M. What are underage smokers worth to Australian tobacco companies? *Aust NZ J Public Health* 2003;**27**:360–1.

534   Doctors told to smoke in private. *The Australian* 26 Oct 1970 (http://tobacco.health.usyd.edu.au/site/gateway/docs/nid/AUS19701026.pdf).

535   Young JM, Ward JE. Declining rates of smoking among medical practitioners. *Med J Aust* 1997;**167**:232.

536   Fong GT, Hammond D, Laux FL et al. The near-universal experience of regret among

smokers in four countries: findings from the International Tobacco Control Policy Evaluation Survey. *Nicotine Tob Res* 2004;**6**(Suppl. 3):S341–51.

537 Thornton DE. [Memo to C. Ayers enclosing a note "The Product in 1980" (RET/JP/46J)]. 13 Jan 1976. British American Tobacco (http://tobaccodocuments.org/ness/37664.html).

538 Whist A. [Memo to R.W. Murray]. 17 Apr 1984. Philip Morris (http://legacy.library.ucsf.edu/tid/uot24e00).

539 Borland R, Yong HH, Cummings KM et al. Determinants and consequences of smoke-free homes: findings from the International Tobacco Control (ITC) Four Country Survey. *Tob Control* 2006;**15**(Suppl. 3):iii42–50.

540 Kornegay HR. Horace Kornegay speech Tobacco & Allied Industries Division of the American Jewish Committee. 11 Dec 1979. Tobacco Institute (http://legacy.library.ucsf.edu/tid/qlp92f00).

541 Alamar B, Glantz SA. Effect of increased social unacceptability of cigarette smoking on reduction in cigarette consumption. *Am J Public Health* 2006;**96**:1359–63.

542 Nixon S. No smoking on the job if you work at Philip Morris. *Sydney Morning Herald* 26 Nov 2002:3 (http://tobacco.health.usyd.edu.au/site/gateway/docs/nid/SMH20021126.pdf).

543 Jarvis MJ, Foulds J, Feyerabend C. Exposure to passive smoking among bar staff. *Br J Addict* 1992;**87**:111–13.

544 Chapman S. Tobacco industry memo reveals passive smoking strategy. *BMJ* 1997;**314**:1569.

545 Nemery B, Piette D. The hot air on passive smoking: experts who evaluated studies seem not to have had relevant experience. *BMJ* 1998;**317**:348.

546 Barnoya J, Glantz S. Tobacco industry success in preventing regulation of secondhand smoke in Latin America: the "Latin Project". *Tob Control* 2002;**11**:305–14.

547 Philip Morris. Worldwide Regulatory Affairs 1995 original budget: draft. 26 Oct 1994. Philip Morris (http://legacy.library.ucsf.edu/tid/tep94c00).

548 Trotter L, Wakefield M, Borland R. Socially cued smoking in bars, nightclubs, and gaming venues: a case for introducing smoke-free policies. *Tob Control* 2002;**11**:300–4.

549 Walls T. CAC presentation number 4, Tina Walls: introduction. 8 Jul 1994. Philip Morris (http://legacy.library.ucsf.edu/tid/vnf77e00).

550 Shiell A, Chapman S. The inertia of self-regulation: a game-theoretic approach to reducing passive smoking in restaurants. *Soc Sci Med* 2000;**51**:1111–19.

551 Harper T. Smoking and gambling: a trance inducing ritual. *Tob Control* 2003;**12**:231–3.

552 US Department of Health and Human Service. *The Health Consequences of Involuntary Exposure to Tobacco Smoke: a Report of the Surgeon General.* Rockville, MD: Dept of Health and Human Services, 2006 (http://www.surgeongeneral.gov/library/secondhandsmoke/report/executivesummary.pdf).

553 US Department of Health and Human Service. *The Health Consequences of Involuntary Exposure to Tobacco Smoke: a Report of the Surgeon General.* Atlanta, GA: US Dept of Health and Human Service, 2006 (http://www.surgeongeneral.gov/library/secondhandsmoke/report).

554 Anon. Goa to ban smoking in public from Oct 2. *Deccan Herald* (India), Sep 1999:12.

555 Mullender R. Liberal tolerance, the proportionality principle, and qualified consequentialism. Newcastle Law School Working Papers; 2000/04. Newcastle upon

Tyne: Newcastle Law School, 2000 (http://www.ncl.ac.uk/nuls/research/wpapers/mullender1.html#fn9).

556 Celermajer DS, Adams MR, Clarkson P et al. Passive smoking and impaired endothelium-dependent arterial dilatation in healthy young adults. *N Engl J Med* 1996;**334**:150–4.

557 Raitakari OT, Adams MR, McCredie RJ et al. Arterial endothelial dysfunction related to passive smoking is potentially reversible in healthy young adults. *Ann Intern Med* 1999;**130**:578–81.

558 Chapman S, Wutzke S. Not in our back yard: media coverage of community opposition to mobile phone towers – an application of Sandman's outrage model of risk perception. *Aust NZ J Public Health* 1997;**21**:614–20.

559 Covello VT. Informing people about risks from chemicals, radiation, and other toxic substances: a review of obstacles to public understanding and effective risk communication. In: Leiss W (ed.) *Prospects and Problems in Risk Communication*. Waterloo, Ontario: University of Waterloo Press, 1989:1–49.

560 Sanner T. Air pollution from cigarette smoking and gasoline cars with catalytic converter. *Abstract for the 8th World Conference on Tobacco or Health, Buenos Aires, Argentina; 30 March–3 April 1992*. Abstract 330; 1992.

561 Wooden M, Bush R. Smoking cessation and absence from work. *Prev Med* 1995;**24**:535–40.

562 Borland R, Cappiello M, Owen N. Leaving work to smoke. *Addiction* 1997;**92**:1361–8.

563 Gray NJ. The case for smoker-free workplaces. *Tob Control* 2005;**14**:143–4.

564 Shaw M, Dorling D, Smith GD. Mortality and political climate: how suicide rates have risen during periods of Conservative government, 1901–2000. *J Epidemiol Community Health* 2002;**56**:723–5.

565 Page A, Morrell S, Taylor R. Suicide and political regime in New South Wales and Australia during the 20th century. *J Epidemiol Community Health* 2002;**56**:766–72.

566 The Fred Hollows Foundation (http://www.hollows.org).

567 Invernizzi G, Ruprecht A, De Marco G et al. Residual tobacco smoke: measurement of its washout time in the lung and of its contribution to environmental tobacco smoke. *Tob Control* 2007;**16**:29–33.

568 Arbes SJ Jr, Gergen PJ, Elliott L et al. Prevalences of positive skin test responses to 10 common allergens in the US population: results from the third National Health and Nutrition Examination Survey. *J Allergy Clin Immunol* 2005;**116**:377–83.

569 Bornschein S, Hausteiner C, Zilker T et al. Psychiatric and somatic disorders and multiple chemical sensitivity (MCS) in 264 "environmental patients". *Psychol Med* 2002;**32**:1387–94.

570 Yano E. Japanese spousal smoking study revisited: how a tobacco industry funded paper reached erroneous conclusions. *Tob Control* 2005;**14**:227–33; discussion 233–5.

571 Philip Morris. Corporate Affairs plan: Philip Morris (Australia) Limited. 19 Oct 1992. Philip Morris (http://legacy.library.ucsf.edu/tid/fgw48e00).

572 Turner A, Asian Tobacco Council. Tobacco: the battle for social acceptance: [speech given to the Sixth World Tobacco Exhibition & Symposium at the Vienna Messelgelande, Austria, 22–25 October 1990]. 22 Oct 1990. R.J. Reynolds (http://legacy.library.ucsf.edu/tid/mfk43d00).

573 Stockdale B. Australia trip: topline learning (highly restricted market). 12 Feb 1997. R.J. Reynolds (http://legacy.library.ucsf.edu/tid/ads90d00).

574 Philip Morris International Management SA. The China National Tobacco Corporation and Philip Morris International announce the establishment of a long-term strategic cooperative partnership, 21 December. 2005 (http://www.philipmorrisinternational.com/PMINTL/pages/eng/press/pr_20051221.asp).

575 Herring HB. Signs of bygone days. *The New York Times* 25 Apr 1999:Sec. 4, 2.

576 British American Tobacco. The vanishing media. 1978. British American Tobacco (http://tobacco.health.usyd.edu.au/site/gateway/docs/pdf2/pdf/BAT500062147_2159.PDF).

577 Slade J. The pack as advertisement. *Tob Control* 1997;**6**:169–70.

578 Joy R. Regulations create design limitations. *World Tobacco* 1992, May:17.

579 Koten J. Tobacco marketer's success formula: make cigarettes in smoker's own image. *Wall Street Journal* 1980, 29 Feb:22.

580 Cunningham R, Kyle K. The case for plain packaging. *Tob Control* 1995;**4**:80–6.

581 Carter SM. New frontier, new power: the retail environment in Australia's dark market. *Tob Control* 2003;**12**(Suppl. 3):iii95–101.

582 Carter SM. Going below the line: creating transportable brands for Australia's dark market. *Tob Control* 2003;**12**(Suppl. 3):iii87–94.

583 Carter SM. The Australian cigarette brand as product, person, and symbol. *Tob Control* 2003;**12**(Suppl. 3):iii79–86.

584 Byrnes H. Fashion's smoking gun: top designers' functions sponsored by cigarette company. *Sun-Herald* (Sydney, NSW), 11 Aug 2002:3.

585 Harper T. Marketing life after advertising bans. *Tob Control* 2001;**10**:196–8.

586 Carter S. Worshipping at the Alpine altar: promoting tobacco in a world without advertising. *Tob Control* 2001;**10**:391–3.

587 Terazono E. Sociable smoking. *Financial Times (FT.Com)* (London) 26 Jan 2004.

588 Rimmer L. *BAT in its Own Words: an Alternative British American Tobacco Social Report*. London: Action on Smoking and Health UK; Christian Aid and Friends of the Earth, 2005 (http://www.foe.co.uk/resource/reports/bat2005.pdf).

589 Sepe E, Ling PM, Glantz SA. Smooth moves: bar and nightclub tobacco promotions that target young adults. *Am J Public Health* 2002;**92**:414–19.

590 Sepe E, Glantz SA. Bar and club tobacco promotions in the alternative press: targeting young adults. *Am J Public Health* 2002;**92**:75–8.

591 Mekemson C, Glantz SA. How the tobacco industry built its relationship with Hollywood. *Tob Control* 2002;**11**(Suppl. 1):i81–91.

592 Maxwell H. Draft speech for Hamish Maxwell marketing meeting, 24 June. 24 Jun 1983. Philip Morris (http://legacy.library.ucsf.edu/tid/nyz24e00).

593 McGinn JA. Unique product placement early contract renewal. 27 May 1986. American Tobacco Company (http://legacy.library.ucsf.edu/tid/big35f00).

594 Kacirk K, Glantz SA. Smoking in movies in 2000 exceeded rates in the 1960s. *Tob Control* 2001;**10**:397–8.

595 Glantz SA, Kacirk KW, McCulloch C. Back to the future: smoking in movies in 2002 compared with 1950 levels. *Am J Public Health* 2004;**94**:261–3.

596 Charlesworth A, Glantz SA. Smoking in the movies increases adolescent smoking: a review. *Pediatrics* 2005;**116**:1516–28.

597 Sargent JD, Beach ML, Adachi-Mejia AM et al. Exposure to movie smoking: its relation to smoking initiation among US adolescents. *Pediatrics* 2005;**116**:1183–91.

598 Siahpush M. Why is lone-motherhood so strongly associated with smoking? *Aust NZ J Public Health* 2004;**28**:37–42.

599 SmokeFree Movies (http://smokefreemovies.ucsf.edu).

600 Chan WC, Knox FA, McGinnity FG et al. Serious eye and adnexal injuries from fireworks in Northern Ireland before and after lifting of the firework ban: an ophthalmology unit's experience. *Int Ophthalmol* 2004;**25**:167–9.

601 Dhar A. Anbumani unfazed by opposition, to go ahead with smoking ban. *The Hindu* (India) 19 Jun 2005 (http://www.hindu.com/2005/06/19/stories/2005061906561000.htm).

602 Ganiwijaya T, Sjukrudin E, De Backer G et al. Prevalence of cigarette smoking in a rural area of West Java, Indonesia. *Tob Control* 1995;**4**:335–7.

603 Masalski KW. *Examining the Japanese History Textbook Controversies*. Bloomington: National Clearinghouse for US-Japan Studies, East Asian Studies Center, Indiana University, 2001 (http://www.indiana.edu/~japan/Digests/textbook.html).

604 Tyas SL, Pederson LL. Psychosocial factors related to adolescent smoking: a critical review of the literature. *Tob Control* 1998;**7**:409–20.

605 Deshmukh S. Smoke screen. *Bombay Times* 11 Feb 2005 (http://timesofindia.indiatimes.com/articleshow/1018681.cms).

606 Shields DL, Carol J, Balbach ED et al. Hollywood on tobacco: how the entertainment industry understands tobacco portrayal. *Tob Control* 1999;**8**:378–86.

607 SmokeFree Movies. *The Solution* (http://smokefreemovies.ucsf.edu/solution/index.html).

608 British American Tobacco. *Social Report*. London: BAT, 2005 (http://www.bat.com/OneWeb/sites/uk__3mnfen.nsf/vwPagesWebLive/C1256E3C003D3339C125715A004FA7D8?opendocument&SID=&DTC=).

609 Wroe D. Tobacco ad campaign angers MPs. *The Age* (Melbourne, Vic) 17 May 2004:5.

610 Lembo L. PM-USA funding for social projects. 16 Sep 1988. Philip Morris (http://tobaccodocuments.org/landman/2044927615–7616.pdf).

611 Stossel J. Big talk and big tobacco: cigarette maker spends big money publicizing its good deeds. *ABC News '20/20': Give Me a Break* (USA) 9 Feb 2001.

612 Anon. BAT Korea aims to surpass 16% market share. *Korea Herald* 25 May 2006.

613 Carter SM. From legitimate consumers to public relations pawns: the tobacco industry and young Australians. *Tob Control* 2003;**12**(Suppl. 3):iii71–8.

614 Cobain I, Leigh D. Tobacco firm has secret North Korea plant: firm with Tories' Ken Clarke on payroll runs factory in country with grim human rights record. *The Guardian* (London) 17 Oct 2005:7.

615 Hirschhorn N. Corporate social responsibility and the tobacco industry: hope or hype? *Tob Control* 2004;**13**:447–53.

616 Chapman S, Shatenstein S. Extreme corporate makeover: tobacco companies, corporate responsibility and the corruption of "ethics". Globalink petition. 2004 (http://petition.globalink.org/view.php?code=extreme).

617 SourceWatch. *Corporate Social Responsibility*. 2006 (http://www.sourcewatch.org/index.php?title=Corporate_social_responsibility).

618 Lexchin J, Bero LA, Djulbegovic B et al. Pharmaceutical industry sponsorship and research outcome and quality: systematic review. *BMJ* 2003;**326**:1167–70.

619 De Angelis C, Drazen JM, Frizelle FA et al. Clinical trial registration: a statement from the International Committee of Medical Journal Editors. *Lancet* 2004;**364**:911–12.

620 Oakland Consultancy. A survey of university policies relating to funding from the tobacco industry. Sep 2000. British American Tobacco (http://bat.library.ucsf.edu/tid/oqj82a99).

621 Policies of Australian universities on funding from the tobacco industry (http://jech.bmjjournals.com/cgi/data/58/5/361/DC1/3).

622 Bero L, Barnes DE, Hanauer P et al. Lawyer control of the tobacco industry's external research program. The Brown and Williamson documents. *JAMA* 1995;**274**:241–7.

623 McKee M. Competing interests: the importance of transparency. *Eur J Public Health* 2003;**13**:193–4.

624 Diethelm PA, Rielle J-C, McKee M. Authors' reply. *Lancet* 2005;**365**:211–12.

625 United States v. Philip Morris, et al. Civil Action No. 1999-2496 amended final opinion issued September 8, 2006 by Judge Gladys Kessler. 2006 (http://www.dcd.uscourts.gov/opinions/2006/Kessler/1999-CV-2496~16:3:44~9-8-2006-a.pdf).

626 Barnes DE, Bero LA. Scientific quality of original research articles on environmental tobacco smoke. *Tob Control* 1997;**6**:19–26.

627 Mauron A, Morabia A, Perneger T et al. Report of the inquiry into the case involving Prof. Ragner Rylander (unofficial translation), Geneva, Sept 6. 2004 (http://www.prevention.ch/rye060904.pdf).

628 Republic and Canton of Geneva. The Judiciary. P/542/01 ACJP/223/03. Decision of the Court of Appeal Criminal Division Hearing of Monday 15 December 2003 (http://www.prevention.ch/ryjue151203.htm).

629 Cummings KM, Morley CP, Horan JK et al. Marketing to America's youth: evidence from corporate documents. *Tob Control* 2002;**11**(Suppl. 1):i5–17.

630 Health Canada. *Canadian Tobacco Use Monitoring Survey.* 2005 (http://www.hc-sc.gc.ca/hl-vs/tobac-tabac/research-recherche/stat/ctums-esutc/2005/index_e.html).

631 Centers for Disease Control and Prevention. *Behavioral Risk Factor Surveillance System – Prevalence Data – Tobacco Use 2005* (http://apps.nccd.cdc.gov/brfss/list.asp?cat=TU&yr=2005&qkey=4394&state=All).

632 Harrison PM, Beck AJ. Prison and jail inmates at midyear 2005. *Bureau of Justice Statistics Bulletin (U.S. Department of Justice, Office of Justice Programs)* 2006 May:1–13 (http://www.ojp.usdoj.gov/bjs/pub/pdf/pjim05.pdf).

633 Belcher JM, Butler T, Richmond RL et al. Smoking and its correlates in an Australian prisoner population. *Drug Alcohol Rev* 2006;**25**:343–8.

634 Okuyemi KS, Caldwell AR, Thomas JL et al. Homelessness and smoking cessation: insights from focus groups. *Nicotine Tob Res* 2006;**8**:287–96.

635 Biener L, Garrett CA, Gilpin EA et al. Consequences of declining survey response rates for smoking prevalence estimates. *Am J Prev Med* 2004;**27**:254–7.

636 Winstanley M, Woodward S, Walker N. Trends in smoking prevalence: smoking rates – adults. In: *Tobacco in Australia: Facts and Issues 1995*, 2nd edn. Carlton South, Vic: Victorian Smoking and Health Program (Quit Victoria), 1995:chap. 1.1 (http://www.quit.org.au/quit/FandI/fandi/c01s1.htm).

637 Mendez D, Warner KE, Courant PN. Has smoking cessation ceased?: expected trends in the prevalence of smoking in the United States. *Am J Epidemiol* 1998;**148**:249–58.

638 Nelson DE, Giovino GA, Emont SL et al. Trends in cigarette smoking among US physicians and nurses. *JAMA* 1994;**271**:1273–5.

639 Siahpush M, Borland R. Socio-demographic variations in smoking status among Australians aged > or = 18: multivariate results from the 1995 National Health Survey. *Aust NZ J Public Health* 2001;**25**:438–42.

640 Siahpush M, Heller G, Singh G. Lower levels of occupation, income and education are strongly associated with a longer smoking duration: multivariate results from

the 2001 Australian National Drug Strategy Survey. *Public Health* 2005;**119**: 1105–10.

641 Ivers RG. An evidence-based approach to planning tobacco interventions for Aboriginal people. *Drug Alcohol Rev* 2004;**23**:5–9.

642 Lasser K, Boyd JW, Woolhandler S et al. Smoking and mental illness: a population-based prevalence study. *JAMA* 2000;**284**:2606–10.

643 Stewart MJ, Brosky G, Gillis A et al. Disadvantaged women and smoking. *Can J Public Health* 1996;**87**:257–60.

644 Smith EA, Offen N, Malone RE. What makes an ad a cigarette ad?: commercial tobacco imagery in the lesbian, gay, and bisexual press. *J Epidemiol Community Health* 2005;**59**:1086–91.

645 Balbach ED, Gasior RJ, Barbeau EM. R.J. Reynolds' targeting of African Americans: 1988–2000. *Am J Public Health* 2003;**93**:822–7.

646 Trinidad DR, Messer K, Gilpin EA et al. The Californian Tobacco Control Program's effect on adult smoking. 3: similar effects for African-Americans across states. *Tob Control* (in press).

647 Gautier A. *Baromètre santé médecins/pharmaciens 2003*. Paris: INPES, 2005.

648 Twardella D, Brenner H. Lack of training as a central barrier to the promotion of smoking cessation: a survey among general practitioners in Germany. *Eur J Public Health* 2005;**15**:140–5.

649 Pizzo AM, Chellini E, Grazzini G et al. Italian general practitioners and smoking cessation strategies. *Tumori* 2003;**89**:250–4.

650 Hay DR. Cigarette smoking by New Zealand doctors and nurses: results from the 1996 population census. *NZ Med J* 1998;**111**:102–4.

651 Maziak W, Mzayek F, Asfar T et al. Smoking among physicians in Syria: do as I say not as I do. *Ann Saudi Medicine* 1999;**19**:253–6.

652 Estudio De Actitudes, Creencias Y Prevalencia De Consumo De Tabaco Entre Los Médicos Uruguayos. Paper presented at the 12th World Conference on Tobacco or Health, Helsinki, Finland, 2003.

653 Taylor NS, Standen PJ, Cutajar P et al. Smoking prevalence and knowledge of associated risks in adult attenders at day centres for people with learning disabilities. *J Intellect Disabil Res* 2004;**48**:239–44.

654 Chapman S. *The Lung Goodbye: Tactics for Counteracting the Tobacco Industry in the 1980s*, 2nd edn. Sydney: Consumer Interpol, 1986.

655 Pertschuk M, Wilbur P. *Media Advocacy: Reframing Public Debate*. Washington, DC: The Benton Foundation, 1991.

656 Advocacy Institute. *Getting Through to the Front Page*. Washington, DC: Advocacy Institute.

657 Hallin DC. Sound bite news: television coverage of elections 1968–1988. *J Commun* 1992;**42**:5–24.

658 Center for Media and Public Affairs. *The Incredible Shrinking Soundbite* (http://www.cmpa.com/pressReleases/index.htm).

659 Burrows DS. Young adult smokers: strategies and opportunities. 29 Feb 1984. R.J. Reynolds (http://legacy.library.ucsf.edu/tid/ftc49d00).

660 Slavitt JJ. TI youth initiative. 12 Feb 1991. Philip Morris (http://legacy.library.ucsf.edu/tid/sjl19e00).

661 Alinsky SD. *Rules for Radicals*. New York: Vintage, 1972.

662 Offen N, Smith EA, Malone RE. The perimetric boycott: a tool for tobacco control advocacy. *Tob Control* 2005;**14**:272–7.

663 Offen N, Smith EA, Malone RE. From adversary to target market: the ACT-UP boycott of Philip Morris. *Tob Control* 2003;**12**:203–7.

664 Peto R, Lopez AD. The future worldwide health effects of current smoking patterns [press release 2 Aug]. University of Oxford, Clinical Trial Service Unit & Epidemiological Studies Unit, 2000 (http://www.ctsu.ox.ac.uk/pressreleases/2000-08-02/the-future-worldwide-health-effects-of-current-smoking-patterns).

665 Gribben R. BAT man who answered the call for help. *Daily Telegraph* (Great Britain) 1 Jul 1993:4.

666 O'Connor AM, Stacey D, Entwistle V et al. Decision aids for people facing health treatment or screening decisions. *Cochrane Database Syst Rev (2)* 2003:CD001431.

667 Wallace C, Leask J, Trevena LJ. Effects of a web based decision aid on parental attitudes to MMR vaccination: a before and after study. *BMJ* 2006;**332**:146–9.

668 Barratt A, Trevena L, Davey HM et al. Use of decision aids to support informed choices about screening. *BMJ* 2004;**329**:507–10.

669 Borthwick C. Not a single vote: the politics of public health – an interview with Michael Wooldridge. *Health Prom J Austr* 2002;**13**:2.

670 Chapman S. Public health advocates: political lap dogs or rottweilers? *Health Prom J Austr* 2002;**13**:250–1.

671 Wachter RM. AIDs, activism, and the politics of health. *N Engl J Med* 1992;**326**: 128–33.

672 Hippocratic corpus, decorum. In: Reiser SJ, Dyck AF, Curran W (eds) *Ethics in Medicine: Historical Perspectives and Contemporary Concerns*. Cambridge, MA: MIT Press, 1977:7.

673 Osler WR. *Aequanimitas with other Addresses to Medical Students, Nurses and Practitioners of Medicine*. Philadelphia: P. Blakiston's Son & Co, 1904.

674 DeVries WC. The physician, the media, and the "spectacular" case. *JAMA* 1988;**259**:886–90.

675 Chapman S. "It is possible he is a kind of nut": how the tobacco industry quietly promoted Dr William Whitby. *Tob Control* 2003;**12**(Suppl. 3):iii4–6.

676 Mackay J, Eriksen M, Shafey O. *The Tobacco Atlas*. Atlanta, GA: American Cancer Society, 2006:26 (http://www.cancer.org/downloads/AA/TobaccoAtlas04.pdf).

677 Muggli ME, Hurt RD. Tobacco industry strategies to undermine the 8th World Conference on Tobacco or Health. *Tob Control* 2003;**12**:195–202.

678 Pertschuk M. *Getting the Message Right: Using Formative Research, Polling and Focus Group Insights on the Cheap*. Blowing away the smoke: a series of advanced media advocacy advisories for tobacco control advocates, no. 3. Washington: Advocacy Institute, 1997. (http://www.strategyguides.globalink.org/docs/blowing_smoke3.doc).

679 Bloom J. Fear and irony on Tobacco Road: notes from the Fourth Tobacco International Exhibition and Conference. *Tob Control* 1993;**2**:46–9.

680 Delvecchio J. Peanut butter recall widened in health scare. *Sydney Morning Herald* 27 Jun 1996:3.

681 ABC. ABC Radio National Perspective 3 Dec 2001: [lung cancer vaccines]. ABC. 2001 (http://www.abc.net.au/rn/perspective/stories/2001/431153.htm#).

682 Spitzer E. UPS joins effort to reduce youth smoking: Spitzer praises company, urges congress to compel the postal service to take similar steps. Office of New York State Attorney General. 2005 (http://www.oag.state.ny.us/press/2005/oct/oct24a_05.html).

683 DHL agrees to stop delivery of cigarettes. Tobacco Public Policy Center at Capital University Law School. 2005 (http://www.law.capital.edu/Tobacco/News/2005/20050705MiscellaneousNews2.asp).

684   Spitzer E. Fedex to strengthen policies restricting cigarette shipments: all major package delivery companies have now joined effort to reduce youth smoking. Office of New York State Attorney General. 2006 (http://www.oag.state.ny.us/press/2006/feb/feb07a_06.html).

685   Chapman S. Advocacy in action: extreme corporate makeover interruptus: denormalising tobacco industry corporate schmoozing. *Tob Control* 2004;**13**:445–7.

686   Chapman S, Dominello A. A strategy for increasing news media coverage of tobacco and health in Australia. *Health Promot Int* 2001;**16**:137–43.

687   Liberman J, Borland R. Australia: lawyers ponder tobacco firms' criminal liability. *Tob Control* 2001;**10**:205.

688   Bauman A, Chen XC, Chapman S. Protecting children in cars from tobacco-smoke. *BMJ* 1995;**311**:1164.

689   Griffin R. Tobacco chief was forced out of Glaxo. *Sunday Business (UK)* 18 Mar 2001 (http://www.ash.org.uk/html/conduct/html/bonham.html).

690   Blum A. Cowboys, cancer, kids, and cash flow: the 1992 Philip Morris annual meeting. *Tob Control* 1992;**1**:134–7.

691   INFACT. Tobacco giant Philip Morris/Altria changes location of annual shareholders' meeting in face of growing public pressure. Corporate Accountability International. 2004 (http://www.stopcorporateabuse.org/cms/page1180.cfm).

692   Wilson DH, Wakefield MA, Esterman A et al. 15's: they fit in everywhere – especially the school bag: a survey of purchases of packets of 15 cigarettes by 14 and 15 year olds in South Australia. *Community Health Stud* 1987;**11**:16s–20s.

693   Wright T. What the people think: maybe she is, maybe not. *Sydney Morning Herald* 24 Aug 1995:4.

694   Wigand J. The Insider: its effect on the public. *Tob Control* 2001;**10**:292.

695   Farone WA. Harm reduction: 25 years later. *Tob Control* 2002;**11**:287–8.

696   Liberman J. The shredding of BAT's defence: McCabe v. British American Tobacco Australia. *Tob Control* 2002;**11**:271–4.

697   Holtz A. Tobacco whistleblowers get warm reception at health meeting. Reuters Health at CancerPage.com. 2000 (http://cancerpage.com/news/article.asp?id=1478).

698   Levin M. Who's behind the building door? *The Nation (USA)* Aug 9–16 1993: 168–71.

Index